MARGERY KEMPE'S SPIRITUAL MEDICINE

MARGERY KEMPE'S SPIRITUAL MEDICINE

Suffering, Transformation and the Life-Course

Laura Kalas

D. S. BREWER

First published 2020
D. S. Brewer, Cambridge
Paperback edition 2023

ISBN 978-1-84384-554-6 hardback
ISBN 978-1-84384-684-0 paperback

D. S. Brewer is an imprint of Boydell & Brewer Ltd
PO Box 9, Woodbridge, Suffolk IP12 3DF, UK
and of Boydell & Brewer Inc.
668 Mt Hope Avenue, Rochester, NY 14620–2731, USA
website: www.boydellandbrewer.com

A CIP catalogue record for this book is available
from the British Library

The publisher has no responsibility for the continued existence or accuracy of URLs for
external or third-party internet websites referred to in this book, and does not guarantee
that any content on such websites is, or will remain, accurate or appropriate

This publication is printed on acid-free paper

Typeset by www.thewordservice.com

For my parents, Anne and Paul Kalas

Contents

List of Illustrations		ix
Acknowledgements		xi
Abbreviations		xiii
Note on Editions and Translations		xiv
Introduction		I
I	Bleeding the Tears of Melancholia	29
2	'Þe mukke' of Marriage and the Sexual Paradox	59
3	Lost Blood of the Middle Age: Surrogacy and Fecundity	97
4	*Margery Medica*: The Healing Value of Pain Surrogacy	127
5	The Passion of Death Surrogacy	161
6	Senescent Reproduction: Writing Anamnestic Pain	183
Afterword / Afterlife		211
Glossary of Medical Terms		223
Select Bibliography		225
Index		245

Illustrations

Figure 1. The recipe folio: British Library Additional MS 61823, fol. 124v. © The British Library Board. 3

Figure 2. Detail of the recipe folio achieved using multispectral imaging technology: British Library Additional MS 61823, fol. 124v. © The British Library Board. 4

Figure 3. Detail of the bottom of the recipe folio achieved using multispectral imaging technology: British Library Additional MS 61823, fol. 124v. © The British Library Board. 4

Figure 4. The medicinal sweets recreated by Theresa Tyers. Photograph: Theresa Tyers. 5

Figure 5. 1437–8 Trinity Guild account roll (KLBA, KL/C 38/16). Photograph: Laura Kalas. Credit to the King's Lynn Borough Archives. 214

Figure 6. Detail of Margery Kempe's entry in the 1437–8 Trinity Guild account roll (KLBA, KL/C 38/16). Photograph: Laura Kalas. Credit to the King's Lynn Borough Archives. 214

Figure 7. 1438–9 Trinity Guild account roll (KLBA, KL/C 38/17). Photograph: Laura Kalas. Credit to the King's Lynn Borough Archives. 215

Figure 8. Detail of Margery Kempe's entry in the 1438–9 Trinity Guild account roll (KLBA, KL/C 38/17). Photograph: Laura Kalas. Credit to the King's Lynn Borough Archives. 215

Figure 9. Photograph from excavations in the Saturday market place at King's Lynn, showing part of the charnel house beneath the chapel of St John, where human burials were discovered. Photograph: Clive Bond, September 2014. 218

The author and publisher are grateful to all the institutions and individuals listed for permission to reproduce the materials in which they hold copyright. Every effort has been made to trace the copyright holders; apologies are offered for any omission, and the publisher will be pleased to add any necessary acknowledgement in subsequent editions.

Edge

The woman is perfected.
Her dead

Body wears the smile of accomplishment,
The illusion of a Greek necessity

Flows in the scrolls of her toga,
Her bare

Feet seem to be saying:
We have come so far, it is over.

Each dead child coiled, a white serpent,
One at each little

Pitcher of milk, now empty.
She has folded

Them back into her body as petals
Of a rose close when the garden

Stiffens and odors bleed
From the sweet, deep throats of the night flower.

The moon has nothing to be sad about,
Staring from her hood of bone.

She is used to this sort of thing.
Her blacks crackle and drag.

Sylvia Plath

al shal be wele, and al shall be wele, and all manner thing shal be wele.

Julian of Norwich

Acknowledgements

This book has materialised at a life moment that resonates curiously with the medieval women of a similar age and stage whose tenacity, persistence, and textual production inspired my return to academia with the same impulse to grow, and to write. That I have been given the chance to flourish in an academic career is something for which I will always be grateful, and I am indebted to my colleagues at Swansea University for giving me the opportunity to do that.

It is hard to express how much I owe to Liz Herbert McAvoy, who, through her feminist, intellectual, and mentoring principles, has been with me on my academic journey, quite literally, every step of the way. Liz has shown extraordinary guidance, scrupulousness, and care, and her support – in more ways than I can possibly say here – has been utterly invaluable. I hope that I might one day do justice to her remarkable mentorship and scholarly example, and I am proud to be able to call her a friend and colleague. In many ways, this book is for her.

My thanks are also due to the many other inspirational scholars who have guided and supported me over the past few years. During my time at the University of Exeter, Eddie Jones was a superlative doctoral supervisor and his continued encouragement and patience as I learned the academic ropes once again was hugely appreciated. Thanks must also go to Catherine Rider for setting me on the medieval medical path as my second supervisor, and to the English department at Exeter, who supported me in my postdoctoral ambitions. I am indebted also to Vincent Gillespie for his meticulous engagement with my work as external examiner, and for his continuing support of my career aspirations. I also owe thanks to Naoë Kukita Yoshikawa for her support and enthusiasm for my work, and the sharing of her own, and to Diane Watt, for her supreme scholarly example, advice, and valiant willingness to work with me.

I am lucky to have generous colleagues and friends at Swansea University who have welcomed me to the college and offered insightful critiques of my work-in-progress. Thanks are due to Roberta Magnani for her wonderful support and friendship, to Trish Skinner, Alison Williams, and Chris Pak for their reading of draft material, and to Alice Barnaby for her unfailing support as Head of Department. Many others have given me invaluable feedback on drafts of this and other publications, along with words of much-needed encouragement in the final stages of this book's production: Sarah Salih, Lucy Allen, the great team that is the Gender and Medieval Studies Group, the anonymous readers of my manuscript for their thoughtful critiques, and my Margery Kempe 'partner in crime', Laura Varnam, whose wisdom and friendship I value greatly. Any errors in this manuscript of course remain my own.

The discovery of the contents of the recipe from the Margery Kempe manuscript has been a joy to reveal, and possible only with the help of several individuals. My thanks go to Andrea Clarke at the British Library for allowing me access to the manuscript, to the British Library imaging scientist, Christina Duffy, for providing me with the multispectral images, and to Daniel Wakelin, Eddie Jones, Susan Maddock, Laura Varnam, and Paul Acker for their help in interpreting the handwriting and enabling me to arrive at a transcription. I am also grateful to Theresa Tyers for taking on the unenviable task of recreating the medicinal sweets in an impressively authentic manner.

Considerable thanks are due to my editor, Caroline Palmer of Boydell & Brewer, for having faith in my book, even as it became as effusive as Margery Kempe herself, and for her patience and support while I completed the manuscript during turbulent times. The production team at Boydell have been remarkable in their professionalism and efficiency, and I thank them for that. I am also appreciative of those in King's Lynn – Kempe's home-town – for supporting my work. Thanks go to Luke Shackell and the King's Lynn Borough Archives; the Revd Canon Christopher Ivory of King's Lynn Minster; Paul Richards; Clive Bond, for inviting me to speak about Margery Kempe at the 2017 King's Lynn Festival; and the team at the True's Yard Museum for inviting me to be involved with the community performance of Elizabeth MacDonald's dramatization of Kempe's life, Skirting Heresy, in 2018, and the children's-book initiative in 2019. Indeed, I am grateful to Liz MacDonald for her interest in and support of my work on Kempe, and for sharing her own work with me.

My final debt of gratitude is to my friends and family, who have championed me and listened tirelessly as I babble about all things medieval. To friends old and new, for your love and laughs, and to Tony McAvoy, for the hospitality, kindness, and sustaining beverages, especially during the final stages of this manuscript's completion. To my parents, Anne and Paul Kalas, who have supported me beyond measure in every possible way, including many years of enforced familiarity with the medieval streets of Canterbury, and whose love and backing continues to mean the world. To my wonderful and supportive sister, Lou Lou, for the 'mers', wine, and general loveliness, and to my sorely missed grandparents, Stella and Russell Pooley, whose memory and love are forever imbricated in this book. Finally, to my boys, Oliver and Jasper, who remain my proudest achievement, for their dry wit and banter, incessant requests for snacks, and for talking to me occasionally. You are all my reason for rising in the morning, and this book is for you all, with love.

Abbreviations

BL	British Library, London
BMK	*The Book of Margery Kempe*
EETS	Early English Text Society
e.s.	Extra Series
o.s.	Original Series
OED	*Oxford English Dictionary*
s.s.	Supplementary Series
MED	*Middle English Dictionary*, ed. Hans Kurath and S.M. Kuhn (Ann Arbor: University of Michigan Press; London: Oxford University Press, 1952–) https://quod.lib.umich.edu/m/middle-english-dictionary/dictionary
n.s.	New Series
PL	Patrologia Latina, ed. J.-P. Migne, 221 vols (Paris, 1844–64)
TEAMS	The Consortium for the Teaching of the Middle Ages

Note on Editions and Translations

The edition used throughout is *The Book of Margery Kempe*, EETS o.s. 212, ed. Sanford Brown Meech and Hope Emily Allen (London: Oxford University Press, 1997, unaltered reprint). Page numbers appear parenthetically in the text; all italic emphases are my own. All quotations from the Bible in English are from the Douay–Rheims version: <http://www.drbo.org/>.

The poem 'Edge', printed above on p. xiii, is from *The Collected Poems of Sylvia Plath*, ed. Ted Hughes © 1960, 1965, 1971, 1981 by the Estate of Sylvia Plath. Editorial material © 1981 by Ted Hughes. Reprinted by permission of HarperCollins Publishers and Faber and Faber Ltd.

Introduction

For fly[ ] take [   ]
Sugyr candy Sugur plate Sugur wyth
Annes sed fenkkell sed notmikis Synamum
Genger Comfetis and licoris Bett them to
Gedyr in a morter and sett them in all maner
of metis and drynkis and dry frist & last et yt

[ ]ger candy sug[?u]r pla[?te]¹

This book begins, *mutatis mutandis*, at its end: a mystery solved; a body
healed. The hastily written, faded recipe, hidden on the final folio of BL
Additional MS 61823, *The Book of Margery Kempe*, has puzzled scholars of Kempe since the rediscovery of the manuscript in 1934, lingering in a tantalising lacuna of illegibility (Figure 1).² Perhaps aptly, the
British Library's multispectral imaging equipment – the same technology
employed in space exploration to capture data about the earth's surface and
the universe, that is, Creation itself – has enabled the faded handwriting
of the manuscript's recipe to be deciphered (Figures 2 and 3).³ The recipe,
annotated by a late fifteenth- or early sixteenth-century reader, probably

---

¹ Translation: 'For fly[ ] take [   ] / Sugar candy, sugar plate, sugar with /
Aniseed, fennel seed, nutmeg, cinnamon, / Ginger comfetes and licorice. Beat them
/ together in a mortar and make them in all / manner of food and drinks and dry first
and last eat it. / [Sugar candy, sugar plate]'. The top line of the recipe is unclear, but
the word 'fly' may indicate 'flux'. If so, the rest of the recipe is unlikely to be connected
to the top line, since the nature of the hot, dry ingredients indicates a remedy for a
phlegmatic disorder of the stomach.
² I am indebted to Andrea Clarke at The British Library for allowing me access to
the manuscript; to Christina Duffy, Imaging Scientist at The British Library, for
providing me with the multispectral images of the folio, and to the British Library
Board. My very grateful thanks go to Eddie Jones, Daniel Wakelin, Susan Maddock,
Laura Varnam, and Paul Acker for their help in transcribing the recipe. All errors in
transcription remain my own.
³ A multispectral image captures data within specific wavelength ranges across the elec-
tromagnetic spectrum and allows the extraction of additional information that the
human eye fails to capture with its receptors for red, green and blue. It was originally
developed for space-based imaging and is still used by NASA. See, for example, Mary
Pagnuttia et al., 'Radiometric characterization of IKONOS multispectral imagery',
Remote Sensing of Environment, 88 (2003), 53–68.

in a monastic context, is for medicinal sweets: curative digestives known as 'dragges' that were commonly used remedies for digestion, employed to dry and warm a cold, phlegmatic stomach.[4] It calls for plentiful sugar, itself considered medicinal in the Middle Ages, and the luxuriant spices of aniseed, fennel seed, nutmeg, cinnamon, ginger, and liquorice. Given Kempe's attendance at many meals with 'worthy' folk, it is inconceivable that she would not herself have eaten dragges. The Middle English translation of Bartholomaeus Anglicus's *De proprietatibus rerum* (written c. 1240), a medical text that circulated widely in the fourteenth century, notes that sweet flavours are pure 'by kynde [nature]' and beneficial for bodily health. Sweetness is restorative, softening the body with moisture: it 'restoreþ in þe body þinge þat is lost, and most conforteþ feble vertues and spirites, and norissheþ speciallich all þe membres'.[5] The spiced sweetness of the recipe is, then, at once therapeutic, sensory, symbolic, and salvific, since the moral properties of food were also imbricated with its ingestion in medieval culture. By consuming a foodstuff, one would acquire some of its associated properties (the Eucharistic wafer, for example).[6] As a medico-religious addendum by one scribal reader, the recipe functions as a means of enhancing – or at least acknowledging – the medical subtext of the *Book*, itself an object of healing potential for subsequent readers who are edified by the unfolding of Margery Kempe's spiritual journey. It is, then, a metonymy for Kempe's own spiritual healing. This healing is inscribed both by the Proem's amanuensis and by Kempe, the designated 'creatur' of the *Book*, who, as a part of the Creation largely beyond her earthly prescience, *sees* in glimpses, like the multispectral snapshots of the twenty-first-century universe.

---

[4] For a detailed exploration of the recipe's genesis, ingredients, purpose, and spiritual semiosis, see Laura Kalas Williams, 'The *Swetenesse* of Confection: A Recipe for Spiritual Health in London, British Library, Additional MS 61823, *The Book of Margery Kempe*', *Studies in the Age of Chaucer*, 40 (2018), 155–90. Short passages from the article are replicated in this study. An adapted section from Chapter 1 appears also appears in the article '"Slayn for Goddys lofe": Margery Kempe's Melancholia and the Bleeding of Tears', *Medieval Feminist Forum: A Journal of Gender and Sexuality*, 52:1 (2016), 84–100. Thanks are due to the editorial boards of *SAC* and *MFF* for allowing the use of the material in this book.

[5] *On the Properties of Things: John Trevisa's Translation of Bartholomaeus Anglicus De proprietatibus rerum*, 2 vols, ed. M.C. Seymour (Oxford: Oxford University Press, 1975), vol. 2, p. 1307.

[6] C.M. Woolgar, 'Food and the Middle Ages', *Journal of Medieval History*, 36 (2010), 1–19 (p. 8).

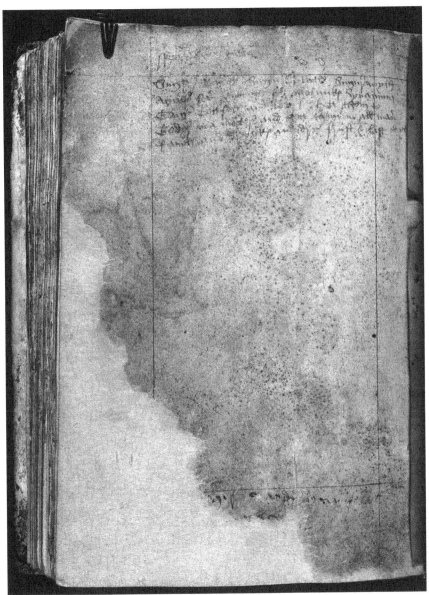

Figure 1. The recipe folio: British Library Additional MS 61823, fol. 124v.

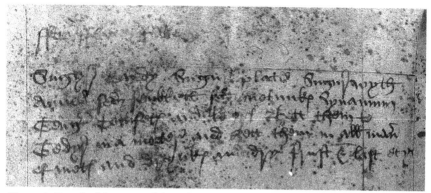

Figure 2. Detail of the recipe folio achieved using multispectral imaging technology: British Library Additional MS 61823, fol. 124v.

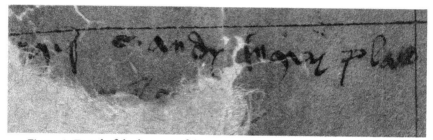

Figure 3. Detail of the bottom of the recipe folio achieved using multispectral imaging technology: British Library Additional MS 61823, fol. 124v.

The interaction of the medieval and postmodern technologies involved in rendering visible the recipe on the page – the medieval codex and the multispectral imaging technology that unveils the past in the present – resonates with the *Book*'s own achronicity, revealing the type of 'heterogeneous temporal experience' signalled by Carolyn Dinshaw, like Kempe's own mystical dissolution of time and space.[7] This 'asynchronous *now*' of the *Book*, as Dinshaw puts it, was made literal in 2018 when the medieval recipe was recreated and Kempe scholars sampled the resulting spiced sweets, a further way through which twenty-first-century readers encountered the past, 'tasting' Kempe's world (Figure 4).[8] Moreover, the annotated recipe chimes with the persistent tendency in scholarly responses to the *Book* to medicalise, or pathologise,

[7] Carolyn Dinshaw, *How Soon is Now? Medieval Texts, Amateur Readers, and the Queerness of Time* (Durham and London: Duke University Press, 2012), p. 5.

[8] Dinshaw, *How Soon is Now?*, p. 117. The sweets' resurrection was thanks to Theresa Tyers, who painstakingly recreated the ingredients and 'dragges' for the landmark conference 'Margery Kempe Studies in the Twenty-First Century', organised by myself and Laura Varnam, held at University College, Oxford, 5–7 April 2018.

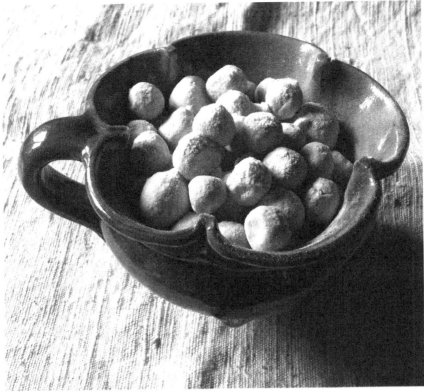

Figure 4. The medicinal sweets recreated by Theresa Tyers.

Kempe's particular form of spirituality.[9] In her Prefatory Note to the 1940 EETS edition, Hope Emily Allen described Kempe as 'largely limited by her constitutional difficulties'. She was, she stated, 'petty, neurotic, vain, illiterate, physically and nervously over-strained; devout, much-travelled, forceful and talented', and Allen hoped that the EETS volume would 'aid the professional psychologist who later will doubtless pronounce at length on Margery's type of neuroticism' (lxiv–lxv). Many have done just that, of course. But while Allen concedes Kempe's tenacity as well as her supposed congenital 'difficulties',

---

[9] The recipe was added by a late fifteenth- or early sixteenth-century reader of the *Book*, according to Sanford Brown Meech, *BMK*, p. xliv. Little has been written about the recipe itself. It is mentioned in Kelly Parsons, 'The Red Ink Annotator of *The Book of Margery Kempe* and His Lay Audience', in *The Medieval Professional Reader at Work: Evidence from Manuscripts of Chaucer, Langland, Kempe, and Gower*, ed. Kathryn Kerby-Fulton and Maidie Hilmo (Victoria: English Literary Studies, University of Victoria, 2001), pp. 143–216 (pp. 153–4); and Johanne Paquette, 'Male Approbation in the Extant Glosses to the Book of Margery Kempe', in *Women and the Divine in Literature before 1700: Essays in Memory of Margot Louis*, ed. Kathryn Kerby-Fulton (Victoria: ELS Editions, 2009), pp. 153–69 (p. 158). Gail McMurray Gibson speculated that the recipe could be for a caudle in *Theatre of Devotion: East Anglian Drama and Society in the Late Middle Ages* (Chicago and London: University of Chicago Press, 1989), p. 51.

subsequent diagnostic readings of Kempe have tended towards the pejorative, marginalising her or framing her insistence upon a bodily experience of God as inferior to the more theologically sophisticated meditations of her mystical contemporaries. But what happens if we read the *Book* not only through the psychology of the 'now', but in the light of medical writings of the 'then'? What if the ubiquitous doctrine of *Christus medicus*, or Christ the Physician, shapes Kempe's life-course more venously than previously acknowledged? Might not such understandings transform our insight into Margery Kempe's mystical experience and its articulation in her world and her text?

This book is concerned with the interactions of medicine, mysticism, life cycle, and (re)production, and with Margery Kempe's negotiation of the painful inheritance of female flesh. In offering a new way of reading the *Book* as a narrative of Kempe's *own* engagement with and use of the medical paradigms of which she has previously been a passive subject, I argue for a turn from the pathologisation that has hitherto reduced her to a historical figure of perplexing disorder. The book also explores the surrogacy hermeneutic that I see as a central *modus operandi* for Kempe's devotional and healing practices, that is, the substitutional activities that she undertakes, both mystically and socially, and which are authorised in the locus of the post-reproductive maternal body. Furthermore, it examines the melancholic mourning phenomena that underlie the operations in the *Book* as Kempe seeks a 'truth' in her quest to *know* God via an epistemology of pain and suffering. That journey begins with the inversion of health as she suffers great bodily sickness as a trigger for spiritual transformation, a trajectory inscribed by the clerical author of the Proem as a primary structuring device:

> [God] *turnyd helth in-to sekenesse*, prosperyte in-to aduersyte, worship in-to repref, & love in-to hatered. Thus *alle þis thyngys turning vp-so-down*, þis creatur which many ʒerys had gon wyl & euyr ben vnstable was parfythly drawen & steryd to entren þe way of hy perfeccyon, whech parfyth wey Cryst owr Savyowr in hys propyr persoone examplyd. Sadly he trad it & dewly he went it beforn. Than þis creatur, of whom thys tretys thorw þe mercy of Ihesu schal schewen in party þe leuyng, towched be þe hand of owyr Lord wyth grett bodyly sekenesse, wher-thorw sche lost reson & her wyttes a long tyme tyl *owr Lord be grace restoryd her a-geyn, as it schal mor openly be shewed aftyrward* (1–2, my emphases).

Margery Kempe's spiritual and medical restoration thus forms a central hermeneutic of the 'schort tretys and a comfortabyl' that is the *Book*. It is 'owr Lord be grace [that] restoryd her a-geyn' – her physician, God, the healer of her body and soul.[10] The Fourth Lateran Council of 1215 had stipulated the primacy of the priest over the physician, stating that:

---

[10] On the interplay of medicine and religion in the Middle Ages see 'Medical Discourse in Premodern Europe', Special Issue, ed. Marion Turner, *Journal of Medieval and Early Modern Studies*, 46 (2016); *Medicine, Religion and Gender in Medieval Culture*, ed. Naoë

[we] command physicians of the body, when they are called to the sick, to warn and persuade them first of all to call in physicians of the soul so that after their spiritual health has been seen to they may respond better to medicine for their bodies, for when the cause ceases so does the effect.[11]

The interplay of medicine and religion, made scholastic in the universities of Italy and France and later disseminated to England, is evidenced locally in Bishop's Lynn (now King's Lynn) – Margery Kempe's home town in Norfolk – by records of religious and medical treatises. The Hospital of St Mary Magdalen in Lynn contained a *Liber vitae* which listed its twelve brethren and sisters and the names of visitors and patrons to be prayed for.[12] Conversely, a thirteenth-century book of miscellaneous *medica* – Oxford, Bodleian Library, MS Ashmole 1398 – was held at the Carmelite convent at Lynn.[13] Margery Kempe was closely connected to both the Dominican and Carmelite Orders in Lynn, and the Carmelite friar Master Aleyn was a particular admirer of Kempe and is likely to have impressed both his medical and theological learning upon her.

The phenomena of pain and mysticism and their ontological connection form a further foundation for my present exploration as specific derivatives of the broader medico-religious context in which this book sits. Like mystical experience, pain is extra-linguistic, intangible, esoteric, and always 'other'. Joanna Bourke's argument that pain is a self-authenticating phenomenon, not an 'it' in the body – or an entity in itself – but a 'type of event', is a useful way of thinking about the articulation of pain in *The Book of Margery Kempe*, particularly since Kempe persistently conflates physical pain and psychological or spiritual suffering, employing the term 'peyne' interchangeably. Bourke, then, challenges Elaine Scarry's essentialising of pain as an 'ontological fallacy', asserting that Scarry mistakenly treats 'metaphoric ways of conceiving suffering … as descriptions of an actual entity'.[14] The problematics

---

Kukita Yoshikawa (Cambridge: D.S. Brewer, 2015); Daniel McCann, *Soul-Health: Therapeutic Reading in Later Medieval England* (Cardiff: University of Wales Press, 2018); 'Medieval and Early Modern Literature, Science and Medicine', ed. Rachel Falconer and Denis Renevey, *Swiss Papers in English Language and Literature*, 28 (Tübingen: Gunter Narr, 2013); Louise Bishop, *Words, Stones, Herbs: The Healing Word in Medieval and Early Modern England* (New York: Syracuse University Press, 2007); and *Religion and Medicine in the Middle Ages*, ed. Peter Biller and Joseph Ziegler (Woodbridge: York Medieval Press, 2001).

[11] From The Fourth General Council of the Lateran, 1215 AD., decree 22, in *Papal Encyclicals Online* <http://www.papalencyclicals.net> [accessed 8th May 2016].

[12] *Medieval Libraries of Great Britain: A List of Surviving Books*, ed. Neil Ker, 2nd edn (London: Butler and Tanner, 1964), p. 127. The *Liber* is now held at Norwich in the Norfolk and Norwich Record Office, B-L ixb. On spiritual and medical care in medieval hospitals see Carole Rawcliffe, *Medicine for the Soul: The Life, Death and Resurrection of an English Medieval Hospital, St Giles's, Norwich, c. 1249–1550* (Stroud: Sutton, 1999); and *The Medieval Hospital and Medical Practice*, ed. Barbara S. Bowers (Aldershot: Ashgate, 2007).

[13] Ker, *Medieval Libraries*, p. 127.

[14] Joanna Bourke, *The Story of Pain: From Prayer to Painkillers* (Oxford: Oxford University Press, 2014), pp. 3–5. Elaine Scarry, *The Body in Pain* (New York, Oxford: Oxford University Press, 1985).

of definition resist satisfactory resolution, particularly when one is attempting to transfer modern categories of pain, psychology, biology, and neuroscience to the texts of the Middle Ages. But I do not think that the distinction between pain and suffering need necessarily be rendered as binary. This book will employ the terms *pain*, *suffering*, and *tribulation* as multivalent nuances of the same overarching experience because Kempe herself uses the term *peyne* metaphorically, spiritually, and literally, and because, in the medieval imaginary, the signifiers of corporeal, spiritual, and social 'suffering' always return to the same signified teleology: God.

The cultural framework of Margery Kempe's experience of pain is predicated upon her interpretation of events and their relationship to God's plan for her life. Indeed, pain is argued by Javier Moscoso to be 'incomprehensible without this duality between the unified form of experience and the cultural modulation that allows the breaking of the (supposedly objective) correspondence between physiological pain and its subjective expression'.[15] The present study of medicalised spirituality and the synchronic spiritualisation of medicine thus offers a fresh way of approaching Kempe's mystical body-in-pain and aims to further our understanding of the *Book* as a product of the micro/macrocosmic concept of the universe and human experience in the medieval imaginary. It will not hide from Kempe's sense of her embodied, female, maternal 'essence', experienced subjectively (and abjectly); at the same time it will explore the medico-cultural *construction* of that same female flesh as diseased and disordered. Through a broadly interpreted framework of the life-course, the book shows how Margery Kempe utilises that very socio-biological matrix to transition, transform, and repurpose herself, within an overarching surrogacy hermeneutic and towards a transcendent encounter with God. My approach is, moreover, part of a necessary project in aligning modern methodologies more holistically with the pre-Cartesian conception of the integrated body–soul dynamic, since, whether perceived through her 'bodily' or 'gostly' eye, mystical and painful experience for Margery Kempe is always equally and 'verily' authentic.

Towards a Medicalised Hermeneutic of Spirituality

The reframing of Margery Kempe's mystical body that this project seeks to achieve occurs within a growing corpus of scholarship that has taken multiple turns, not least the retrospective diagnoses that were favoured in the medicalised studies of the 1980s and 1990s.[16] Among these, Richard Lawes argued that Kempe's 'symptoms' indicate a depressive psychosis in the puerperium,

---

[15] Javier Moscoso, *Pain: A Cultural History*, trans. Sarah Thomas and Paul House (Basingstoke: Palgrave Macmillan, 2012), pp. 6–8.

[16] See Diane Watt's very useful online bibliography on Margery Kempe criticism: 'Margery Kempe', *Oxford Bibliographies Online* <DOI: 10.1093/obo/9780199846719-0034>.

along with temporal-lobe epilepsy or psychomotor epilepsy, considering the *Discretio spirituum* of the Middle Ages as similar to modern psychiatry since both systems recognise the patterns of inner experience.[17] Further 'diagnoses' include Hope Phyllis Weissman's Freudian interpretation of Kempe's tears as a productively utilised facet of a 'conversion hysteric'; and other studies that conceptualise the first childbirth episode as an example of postpartum depression or psychosis.[18] Wendy Harding interpreted Kempe's behaviours as mimicking the pains of birthing, while other pathologies have included Tourette's Syndrome and the psychological advantages of 'hysteria'.[19] Such approaches followed early and mid-twentieth-century psychoanalytical responses to the *Book*, which mainly dismissed Kempe as pathologically disordered.[20] The historicist approaches that have dominated Kempe scholarship in more recent years have continued the debate over the form of authorship that the *Book* takes, building on John Hirsch's stance that the scribe is the author of the text. Lynn Staley's important intervention drew a distinction between Kempe the author, Margery, her fictional creation, and the scribe as a literary trope. Nicholas Watson conversely regards Kempe as the author in a 'positivistic

---

[17] Richard Lawes, 'The Madness of Margery Kempe', in *The Medieval Mystical Tradition in England, Ireland and Wales, Exeter Symposium VI, Papers Read at Charney Manor, July 1991*, ed. Marion Glasscoe (Cambridge: D.S. Brewer, 1999), pp. 147–68; and 'Psychological Disorder and the Autobiographical Impulse in Julian of Norwich, Margery Kempe and Thomas Hoccleve', in *Writing Religious Women: Female Spiritual and Textual Practices in Late Medieval England*, ed. Denis Renevey and Christiania Whitehead (Cardiff: University of Wales Press, 2000), pp. 217–43.

[18] See Hope Phyllis Weissman, 'Margery Kempe in Jerusalem: *Hysterica Compassio* in the Late Middle Ages', in *Acts of Interpretation: The Text in Its Contexts, 700–1600, Essays on Medieval and Renaissance Literature*, ed. Mary J. Carruthers and Elizabeth D. Kirk (Oklahoma: Pilgrim Books, 1982), pp. 201–17; Maureen Fries, 'Margery Kempe', in *An Introduction to The Medieval Mystics of Europe*, ed. Paul E. Szarmach (Albany: State University of New York Press, 1984), pp. 217–35; and Mary Hardman Farley, 'Her Own Creatur: Religion, Feminist Criticism, and the functional Eccentricity of Margery Kempe', *Exemplaria*, 11 (1999), 1–21. On the risks of retrospective diagnoses see Piers D. Mitchell, 'Retrospective Diagnosis and the Use of Historical Texts for Investigating Disease in the Past', *International Journal of Paleopathology*, 1 (2011), 81–8; and Juliette Vuille, '"Maybe I'm Crazy?" Diagnosis and Contextualisation of Medieval Female Mystics', in *Medicine, Religion and Gender in Medieval Culture*, ed. Yoshikawa, pp. 103–20.

[19] Wendy Harding, 'Medieval Women's Unwritten Discourse on Motherhood: A Reading of Two Fifteenth Century Texts', *Women's Studies*, 21 (1992), 197–209; Nancy P. Stork, 'Did Margery Kempe suffer from Tourette's Syndrome?', *Mediaeval Studies*, 59 (1997), 261–300; and Becky R. Lee, 'The Medieval Hysteric and the Psychedelic Psychologist: A Revaluation of the Mysticism of Margery Kempe in the Light of the Transpersonal Psychology of Stanislav Grof', *Studia Mystica*, 23 (2002), 102–26.

[20] For early accounts of Kempe's 'disordered' spirituality, see Herbert Thurston, 'Margery the Astonishing', *The Month*, 168 (1936), 446–56; David Knowles, *The English Mystical Tradition* (London: Burns and Oates, 1961), pp. 138–50; and Wolfgang Riehle, *The Middle English Mystics*, trans. Bernard Standring (London: Routledge and Kegan Paul, 1981), p. 96. More recently, Riehle has 'come to recognize [Kempe's] importance', in *The Secret Within: Hermits, Recluses, and Spiritual Outsiders in Medieval England* (Icatha and London: Cornell University Press, 2014), p. 280.

attitude to some of the text's historical claims'.[21] New historical discoveries have deepened our understanding of the *Book*'s genesis. Sebastian Sobecki's uncovering of evidence in Gdansk corroborates the theory that Margery Kempe's son was the first scribe, and Robert Spryngolde the revising, clerical scribe. Anthony Bale has traced Richard Salthouse (inscribed at the end of the *Book* in the lines 'Jhesu mercy quod Salthows') as a monk at the powerful Benedictine cathedral priory in Norwich, persuasively arguing that he was the copier of the original manuscript, and most likely writing in Norwich – one of the most wealthy and prestigious religious houses of Europe.[22] Bale's work has significant implications for the source of the recipe's annotation, since a wealthy Norwich monastic context would explain the expensive ingredients of the 'dragges', and its reception in a location of theological and medical education resonates further with this volume's central concern to illuminate the medico-religious operations that underlie the *Book*'s presentation of physio-spiritual health.

The *Book*'s very capaciousness and resistance to definition are reflected in the expansiveness of its critical avenues, not least those that have situated Kempe as an authorised holy woman: as saint, pious exemplar, and as part of a much broader female devotional and European context than was previously recognised.[23] The work of Sarah McNamer in foregrounding the

[21] See Clarissa W. Atkinson, *Mystic and Pilgrim: The Book and the World of Margery Kempe* (Ithaca: Cornell University Press, 1983); Anthony Goodman, *Margery Kempe and Her World* (London: Longman, 2002); John C. Hirsch, 'Author and Scribe in *The Book of Margery Kempe*', *Medium Aevum*, 44 (1975), 145–50; Lynn Staley Johnson, 'The Trope of the Scribe and the Question of Literary Authority in the Works of Julian of Norwich and Margery Kempe', *Speculum*, 66 (1991), 820–38; Staley, *Margery Kempe's Dissenting Fictions* (Philadelphia: Pennsylvania State University Press, 1994); and Nicholas Watson, 'The Making of *The Book of Margery Kempe*', in *Voices in Dialogue: Reading Women in the Middle Ages*, ed. Linda Olson and Kathryn Kerby-Fulton (Notre Dame: University of Notre Dame Press, 2005), pp. 395–434 (p. 397). For readings of collaborative authorship see Ruth Evans, 'The Book of Margery Kempe', in *A Companion to Medieval English Literature and Culture, c. 1350–c. 1500*, ed. Peter Brown (Oxford: Blackwell, 2007), pp. 507–21; and Felicity Riddy, 'Text and Self in *The Book of Margery Kempe*', in *Voices in Dialogue*, ed. Olson and Kerby-Fulton, pp. 435–53. On the autobiography of the *Book* see Janel M. Mueller, 'Autobiography of a New Creature: Female Spirituality, Selfhood, and Authorship in *The Book of Margery Kempe*', in *Women in the Middle Ages and Renaissance*, ed. Mary Beth Rose (Syracuse: Syracuse University Press, 1986), pp. 155–71.

[22] Sebastian Sobecki, '"The writyng of this tretys": Margery Kempe's Son and the Authorship of Her Book', *Studies in the Age of Chaucer*, 37 (2015), 257–83; and Anthony Bale, 'Richard Salthouse of Norwich and the Scribe of *The Book of Margery Kempe*', *Studies in the Age of Chaucer*, 52 (2017), 173–87 (p. 177).

[23] On sainthood, see Gail McMurray Gibson, 'St Margery: "The Book of Margery Kempe"', in *Equally in God's Image: Women in the Middle Ages*, ed. Julia Bolton Holloway, Joan Bechtold, and Constance S. Wright (New York: Peter Lang, 1990), pp. 144–63; Diane Watt, *Medieval Women's Writing: Works by and for Women, 1100–1500* (Cambridge: Polity, 2007), pp. 116–35; Katherine J. Lewis, 'Margery Kempe and Saint Making in Later Medieval England', in *A Companion to 'The Book of Margery Kempe'*, ed. John H. Arnold and Katherine J. Lewis (Cambridge: D.S. Brewer, 2004), pp. 195–215; Rebecca Krug,

'insistent feminization' of spirituality during the so-called 'affective turn' of the later Middle Ages has inspired scrutiny of the role of affect and emotion in female spirituality, something that is taken up by Rebecca Krug in her book-length study of Kempe which brings to the fore the spiritual comfort offered by devotional writing and community and Kempe's inherent contribution.[24] Indeed, that devotional community is increasingly understood to be Europe-wide, indicating how Kempe's affective and bodily inflected form of spirituality was greatly influenced by her Continental antecedents and contemporaries, through texts that circulated in England and were read to her by her confessors.[25] The pioneering work of Caroline Walker Bynum has been central to much of our understanding of medieval religious women and their embodiment, while other scholars have specifically uncovered the cruciality of Margery Kempe's own bodily types of devotion.[26] McNamer has

'Margery Kempe', in *The Cambridge Companion to Medieval English Literature, 1100–1500*, ed. Larry Scanlon (Cambridge: Cambridge University Press, 2009), pp. 217–28; and Krug, 'The Idea of Sanctity and the Uncanonised life of Margery Kempe', in *The Cambridge Companion to Medieval English Culture*, ed. Andrew Galloway (Cambridge: Cambridge University Press, 2011), pp. 129–46. On authority and exemplarity see Naoë Kukita Yoshikawa, *Margery Kempe's Meditations: The Context of Medieval Devotional Literature, Liturgy, and Iconography* (Cardiff: University of Wales Press, 2007); Carolyn Dinshaw, *Getting Medieval: Sexualities and Communities, Pre- and Postmodern* (Durham, NC: Duke University Press, 1999), pp. 143–82; and Laura Varnam, 'The Importance of St Margaret's Church in *The Book of Margery Kempe*: A Sacred Place and an Exemplary Parishioner', *Nottingham Medieval Studies*, ed. Joanna Martin and Rob Lutton, 61 (2017), pp. 197–243.

24 Sarah McNamer, *Affective Meditation and the Invention of Medieval Compassion* (Philadelphia: University of Pennsylvania Press, 2010), p. 11; Rebecca Krug, *Margery Kempe and the Lonely Reader* (Ithaca and London: Cornell University Press (2017).

25 See Diane Watt, 'Before Margery: *The Book of Margery Kempe* and Its Antecedents', and Naoë Kukita Yoshikawa and Liz Herbert McAvoy, 'The Intertextual Dialogue and Conversational Theology of Mechthild of Hackeborn and Margery Kempe', both in *Encountering The Book of Margery Kempe*, ed. Laura Kalas and Laura Varnam (Manchester: Manchester University Press, forthcoming). See also 'Women's Literary Culture & Late Medieval English Writing', Special Issue, ed. Liz Herbert McAvoy and Diane Watt, *The Chaucer Review*, 51 (2016); and Naoë Kukita Yoshikawa, 'Mysticism and Medicine: Holy Communion in the *Vita of Marie d'Oignies* and *The Book of Margery Kempe*', in 'Convergence / Divergence: The Politics of Late Medieval English Devotional and Medical Discourses', Special Issue, ed. Denis Renevey and Naoë Kukita Yoshikawa, *Poetica*, 72 (2009), 109–22. Some prior work on the Continental tradition includes: Gunnel Cleve, 'Margery Kempe: A Scandinavian Influence on Medieval England', and Susan Dickman, 'Margery Kempe and the Continental Tradition of the Pious Woman', both in *The Medieval Mystical Tradition in England: Papers Read at Dartington Hall, July 1984*, ed. Marion Glasscoe (Cambridge: D.S. Brewer, 1984), pp. 163–75 and pp. 150–68 respectively; and Janet Dillon, 'Holy Women and Their Confessors or Confessors and Their Holy Women?: Margery Kempe and Continental Tradition', in *Prophets Abroad: The Reception of Continental Holy Women in Late-Medieval England*, ed. Rosalynn Voaden (Cambridge: D.S. Brewer, 1996), pp. 115–40.

26 See Caroline Walker Bynum, *Holy Feast and Holy Fast: The Religious Significance of Food to Medieval Women* (Berkeley: University of California Press, 1987); and *Fragmentation and Redemption: Essays on Gender and the Human Body in Medieval Religion* (New York: Urzone, 1989). On Margery Kempe and corporeal spirituality see Liz Herbert McAvoy,

argued that the later medieval 'rise of compassionate devotion to the suffering Christ', and the performance of compassion 'in the private drama of the heart that [devotional] texts stage – is to feel like a woman'.[27]

Much of this book engages with the environs of compassion, but more than that, it argues for the way in which Margery Kempe's own sense of a deeply feminine self is enacted not in the 'private drama of the heart', but in the very public, explosive demonstration of her piety, even as it emanates from an inner affectivity. McNamer posits that the 'presumed dominance of medical theory in the Middle Ages' overlooks the possibility that the performance of an emotion via the 'scripted' medieval texts that she explores might, conversely, '*create* that state of mind'.[28] Kempe does not neatly follow such scripted devotions, however. Never escaping from her compulsive instinct to *show* how she *feels*, her religiosity persistently attends to her mystical body, utilising and repurposing her female, post-reproductive maternity through operations of spiritual surrogacy that facilitate a manner of devotion that is both radical in its power and familiar in its socio-biological context. The ontology of female flesh that originates in the Garden of Eden sets up woman-embodied as a symbol of sinful fallibility, forever tainted with the promise that God 'will multiply [her] sorrows, and [her] conceptions' (Genesis 3:16). But that promise of indefinite pain, through the Original Sin that renders all of humankind thereafter inherently 'diseased', is also resolved through that self-same maternity to which I here turn: for although Eve will bear children 'in sorrow', she will also be the mother of redemption through the power of her 'seed' to crush all evil via the eventuality of Christ's foretold birth.[29] This is, I suggest in this book, a central facet of Margery Kempe's devotional praxes, as she embodies the pains of Eve's sorrows and of Mary's pierced heart, encased as those women are in the maternal matrices of their bodies, but synchronically empowered to 'crush' evil in the salvific potential of that same corporeality. The scholarly avenues that this book unites, therefore, are the medico-somatic significations of spirituality in the Middle Ages, engaging with the tangled issue of female pathologisation and the work of corporeal feminism in showing how medieval religious women's experience of embodied spirituality is at once empowering and abject, through a focus on female sexuality, flesh, and its concomitant cultural medicalisation.

The diversity of critical approaches is testament to the myriad passageways through which the *Book* invites us to slip. However, several coexisting strands

---

Authority and the Female Body in the Writings of Julian of Norwich and Margery Kempe (Cambridge: D.S. Brewer, 2004); Karma Lochrie, *Margery Kempe and Translations of the Flesh* (Philadelphia: University of Pennsylvania Press, 1991); and Kathy Lavezzo, 'Sobs and Sighs Between Women: The Homoerotics of Compassion in *The Book of Margery Kempe*', *Premodern Sexualities*, ed. Louise Fradenburg and Carla Freccero (New York and London: Routledge, 1996), pp. 175–98.
[27] McNamer, *Affective Meditation*, pp. 2–3.
[28] My emphasis. Ibid., p. 13.
[29] See Genesis 3:15–16.

of entry – the ontology of female flesh, the medicalisation of Kempe's spirituality, the ethics of a maternal theology – have opened up a space for this project, which argues that the *Book* can be better understood through a medical humanities approach driven not by modern understandings but by *medieval* medical discourse. This aligns with Anthony Bale's recent comment that 'Kempe should not be dismissed as either ill or eccentric but read as a product of her times'.[30] Moreover, whilst scholarship has widely considered the diagnostic potentialities of Kempe's boisterous form of religiosity, little has been written on the *peyne* that she so frequently describes, the paradigms of sickness and health during the life-course, or the *Book's* insistence on a surrogacy hermeneutic based upon a poetics of reproductivity – of natality, even – which I here explicate. These notions draw together the approaches of historicism, pathology, and embodied female spirituality, to offer a fresh exploration of *The Book of Margery Kempe* in its medicalised, phenomenological contexts.

Embodying Pain through the Life-Course

One of the most stark examples of Margery Kempe's insistent corporeality is her offer to be driven in a cart, in naked humiliation, for God's love:

> And I wolde, Lord, for þi lofe be leyd nakyd on an hyrdill, alle men to won-deryn on me for þi lofe, so it wer no perel to her sowlys, & þei to castyn slory & slugge on me, & be drawyn fro town to town euery day my lyfe-tyme, ȝyf þu wer plesyd þerby & no mannys sowle hyndryd, þi wil mote be fulfillyd & not myn (184).[31]

That she is willing to suffer her exposed body to be abused, sullied, and shamed 'euery day my lyfe-tyme' for God illustrates how it is through her raw and human physicality that she seeks transcendence. While her painful suffering and embodied spirituality through the life cycle are my primary foci in this book, to avoid the binary reductivism of women with matter and the body and men with spirit and society I prioritise Margery Kempe's subjective and spiritual *experience* as it is memorialised in the *Book*, her somatic adaptations and transformations from virgin to wife, from young woman to

---

[30] Anthony Bale, *The Book of Margery Kempe* (Oxford: Oxford University Press, 2015), pp. xi and xxxiii. On the medical humanities and the Middle Ages see 'Medievalism and the Medical Humanities', Special Issue, ed. Corinne Saunders and Jamie McKinstry, *Postmedieval*, 8 (2017). See also *Medical Humanities: An Introduction*, ed. Thomas R. Cole, Nathan S. Carlin, and Ronald A. Carson (Cambridge: Cambridge University Press, 2015); and *Medicine, Health and the Arts: Approaches to the Medical Humanities*, ed. Victoria Bates, Alan Bleakley, and Sam Goodman (London and New York: Routledge, 2014).
[31] MED s.v. hirdel: A frame or lattice of interwoven twigs, crossed wooden bars; d.) used for the sides of a cart, f.) used as a sledge on which criminals are taken to execution.

mother, and from sickness to health.[32] To overcome tribulation Kempe, I suggest, manoeuvres fluidly and adaptively, utilising her body to reflect the evolving state of her soul. But any attempt to analyse the *Book* through the broad structure of the life cycle is necessarily problematised by its achronicity. As others have acknowledged, Kempe is difficult to categorise or to impose 'order' upon. At the same time as the Christian theology of temporal order is implicit in Kempe's understanding (the creation of the world in seven days; the foretold birth, death and resurrection of Jesus; the day of Final Judgement), and the influence of church liturgy on her religious and mystical experience is clear (as Naoë Kukita Yoshikawa has illuminated), Kempe simultaneously explodes out of those very limits: she breaks the social codes of behaviour in church, allows her female body to *react* at will, and recounts her life events 'as þe mater cam to þe creatur in mend', rather than allowing the imposition of the conventional format of a 'life' upon those events.[33] Indeed, as Patricia Skinner has argued, while a linear progression through a supposed life-course is always 'disturbed and disrupted by the actualities of medieval women's lives', a 'genuinely feminist project needs to allow for similarities and shared experience between women to emerge, or for hitherto unnoticed female spaces to be apparent in the medieval landscape, overlooked because they occur only as fragmentary details in widely disparate sources'.[34] Margery Kempe has been in no way 'overlooked', of course. But in utilising the broad framework of the life-course in this book, I aim to show the ways in which Kempe both adheres to and deviates from such paths, as she persists in her own idiosyncratic navigation through earthly and mystical experience and moves in and out of linear time. In this way, the life-cycle approach is by no means a rigid methodology, and is deviated from deliberately in Chapters 1 and 5 to illustrate how her melancholic fixation on the Christic body-in-pain intersects all other life moments.

Characteristically, however, Margery Kempe does conform to many life-course conventions. Born c. 1373, she is married and pregnant at twenty, takes a vow of chastity in 1413, aged forty, and makes her final, holy journey in 1433, aged sixty. There is a latent symbolism and 'wholeness' within her life stages and ages that is suggestive of a distinct rarefaction, the *Book* as an exalted 'life'. Indeed, that Kempe is born in 1373 – the year in which her lifelong role model, Bridget of Sweden, dies – also suggests an uncanny continuity and synchronicity between these two holy women's lives, a mystical

---

[32] On the medieval body, see Caroline Walker Bynum, 'Why All the Fuss about the Body? A Medievalist's Perspective', *Critical Enquiry*, 22 (1995), 1–33. For a challenge to Bynum's 'essentialist' approach, see Kathleen Biddick, 'Genders, Bodies, Borders: Technologies of the Visible', *Speculum*, 68 (1993), 389–418.

[33] Yoshikawa, *Margery Kempe's Meditations*.

[34] Patricia Skinner, 'The Pitfalls of Linear Time: Using the Medieval Female Life Cycle as an Organizing Strategy', in *Reconsidering Gender, Time and Memory in Medieval Culture*, ed. Elizabeth Cox, Liz Herbert McAvoy, and Roberta Magnani (Cambridge: D.S. Brewer, 2015), pp. 13–28 (p. 17).

semiosis, even.[35] But Kempe also violates taxonomies, as Kim Phillips notes: 'established notions of the stages of a woman's life ... do not fit Margery well'.[36] Nevertheless, the ancient connection between the four humours and the Four Ages of Man drawn by medical writers as early as the Pythagoreans is indicative of an early interrelation between physiology and the social life stage. Black bile, associated with a melancholic disposition (and Margery Kempe's dominant humour, as I argue in Chapter 1), is aligned with Autumn – the age of 'manhood' or 'decline', from forty until approximately sixty – the very span of Margery Kempe's most important spiritual evolution. Such correlations between life stage, the seasons, individual physiological constitution, and mystical aptitude thus render a focus on the life-course a useful methodological apparatus for this book in representing the physiological and spiritual shape of Kempe's adult life in the broad sense.

In fact, the *Book*'s achronicity is a mark of agency that supports those who argue (like Watson and myself) for Kempe's position as primary author. The Proem establishes this unreservedly: that 'Sum proferyd hir to *wrytyn* hyr felyngys *wyth her owen handys*' (3) tells us that she must have been literate – that her social station in the esteemed merchant class was reason for the employment of a scribe, as opposed to a lack of education. Moreover, Kempe controls the order and content of the text through her own memorial volition as a woman of some age. The lack of linear chronology is not, then, a failing of the *Book* but rather a stamp of its authenticity; it realises the stream-of-consciousness of a sixty-three-year-old holy woman who may have a depleted calendric recall, but who dictates the narrative in her own way nonetheless:

> Thys boke is not wretyn in ordyr, euery thyng aftyr oþer as it wer don, but lych as þe mater cam to þe creatur in mend whan it schuld be wretyn, for it was so long er it was wretyn þat sche had for-getyn þe tyme & þe ordyr whan thyngys befellyn (5).[37]

Though the third-person designation of 'þis creatur' is a necessary stylistic form given that the *Book is* written down by her priestly amanuensis, we still hear Kempe's voice resound through the 'felyngys & reuelacyons & þe forme

[35] On the connection between Bridget and Margery Kempe, see, for example, Nanda Hopenwasser and Signe Wegener, 'Vox Matris: The Influence of St Birgitta's "Revelations" on *The Book of Margery Kempe*: St Birgitta and Margery Kempe as Wives and Mothers', in *Crossing the Bridge: Comparative Essays on Medieval European and Heian Japanese Women Writers*, ed. Barbara Stevenson and Cynthia Ho (New York: Palgrave, 2000), pp. 61–85.

[36] Kim Phillips, 'Margery Kempe and the Ages of Woman', in *A Companion to 'The Book of Margery Kempe'*, ed. Arnold and Lewis, pp. 17–34 (p. 33). See also Elizabeth Sears, *The Ages of Man: Medieval Interpretations* (Princeton: Princeton University Press, 1986); J.A. Burrow, *The Ages of Man: A Study in Medieval Writing and Thought* (Oxford: Clarendon Press, 1988); and Deborah Youngs, *The Life Cycle in Western Europe, c. 1300–1500* (Manchester: Manchester University Press, 2006).

[37] On memory, see Mary Carruthers, *The Book of Memory: A Study of Memory in Medieval Culture* (Cambridge and New York: Cambridge University Press, 2008).

of her leuyng' (3–4) that make up its content. This book therefore employs the nomenclature Kempe, or Margery Kempe, to reassert her status as a recognised canonical woman writer, eschewing the mythologised 'Margery' that might limit her authority. Indeed, it is something of an irony that critics have debated the extent of Kempe's 'authentic voice' and its partial or total external construction, and yet often continue to enact discourse on the basis of first-name terms. Another central concern of this book, then, is to suggest that the anamnestic quality of the narrative increases its authenticity as a product of human recollection and retrospection. The influence of memory cogni-zance in Kempe's choices of example, order, and emotional response does not detract from the *Book*'s value but rather enhances it as a work crafted by the cognitive pulses of recall – the social and mystical events recounted are them-selves indicative of their affective and spiritual import for her construction and understanding of self. Since these events emerge almost 'by nature' – 'as þe mater cam to þe creatur in mend' – we reach a level of truth in the words as historical relics of Kempe's experience. This is a more crucial issue for a discussion of Book II, whose texture is strikingly different in content and tone from Book I. This is a subject deserving of further scrutiny, which I begin to examine in Chapter 6.[38]

Although this is a study of *The Book of Margery Kempe* through a medieval medical lens, I do not seek to pathologise or to 'diagnose' her recorded expe-riences, but rather to elucidate how the discourse of pain and suffering in the *Book* enables Kempe (and, indeed, her readers) to orient themselves in relation to their physiological and social worlds. References to painful experience in the *Book* are multiple and include the derivations *peyne*, *payn*, *peyned*, and so forth, along with related terms of suffering such as *angwisch*, *dysese*, and to *ponysch* or *labowr*. While my approach to the concept of pain in the *Book* will be broad and I will use the term to encompass all of the variations here, a consideration of what we might surmise as an epistemology of pain is useful in attempting to encapsulate the meaning of pain in the medieval imaginary. As well as the subjective *now* of pain sensation – Scarry's 'unsharable' *it* – the cultural imbrications of the political, social, medical, theological, and spiritual form an important part of how we might understand the medieval experience of pain and suffering. Given the iconographic paradigm of later medieval Christianity during its 'affective turn', with the Christic body-in-pain as a ubiquitous reminder of the need to live and die well, suffering and salvation are inescapable aspects of the human condition.

Kempe couches her spiritual pain in terms of the visceral apprehension of bodily suffering, a perhaps inevitable conflation in the light of the current OED definition of pain, which still prioritises denotations of 'punishment, penalty', and suffering in 'hell and purgatory' over physical anguish – an

---

[38] This is also something taken up by Katherine Lewis in 'Margery Kempe, Oral History and the Value of Intersubjectivity', in *Encountering The Book of Margery Kempe*, ed. Kalas and Varnam (forthcoming).

'unpleasant or agonising sensation in the body' – suggesting how cultural constructions of pain continue to be hinged on the connotations of sin and suffering.[39] In contrast, the definition of pain by The International Association for the Study of Pain (IASP) is 'an unpleasant sensory and emotional experience associated with actual or potential tissue damage, or described in terms of such damage'. An important footnote follows that 'pain is always subjective' and that 'each individual learns the application of the word through experiences related to injury in early life'; however, the definition does not allow for the non-sensory or non-neurological experience of emotional or spiritual suffering.[40] Scientists like Patrick Wall, who formulated the influential Gate Control Theory (which proposes that nerve gates in the spinal cord transmit pain signals depending on the brain signals being sent back down), see the mind and body as integrated but nevertheless believe that there is an essence of pain: a 'pure pain' that is accompanied by emotion and individual meaning.[41] However, as Joanna Bourke points out, the IASP definition does allow for emotional pain, given that pain can be '*described* in terms of' tissue damage, thus overcoming the 'myth of two pains'. Indeed, David Biro argues that scientific investigations are beginning to determine how psychological pain appears to 'run on the same neural tracks as physical pain', and that, regardless of its original source or taxonomy, 'Everything is contingent on the *feeling* of pain'.[42] Adopting Esther Cohen and Leona Toker's stance, which 'suspend[s] the distinction between the physical and the emotional pain or at least register[s] the porousness of the dividing line between them', I will suggest that Margery Kempe's understanding of pain – like that of her medieval counterparts – also evades such distinctions.[43] Her *felyngys* in the *Book* are frequently juxtaposed with her *reuelacyons*, emphasising the primacy of the sensory faculties as markers of her mystical prescience; she perceives pain as she *feels* it, as a subjective sensation, as it harbours inside her. This is viewed by Na'ama Cohen-Hanegbi as a culturally internalised mechanism, the intense mental exercises of meditation on Christ's wounds by medieval visionaries showing that 'medieval pain was … understood as a physical phenomenon configured by psychological processes'.[44]

---

39 OED s.v. pain: denotations 1(a), 2, and 3(a) respectively.
40 U. Lindblom et al., 'Pain Terms: A Current List with Definitions and Notes on Usage', *Pain*, 24 (1986), Supplement 1, S1–S226 (p. S217).
41 Patrick Wall, *The Science of Suffering* (London: Weidenfeld and Nicholson, 1999), p. 31. See also Ronald Melzack and Patrick Wall, *The Challenge of Pain* (London: Penguin, 1996). On the interaction of the science and culture of pain see David Morris, *The Culture of Pain* (Berkley and Los Angeles: The University of California Press, 1991).
42 David Biro, 'Is There Such a Thing as Psychological Pain? And Why It Matters', *Culture, Medicine and Society*, 34 (2010), 658–67 (p. 663).
43 Esther Cohen and Leona Toker, 'Introduction', in *Knowledge and Pain*, ed. Esther Cohen, Leona Toker, Manuela Consonni, and Otniel E. Dror (Amsterdam and New York: Rodopi, 2012), pp. vii–xviii (p. viii).
44 Na'ama Cohen-Hanegbi, 'Pain as Emotion: The Role of Emotional Pain in Fifteenth-

Elaine Scarry's work remains influential in considering pain as an exceptional human interior state since, she argues, 'physical pain – unlike any other state of consciousness – has no referential content. It is not *of* or *for* anything. It is precisely because it takes no object that it, more than any other phenomenon, resists objectification in language'. It is the visibility of painful expression that she considers central to its external reception: 'It is not simply accurate but tautological to observe that given any two phenomena, the one that is more visible will receive more attention.' This is because, she writes, 'Physical pain does not simply resist language but actively destroys it, bringing about an immediate reversion to a state anterior to language, to the sounds and cries a human makes before language is learned.'[45] Yet while certainly the expressions of pain in Kempe's *Book* and in other medieval depictions of suffering, like the cries and asceticism of Marie of Oignies (1177–1213) or the self-mortifications of Henry Suso (c. 1295–1366), align with the efficacious visibility and non-verbal clamour of Scarry's theory, I take issue with the notion of pain as a free-floating, non-referential phenomenon, particularly in the context of the highly iconographic Christocentric Middle Ages where, for the mystics at least, the *point* of the pain was that it was for God.[46] The modern nursing tool known as McCaffery's Principle states that 'pain is whatever the experiencing person says it is, existing wherever he [*sic*] says it does'; here pain is defined as self-authenticating, the definition offering an atemporal system better aligned with medieval pain perception.[47] Indeed, as well as being alert to the danger of assuming a 'unique experience' of pain in individuals, Javier Moscoso writes that 'the probability that their experience will be culturally meaningful increases depending on whether it can be imitated or represented … If the sensations do not correspond to any visible or known cause, some problems will arise.' This is a familiar difficulty in the *Book*, as Kempe's boisterous expressions are sometimes perplexing to her spectators.[48] Only those clerics informed of the lives of other affective devotees such as Marie of Oignies understand the discourse at work in Kempe's 'drama' of suffering, and thus attach to it the requisite cultural meaning. In medieval terms, pain is a foundational hermeneutic of devotional participa-

---

Century Italian Medicine and Confession', in *Knowledge and Pain*, ed. Cohen et al., pp. 63–82 (pp. 64–5).

[45] Elaine Scarry, *The Body in Pain*, p. 5, p. 12 and p. 4 respectively.

[46] See *Three Women of Liège: A Critical Edition of and Commentary on the Middle English Lives of Elizabeth of Spalbeek, Christina Mirabilis and Marie d'Oignies*, ed. Jennifer N. Brown (Turnhout: Brepols, 2008). See also Henry Suso, *Heinrich Seuse. Deutsche Schriften*, ed. Karl Bihlmeyer (Stuttgart: W. Kohlhammer, 1907), translated by Frank Tobin in *Henry Suso: The Exemplar, with Two German Sermons* (Mahwah, New Jersey: Paulist Press, 1989).

[47] Margo McCaffery, *Nursing Practice: Theories Related to Cognition, Bodily Pain, and Man–Environment Interactions* (Los Angeles: UCLA Student Store, 1968).

[48] Moscoso, *Pain: A Cultural History*, p. 8. On the scientific and cultural significations and modifications of suffering, see also Robert Fuller, *Spirituality in the Flesh: Bodily Sources of Religious Experience* (Oxford and New York: Oxford University Press, 2008).

tion, simultaneously caused by intense meditation on the suffering Christ and alleviated by his redemptive power. As Ariel Glucklich attests, despite the 'insurmountable privacy of the body in pain', in fact 'the phenomenon of shared pain is extremely pervasive', for otherwise the suffering of the crucified Christ, or the martyrdom of saints, would not mean anything to anyone.[49] The two 'types' of pain that Glucklich identifies – 'disintegrative' (disruptive, devastating, punitive) and 'integrative' (strengthening, situating, affirming) – are apt for understanding Kempe's own unmaking and remaking of self, as she bursts, collapses, erupts, and becomes whole again. Time and again, her suffering is *integrative*, nonetheless, as her journey offers renewed mechanisms for surrogacy, fecundity, and painful productivity.

In medieval medical scholasticism the inherited definitions of pain from the *De interioribus* by Galen (b. c. 129) and later from the *al-Qānūn fī'l-tibb* (*The Canon of Medicine*) by Ibn Sīnā (980–1037; Latinised to Avicenna) meant that patients' pain was categorised according to 'causal and locative principles and not to the painful feeling as described by the patient'.[50] Avicenna extended Galen's classification of four types of pain, establishing the categories as: boring pain, compressing pain, corrosive pain, dull pain, fatigue-pain, heavy pain, incisive pain, irritant pain, itching pain, pricking pain, stabbing pain, tearing pain, tension pain, and throbbing pain.[51] But because medieval physicians focused on the somatic aspects of painful experience, the use of a standardised vocabulary for naming pain 'inevitably cancelled the particular subjective experience of the individual'.[52] The *truth* of a patient's pain, then, was clouded by the terms which medical masters and physicians insisted upon imposing on the sufferers' own descriptions, obscuring the subjective referents in which sufferers like Margery Kempe were imbricated. Esther Cohen notes that pain in the Middle Ages developed from an individual feeling to a social, religious, and cultural phenomenon; 'suffering was not to be dismissed, vanquished, or transcended: suffering was to be felt with an ever-deepening intensity'.[53] Not simply an emotional preoccupation, it was a 'teleological, all-embracing civilizing process' by which 'one could perfect one's self'.[54] This

---

[49] Ariel Glucklich, *Sacred Pain: Hurting the Body for the Sake of the Soul* (Oxford: Oxford University Press, 2001), p. 30 and p. 63.

[50] Fernando Salmón, 'From Patient to Text? Narratives of Pain and Madness in Medical Scholasticism', in *Between Text and Patient: The Medical Enterprise in Medieval and Early Modern Europe*, ed. Florence Eliza Glaze and Brian K. Nance (Florence: Sismel, 2011), pp. 373–95 (p. 381).

[51] Avicenna, *The Canon of Medicine (al-Qānūn fī'l-tibb)*, vol. 1, trans. O. Cameron Gruner and Mazar H. Shah, adapted by Laleh Bakhtiar (Chicago: Kazi Publications, 1999), 10.19, pp. 249–51. The series of five volumes from 'The Great Books of the Islamic World' (series editor Seyyed Hossein Nasr), is the closest English translation of the original Arabic text.

[52] Salmón, 'From Patient to Text', in *Between Text and Patient*, ed. Glaze et al., p. 387.

[53] Esther Cohen, *The Modulated Scream: Pain in Late Medieval Culture* (Chicago and London: University of Chicago Press, 2010), pp. 3–4.

[54] Ibid, p. 4.

was especially the case in the medico-religious imaginary, since Galen had attached hierarchical meaning to the bodily organs in terms of their 'noble' or 'non-noble' nature (the brain, heart, and eyes being noble). The noble organs were considered more sensitive to pain, and since Christ was superior and noble in nature, his pain was most acute. As Christ's humanity and medically perfect complexion were increasingly emphasised from the eleventh century, so he came to stand for the 'greatest possible sensitivity to pain': in medieval culture, to be in pain was to be Christ-like.[55] As Cohen attests, 'pain is good because it is bad'; 'its value is its utility', and it is this utility of pain as a productive force with which this book is concerned, particularly in terms of the knowledge of pain that Kempe acquires on her eschatological journey.[56] This central question – posed by S. Benjamin Fink as '[do] we know pain?' – is one which courses through the veins of this study. Fink argues that to *know* pain requires an understanding of pain as non-homogeneous; it covers a plethora of concepts.[57] For Margery Kempe pain is also multiple in its manifestation, but it is simultaneously singularly constructed around knowing God, knowing her pain, and what is at stake through that suffering.

Julian of Norwich writes that 'the night is cause of oure paine', as the dark and bleak opposition to the light of faith which 'kindly com[es] of oure endless day that is oure fader, God'.[58] But for Julian that pain is purgative and productive: 'This dred doth good, for it helpeth to purge man, as doth bodely sicknesse or such other paine that is not sinne. For all such paines helpe man, if they be patiently taken.'[59] The purgative or cleansing function of pain for Julian as a pseudo-medical activity, eliminating evils from the human body, is a further concern of this book, as it seeks to explore Kempe's wrangling with pain as a series of life events, toward a nexus with God the Physician. In this way the complex removal and distancing of Kempe's interior experience of suffering through the scribal production of the *Book* is a perhaps twofold iteration of *any* attempt to write an individual consciousness of pain. Though that pain can never be truly replicated, my approach is to regard the scribal process as one of the many interpretative responses to Kempe's pain, like those of the priests and parishioners who witness her writhing and sobbing in discomfort or awe, or the physician who takes notes from a patient's description of her pain. In announcing her pain in thunderous and gesticulatory ways, Margery

---

[55] See Esther Cohen, '"If You Prick Us, Do We Not Bleed?": Reflections on the Diminishing of the Other's Pain', in *Knowledge and Pain*, ed. Cohen et al., pp. 25–41 (pp. 26–7).

[56] Cohen, *The Modulated Scream*, p. 4 and 8.

[57] S. Benjamin Fink, 'Knowing Pain', *Knowledge and Pain*, ed. Cohen et al., pp. 1–22 (pp. 10–12).

[58] Julian of Norwich, 'A Revelation of Love', in *The Writings of Julian of Norwich: A Vision Showed to a Devout Woman and A Revelation of Love*, ed. Nicholas Watson and Jacqueline Jenkins (University Park: Pennsylvania State University Press, 2005), Ch. 83, p. 377.

[59] Julian of Norwich, 'A Revelation of Love', in *The Writings of Julian of Norwich*, ed. Watson and Jenkins, ch. 74, p. 355.

Kempe imprints her suffering on her world, in her *Book*, and in the medical records of her physician, Christ, in whose care she is promised to flourish.

The Textual Corpus

The body of medical texts that I employ in this book is rationalised both upon the relevance of the treatises for women's medicine and the circulation of those texts in England in the later Middle Ages, in order to establish, as far as possible, the medico-cultural milieu in which Margery Kempe self-conceptualised and was understood. The important tradition of tribulation texts, originating in the psalm 'He shall cry to me, and I will hear him: I am with him in tribulation, I will deliver him, and I will glorify him', is also alluded to in the *Book*'s Proem – 'of whech tribulacyons sum schal ben schewed aftyr' (6).[60] The tribulation genre is one which offers an obvious lens through which to approach Kempe's experience of suffering, and has been recently explored by Rebecca Krug, but it is not my present concern since my focus is the medicalised discourse in the *Book*'s spiritual signification.[61] By far the most well-known text within such discourse for women's medicine was the so-called *Trotula* ensemble, composed of the 'Liber de sinthomatibus mulierum' (Book on the Conditions of Women), 'De curis mulierum' (On Treatments for Women), and 'De ornatu mulierum' (On Women's Cosmetics). Each text circulated independently in Europe but, by the end of the twelfth century, they were compiled in a single ensemble and entitled *Summa que dicitur 'Trotula'* (*The Compendium Which is Called the 'Trotula'*).[62] Its circulation in England was vast, and vernacular translations appeared from the thirteenth century; these were often addressed to female audiences since women readers more often accessed material in the vernacular. Later medieval translations, however, seem to be intended for male readers.[63] The most widely disseminated text on women's medicine in late medieval England were the gynaecological and obstetrical chapters excerpted from the *Compendium medicinae*, written c. 1240 by Gilbertus Anglicus, known as *The Sekenesse of Wymmen*. Existent in two Middle English versions, the title in Yale Medical Library MS 47 and London, Wellcome Library MS 5650 states, metonymically, that the uterus *is* 'the

---

[60] Psalm 90:15.

[61] Krug, *Margery Kempe and the Lonely Reader*, especially ch. 1. See, for example, *The Twelve Profits of Tribulation*, in *Yorkshire Writers: Richard Rolle of Hampole and His Followers*, ed. Carl Horstmann, 2 vols (London: Swan Sonnenschein, 1896); *The Book of Tribulation*, ed. Alexandra Barratt (Heidelberg: Carl Winter, 1983); and *The Chastising of God's Children and the Treatise of Perfection of the Sons of God*, ed. Joyce Bazire and Eric College (Oxford: Basil Blackwell, 1957).

[62] *The Trotula: A Medieval Compendium of Women's Medicine*, ed. and trans. Monica H. Green (Philadelphia: University of Pennsylvania Press, 2001), pp. xi–xii.

[63] Monica H. Green, 'Making Motherhood in Medieval Medicine: The Evidence from Medicine', in *Motherhood, Religion, and Society in Medieval Europe, 400–1400*, ed. Conrad Leyser and Lesley Smith (Farnham: Ashgate, 2011), pp. 173–203 (p. 174).

sekenesse of wymmen'.[64] Monica Green and Linne Mooney have superseded previous editions in their publication of Cambridge, Trinity College MS R.14.52, fols 107r–135v, which corrects previous misidentifications of the text's Latin source and its relations.[65] The Trinity text was probably produced in the mid-fifteenth century and appears to be addressed directly to women ('that oo woman may help another in hir sikenes'), though, since the number of literate midwives is unknown, it is likely that the text was read aloud to them.[66] Another highly popular gynaecological text which also addresses a female audience is the late fourteenth- or early fifteenth-century treatise *The Knowing of Woman's Kind in Childing*, which has particular similarities with *The Sickness of Women* since both employ extended obstetrical information derived from a late Antique gynaecological text, Musico's *Non omnes quidem*.[67] Written in Middle English prose and apparently translated from French and Latin texts it survives in five manuscripts.[68] Alexandra Barratt has edited two versions of the text in her volume: Oxford, Bodley MS Douce 37, and Cambridge University Library MS Ii.6.33. The Douce version is longer, includes some additional material, is written in a more expansive style, and adopts pseudo-chapter headings. For these reasons I employ the Douce text in this study.

The natural-philosophic text *De secretis mulierum*, falsely attributed to the Dominican theologian Albertus Magnus (d. 1280), is a Latin text composed in Germany in the last quarter of the thirteenth century, perhaps by a student in Albert's circle.[69] The unapologetically misogynistic treatise circulated widely both in Latin and in several vernacular translations (although it was perhaps

---

[64] Monica H. Green, 'Obstetrical and Gynaecological Texts in Middle English', *Studies in the Age of Chaucer*, 14 (1992), 53–88 (pp. 72–4). Editions of the *Sekenesse of Wymmen* include *A Middle English Treatise on Diseases in Women*, Yale Medical Library, Ms. 47 *fols. 60r–71v*, ed. M.R. Hallaert, in *Scripta: Mediaeval and Renaissance Texts and Studies* 8 (Brussels: Omirel, 1982); and, from London, BL, Sloane MS 2463, in *Medieval Women's Guide to Health: The First English Gynecological Handbook*, ed. Beryl Rowland (Kent, Ohio: The Kent State University Press, 1981).

[65] Green and Mooney note how Rowland's edition was not the 'first' English gynaecological handbook, and that at least four other texts antedate it by several decades. *Sickness of Women*, ed. Monica H. Green and Linne R. Mooney, in *Sex, Aging, and Death in Medieval Medical Compendium: Trinity College Cambridge MS R.14.52, Its Texts, Language, and Scribe*, vol. 2, ed. M. Teresa Tavormina (Tempe: Arizona Centre for Medieval and Renaissance Studies, 2006), pp. 455–568 (p. 456, n. 1). For corrections on the Rowland edition see Jerry Stannard and Linda Ehrsam Voigts, 'Review of Beryl Rowland, *Medieval Woman's Guide to Health*', *Speculum*, 57 (1982), 422–6; and Alicia Rodríguez Alvarez, 'The *Sekenesse of Wymmen* Revised', *Manuscripta*, 40 (2000), 157–64.

[66] *Sickness of Women*, pp. 485 and 462.

[67] Ibid., p. 463.

[68] *The Knowing of Woman's Kind in Childing: A Middle English Version of Material Derived from the Trotula and Other Sources*, ed. Alexandra Barratt (Turnhout: Brepols, 2001), p. 1.

[69] Monica Green, '"Traittié tout de mençonges": The *Secrés des dames*, "Trotula", and Attitudes towards Women's Medicine in Fourteenth- and Early-Fifteenth-Century France' (1998), in *Women's Healthcare in the Medieval West*, Monica H. Green (Aldershot: Ashgate, 2000), VI, pp. 146–78 (p. 150).

less well known in England).[70] Various editions were produced, including over fifty printed versions in the fifteenth century, thus the text represents ideas about women and science that permeated the thirteenth- and four-teenth-century scholastic milieu, disseminating through the Church and into popular medicine.[71] As Green notes, by the fourteenth century the practical medical tradition of the *Trotula* texts and the theoretical, natural–philosophical tradition of the *Secretis mulierum* began to collide, 'ultimately becoming so closely allied as to be often indistinguishable'.[72] I therefore include this treatise not because of its particular circulation in England but because it represents ideas that diffused from scholasticism into medicine in Europe, and the con-comitant influence of educated clerics on Kempe's learning. Indeed, it is clear from the *Book* that Margery Kempe's behaviour was pathologised similarly by her onlookers, indicating how these ideas were composite of a wider atmos-phere of pejorative thought about the female body in the Middle Ages. Green has shown how 'evidence for ownership of texts on women's medicine by male clerics and scholars becomes ample by the end of the thirteenth century', and how male interest in 'the secrets of women' grew in the fourteenth.[73] While gynaecological and obstetrical theory and practice were masculinised, and women had 'no claim to the *authoritative knowledge* that distinguished the now professionalised, institutionally sanctioned practices of male physicians, surgeons, barbers, and apothecaries', it was also the case, according to Green, that 'certain kinds of female medical practice never disappeared'.[74] Women still maintained an unrecorded role in the birthing room and held medical authority in the domestic sphere.[75]

In addition to these gynaecological and obstetrical texts, I incorporate further material from ancient and medieval medical writings that shaped the cultural context in which Kempe lived, including the foundational ideas of

---

[70] Although the text is largely composed of natural philosophy, several of the vernacular translations (mostly in France) incorporate additional obstetrical material, addressed to midwives, indicating the interaction of natural philosophy and medicine. See Monica Green, 'Medieval Gynaecological Texts: A Handlist', in *Women's Healthcare in the Medieval West*, Appendix pp. 1–36 (pp. 1–2, n. 3).

[71] Psuedo-Abertus Magnus, *De secretis mulierum: Item de virtutibus herbarum lapidum et animalium* (Amsterdam: J. Janssonius, 1662). *De secretis mulierum, Women's Secrets: A Translation of Pseudo-Albertus Magnus' 'De secretis mulierum' with Commentaries*, ed. Helen Rodnite Lemay (Albany: State University of New York Press, 1992), pp. 1–2.

[72] Green, "Traittié tout de mençonges", in *Women's Healthcare in the Medieval West*, p. 148.

[73] Green, 'Making Motherhood', in *Motherhood, Religion, and Society*, ed. Leyser, p. 182; and Green, *Making Women's Medicine Masculine: The Rise of Male Authority in Pre-Modern Gynaecology* (Oxford: Oxford University Press, 2008), pp. 204–45.

[74] Monica Green, *Making Women's Medicine Masculine*, p. 299 and p. 290.

[75] Ibid., p. 290. For a handlist of all gynaecological texts in western Europe from the fourth to the fifteenth centuries, see Monica Green, 'Appendix: Medieval Gynecological Texts: A Handlist', in *Women's Healthcare in the Medieval West*, pp. 1–36. See also Green, 'Bibliography on Medieval Women, Gender, and Medicine (1985–2009)', *Digital Library of Sciència.cat* (2010), Universitat de Barcelona: <http://www.sciencia.cat/biblioteca/documents/Green_CumulativeBib_Feb2010.pdf>.

the Hippocratic corpus, Galen and Aristotle, and the early Church Fathers. Further works that are central to this book's overarching narrative include the widely circulated works of Constantine the African (d. 1087), who translated Ishāq ibn Imrān's works into the *Viaticum and De melancholia*; Avicenna's *Canon*, which significantly influenced later medieval thought in the West; and the *Summa theologiae* of the Dominican friar and proponent of natural theology Thomas Aquinas (c. 1225–1274). The scientific works of Hildegard of Bingen (1098–1179), notably *Causae et curae* and *Physica*, form a significant contribution to my assimilation of medical ideas about the female body. While Hildegard's medical works had limited direct circulation in England, her writings and ideas were advanced by Bernard of Clairvaux, to whom Hildegard wrote in request of support, and were later disseminated in part via compilations and fragmented excerpts, clearly forming an influential part of 'the great age of Latin mystical writing' in Europe.[76] A Middle English translation of Gilbertus Anglicus's *Compendium medicinae* (c. 1230–40), edited under the title *System of Physic*, and John Trevisa's *On the Properties of Things*, a Middle English translation of Bartholomaeus Anglicus's *De proprietatibus rerum*, further enrich the underlying corpus of scientific texts that, if not directly known by Margery Kempe, would certainly have filtered into her wider cognizance through interaction with the learned clerics and confessors of her daily life.

The Ordyr of thys Boke

The chapters that follow are largely structured around the same methodological trajectory: an initial explication of the medico-religious context is followed by application to and analysis of *The Book of Margery Kempe*. In so doing, I seek to uncover the medical subtext of Kempe's spirituality and to situate that experience within its medieval frame of reference. Chapter 1, 'Bleeding the Tears of Melancholia', explores Margery Kempe's humoral and constitutional disposition as a natural melancholic, a thesis upon which all subsequent chapters are framed, in considering her weeping in its medical context as a teleology of a Christic object-fixation. Establishing Kempe's tears as wounds, caused by her internalisation of the trauma of Christ's crucifixion, the chapter argues for a desire-loss hermeneutic where Kempe experiences totalisation through her retaining of Christ inside her soul. After exploring the possibilities for her onlookers' persistent pathologisation of her weeping based on scientific understanding, I propose an alternative medicalisation, situating Kempe's mysticism within the tradition of melancholia's association with giftedness and affective receptivity and elucidating the dichotomous

---

[76] Barbara Newman, 'Latin and the Vernaculars', in *The Cambridge Companion to Christian Mysticism*, ed. Amy Hollywood and Patricia Z. Beckman (Cambridge: Cambridge University Press, 2012), pp. 225–39 (p. 229).

pain and spiritual advantage of her weeping. In Chapter 2, '"Þe mukke" of Marriage and the Sexual Paradox', the book's focus on the life-course begins through an analysis of Margery Kempe's early adulthood and reproductive years. Focusing on what I have termed the 'pain paradox' of celibacy as inescapably painful, the chapter illuminates Kempe's early married years until her vow of chastity, aged forty. The trauma of her first childbirth, signalling Kempe's 'unmaking' and eventual rebirth through Christ's medicine, functions as a structuring device for the rest of the *Book*. While theological doctrine held virginity as an ultimate state of holiness and freedom from the 'disease' of sin, medical texts contradicted this logic, positing chaste living as causative of pain – a particularly problematic notion for religious women. In considering Kempe's ascetic strategies, the deadly power of the female touch, and the fortifications with which she surrounds herself, the chapter untangles the extent to which her vow of chastity and mystical marriage enable analgesic relief.

Chapter 3, 'Lost Blood of the Middle Age: Surrogacy and Fecundity', is an exegesis of Margery Kempe's middle age in relation to the gendered implications of the 'lost blood' of menstruation and the concomitant ontological shift at menopause: a topic that has, surprisingly, been barely studied. The chapter's focus on her middle age and post-reproductivity – in the sense of both the self-imposed post-reproductive state brought about by her vow of chastity at the age of forty, and, later, the biological state of menopause – concerns the metamorphosis of body and experience at this life stage and Kempe's transformation into an agent of ministry and, particularly, surrogacy, during the intense 'blood piety' of the Middle Ages. In developing the surrogacy hermeneutic that is central to this book, I argue that her actualised reproduction is replaced with alternative, fecund strategies of surrogacy as she utilises previous maternity for the social and mystical substitutions of wet nursing, godparenting, fostering, image-substitution, and pain-bearing as alternative acts of production. As Kempe mystically internalises the suckling of the Christ Child by Mary in her soul, her anachronistic body is transformed into one of new fecundity. Chapter 4, '*Margery Medica*: The Healing Value of Pain Surrogacy', develops the book's focus on Kempe's middle age and surrogacy praxes in relation to her healing strategies as a disciple of *Christus medicus*. Kempe's knowledge of pain is translated to an operation that I term 'pain surrogacy' – that is, her willing receipt and support of pain that does not originate in the self and which, by its very nature, is rooted in the maturing female body. This chapter explores Kempe's capacity to (re)experience, or to *bear*, productive and physical pain for both earthly and divine sufferers. In considering the medieval 'nurse' as a surrogate healing agent, I examine the ways in which her post-reproductivity evolves to a transition from wet nurse, to healing nurse, to healer. Focusing on her healing of women in Rome, her mystical healing and caring interventions, her fixation on 'lepers', the body-soul healing of her adult son, and the caring of her infirm husband, who eventually dies, the chapter concludes at the point of Margery Kempe's metamorphosis, through pain surrogacy, to the 'parfyte' state of widowhood, in domestic liberation and spiritual transcendence.

In Chapter 5, 'The Passion of Death Surrogacy', the life-course paradigm is deliberately lifted in an analysis of Kempe's meditations on the Passion as nevertheless climactic indications of her mystical maturity and eschatological insight. Her predisposition to the black bile of melancholia, mourning, and mystical perspicacity is again evoked through the intense verisimilitude of her Passion visions. The symbiosis of Kempe's pain and Christ's is established early in the *Book*, when his crucified body is mystically located within her own, as he 'schuld be newe crucified in [her]' time and again. Such ascetic profit is emphasised when she is conceived by Christ as a fleshly sacrifice to be consumed and martyred in quasi-Eucharistic substitution: 'Þow xalt ben etyn & knawyn of þe pepul of þe world as any raton knawyth þe stokfysh.' Kempe thus reveals her conceptualisation as a willing sacrificial lamb early in her recollections, deliberately foregrounding her embodiment in vulnerable human flesh at the same time as insisting on the amalgamation of Christ's torture with her own. By comparison with Catherine of Siena's 'mystical death', I argue that Kempe's altered consciousness during the Passion visions is similar to Catherine's temporary physical annihilation. In uncovering the physiological Signs of Death that appear in medical and religious texts, Kempe's own experience of illness, and her role as a death-bed vigilant for her *even cristen*, the chapter argues for the continuation of the surrogacy hermeneutic up until the end of life through her willingness to be a 'death-surrogate' for Christ himself, as her drive for immolation renders her 'dead to the world'. Chapter 6, 'Senescent Reproduction: Writing Anamnestic Pain', moves to the end of the life-course, examining Margery Kempe's old age as a framework for the casting of her entire project, the spiritualisation of her pain, and the *Book* as itself the ultimate surrogate production. As a retrospective, the pain narrative of Kempe's life is an anamnestic production, in the context of her increased authority as an 'elder' in the world. In finally inscribing her life and learning to the manuscript page some twenty years after her conversion, Margery Kempe recalls the memory of her pains – more recently experienced in the events of Book II than Book I – from the perspective of old age. I argue here that we might grasp the *voice* of Margery Kempe particularly urgently in Book II, since, while there is a certain 'saintly box-ticking' subtext at play, the conflation of age, experience, and narrative immediacy brings a particular form of truth to the reader. Since the culturally abject ageing body is, to an extent, diseased by default, Kempe utilises such significations to undertake an *aged asceticism* in her elderly years – the efficacious pain of her cooling, drying, ageing body. In analysing the wise old holy women with whom she identifies, her northern European travel, and her transformation to a sagacious church 'elder', the chapter concludes at her climactic attendance at the Lammastide pardon ceremonies at Syon in 1434, where she is not only validated as a teacher via the important Brigittine connection but is also adopted as 'Modir' by a young man who learns of her pain-given understanding.

In the Afterword I seek to uncover the multiple afterlives of Margery Kempe. Conversely, the printed extracts by Wynkyn de Worde in 1501 erase all autobiographical detail of Kempe's life: 'In no extract is there a single circumstance of the worldly life of Margery.'[77] The narrative arc of this book and its exploration, through Kempe's broad life-course, extrapolates the medical discourse at work in the *Book* to trace the function and utility of painful experience in her eschatological trajectory. The recipe's curative symbolism is thus an apt 'conclusion' in its teleological signalling of Kempe's spiritual healing, and that of her readers, themselves healed by the medicine of the text. The resulting narrative of this study should therefore reorient our understanding of the *Book*, leading us to appreciate it as an example of the centrality of medico-religious discourse in the later Middle Ages. Without such attention to the deep conflation of spiritual and medical semiosis, crucial meanings, particularly about the lived female spiritual experience, remain dormant. While Kempe's suffering mutates as she traverses life and spiritual stages, its final destination is a one-ing with the Christ whose own body-in-pain, suspended in temporal agony, calls to her from the moment of her conversion to the moment when she agrees to write the *Book*, where pain and word somehow collide, and from where she writes her life, in all its painful glory.

---

[77] S.B. Meech, *BMK*, xlvi.

1

Bleeding the Tears of Melancholia

> Mourning is commonly the reaction to the loss of a beloved person or an
> abstraction taking the place of the person, such as fatherland, freedom, an ideal
> and so on. In some people, whom we for this reason suspect of a pathological
> disposition, melancholia appears in place of mourning.[1]

Sigmund Freud's definition of melancholia takes as its focus the loss of a
loved object that, rather than being ultimately relinquished over time as with
the comparable condition of mourning, is retained and internalised by the
sufferer, who then manifests an 'exclusive devotion to mourning'. Not only
does Freud acknowledge our unquestioning acceptance that 'the mood of
mourning [is] a "painful" one', he also suggests that this experience takes on a
metapsychological process: 'this tendency can become so intense that it leads
to a person turning away from reality and holding on to the object through a
hallucinatory wish-psychosis'.[2] Beyond this, the sufferer is subject to a 'detour
of self-punishment' whereby 'the indubitably pleasurable self-torment of
melancholia … signifies the satisfaction of tendencies of sadism and hatred,
which are applied to an object and are thus turned back against the patient's
own person'.[3] The grieving melancholic, then, experiences an uncanny state
of pain and pleasure, reliving and re-experiencing a loss which is at once
agonisingly acute yet also gratifying because it symbolises a means of retaining a connection – a diachronic oneness – with the lost object of desire. The
complex of melancholia, according to Freud, 'behaves like an open wound',
drawing energies towards itself and leaving the self impoverished.[4]

---

[1] Sigmund Freud, *On Murder, Mourning and Melancholia*, trans. Shaun Whiteside (London: Penguin Classics, 2005), p. 203.

[2] Ibid., p. 204.

[3] Ibid., p. 211.

[4] On the psychoanalysis of mourning and melancholia, see Lorraine D. Siggins, 'Mourning: A Critical Survey of the Literature', *International Journal of Psycho-Analysis*, 47 (1966), 14–25; M. Torok, 'The Illness of Mourning and the Fantasy of the Exquisite Corpse' (1968), in *The Shell and the Kernel*, ed. and trans. Nicholas T. Rand (Chicago and London: University of Chicago Press, 1994), pp. 107–24; and Nicholas Abraham and Maria Torok, 'Introjection – Incorporation: Mourning or Melancholia', in *Psychoanalysis in France*, ed. Serge Lebovici and Daniel Widlöcher (New York: International Universities Press), pp. 3–16.

As an open wound, melancholia is therefore strikingly resonant with Judeo-Christian imagery.[5] Amy Hollywood makes the connections between mourning, melancholia, and Christian mysticism explicit in her study of Beatrice of Nazareth and Margaret Ebner, arguing for a pattern that moves:

> from external objects to their internalization by the devout person (the key component of melancholy for both medieval and modern theorists), and then their subsequent re-externalization in and on the body of the believer (the rendering visible of melancholic incorporation whereby the holy person becomes Christ to those around her).[6]

In her discussion of medieval mystical rapture, Hollywood suggests that devotees internalise traumatic memories 'by rendering involuntary, vivid, and inescapable the central catastrophic event of Christian history so that the individual believer might relive and share in that trauma'. She regards 'medieval practitioners of meditation on Christ's Passion' as having 'the desire to inculcate something like traumatic memory [as] theologically justified by a promise: through sharing in the suffering of those who witnessed Christ's death or ... sharing Christ's own pain, one can participate in the salvific work of the cross'.[7]

In this chapter, I want to suggest that Margery Kempe is a crucial example of the interplay between melancholia, mysticism, and medieval medical theory.[8] Her tears, for which she is well known, and which have inspired much scholarship, are usually interpreted as symbolic *expressions* of that mystical experience.[9] However, I offer here what is effectively a reversal of that interpretation: that

---

[5] See Gil Anadjar, *Blood: A Critique of Christianity* (New York: Columbia University Press, 2014), pp. 191–203.

[6] Amy Hollywood, 'Acute Melancholia', *Harvard Theological Review*, 99 (2006), 381–406 (p. 383). See also David Aers, 'The Self Mourning: Reflections on *Pearl*', *Speculum*, 68:1 (1993), 54–73.

[7] Hollywood, 'Acute Melancholia', p. 397.

[8] I am aware of only one example of scholarship which suggests Margery Kempe to be melancholic: Phyllis R. Freeman, Carley Rees Bogarad and Diane E. Sholomskas, 'Margery Kempe, a New Theory: The Inadequacy of Hysteria and Postpartum Psychosis as Diagnostic Categories', *History of Psychiatry*, I (1990), 169–90. However, Freeman et al. argue that Kempe suffers from bipolar disorder, characterised by cycles of melancholia and mania. Juliette Vuille has convincingly argued against this theorem in '"Maybe I'm Crazy?": Diagnosis and Contextualisation of Medieval Female Mystics', in *Medicine, Religion and Gender in Medieval Culture*, ed. Yoshikawa, pp. 103–20.

[9] See Barbara H. Rosenwein, 'Coda: Transmitting Despair by Manuscript and Print', in *Crying in the Middle Ages: Tears of History*, ed. Elina Gertsman (London: Routledge, 2012), pp. 249–66; and Hope Phyllis Weissman, 'Margery Kempe in Jerusalem: *Hysteria Compassio* in the Late Middle Ages', in *Acts of Interpretation*, ed. Carruthers and Kirk, pp. 201–17. See also Karma Lochrie, *Margery Kempe and Translations of the Flesh*, pp. 167–202; and Ellen Ross, '"She wept and cried right loud for sorrow and for pain": Suffering, the Spiritual Journey, and Women's Experience in Late Medieval Mysticism', in *Maps of Flesh and Light: The Religious Experience of Medieval Women Mystics*, ed. Ulrike Wiethaus (Syracuse, N.Y: Syracuse University Press, 1993), pp. 45–59. On the red ink annotator's interest in Kempe's tears see Johanne Paquette, 'Male Approbation in the Extant Glosses to *The Book of Margery Kempe*', in *Women and the Divine in Literature before 1700*, ed. Kerby-Fulton, pp. 153–69.

Kempe's tears are teleologies of a *prior* disposition of melancholia, a condition which, according to medieval medical theory, renders her more receptive and acutely sentient to mystical phenomena and visionary experience. Her weeping, in response to those privileged visions, is thus the inevitable articulation of a melancholic who is unable to relinquish the lost Christic object or stem the grief that lingers as an 'open wound'. This chapter will therefore move forward from Hollywood's analysis by exemplifying the medieval medical theory of melancholia in order ultimately to argue that Margery Kempe's notorious weeping signifies a pseudo-stigmatic woundedness.

According to the medieval theories of the non-naturals and the emotions, as Peregrine Horden has shown, perpetual grief is not conducive to health.[10] Furthermore, George Mora has suggested that Kempe operates in a milieu where a broader notion of social melancholia might be argued to signify a type of cultural dyscrasia.[11] With these socio-medical contexts in mind, the chapter will draw upon scientific understandings to examine the way in which Kempe's onlookers pathologise her weeping in attempts to explain the manner of her devotion. I then explore an alternative medicalisation which argues for a melancholic stasis – a fixation on the crucified Christ – to which Kempe is helplessly subjected. This object-fixation that, according to Thomas Aquinas (c. 1225–1274), is 'difficile cui resisti non potest' (difficult for [anyone] who is unable to resist [it]) leads to the self-fulfilment of melancholia as a constitutional basis for affective receptivity, where physiology creates a predisposition to metaphysical vision.[12] This chapter therefore offers a re-reading of Kempe's *bleeding* tears, which function as ascetic emblems of an outpouring of grief that causes acute pain, but from which she refuses to separate. In bringing into dialogue the complexities of melancholia, mysticism, medical theory, and affective receptivity, this chapter is thus the centre from which the rest of the book spreads in its exploration of physiology and metaphysical rapture, linking the two just as mind and body were unified in the medieval imaginary.

[10] Peregrine Horden, 'A Non-Natural Environment: Medicine without Doctors and the Medieval European Hospital', in *The Medieval Hospital and Medical Practice*, ed. Bowers, pp. 133–45 (pp. 133–6).

[11] George Mora suggests that there was a melancholic atmosphere during the late Middle Ages, born from the Hundred Years' War, the black plague, the decay of Rome, heretical movements, the fall of Constantinople and the Great Schism. See 'Mental Disturbances, Unusual Mental States, and Their Interpretation during the Middle Ages', in *History of Psychiatry and Medical Psychology: With an Epilogue on Psychiatry and the Mind-Body Relation*, ed. Edwin R. Wallace and John Gach (New York: Springer, 2008), pp. 199–223 (p. 212).

[12] Thomas Aquinas, *Summa theologiae*, Iª-IIae q. 41 a. 2. <http://www.ccel.org/ccel/aquinas/summa>. For a study of the connection between physiology and mysticism, see Dyan Elliott, 'The Physiology of Rapture and Female Spirituality', in *Medieval Theology and the Natural Body*, ed. Peter Biller and Alastair J. Minnis (York: York Medieval Press, 1997), pp. 141–73.

Painful Melancholia

Medieval medicine made no particular distinction between mental and physical disorders, and most mental disorders were attributed to physiological causes.[13] Many physiological explanations originated with the Hippocratic corpus and the book *The Sacred Disease*, which rejected supernatural causes of afflictions such as epilepsy, and instead proffered the theory of humoral imbalance. Stephen Medcalf suggests that 'the medieval classification is psychophysical', and that 'a man's character and his body may be seen at the same glance' in a 'narrowing of the gap between inner and outer'.[14] Furthermore, while the mind–body system of the medieval person was thought to be unified and fluid, this 'narrowed gap' can also be applied to the division between heaven and earth: between physical and spiritual phenomena. As Medcalf argues, for example, though Margery Kempe's onlookers question her qualification to discuss the joys of heaven, Kempe's understanding is less disconnected, illustrated by her passing through that fissure via her marriage to the Godhead in Chapter 35 of the *Book*.[15] In relation to some medieval medical theories which propose the female as an inversion of the male, it seems logical for female experience to bridge more 'naturally' that inside–outside divide in the medieval imaginary.[16] Indeed, Kempe envisions events with equal actuality (she sees as 'verily') with her 'gostly eye' as she does with her 'bodily eye'. There is an emphasis on the *truth* of her phenomenological perception that illustrates the heightened receptivity of the melancholic. As such, the argument for Kempe's melancholic diathesis is supported by the complex web of the medieval systems of body–mind, heaven–earth, inner–outer that conflate to indicate what I suggest would have been the glaring appearance of melancholia to Kempe's contemporaries.[17]

The doctrine of the humours stated that illness was caused by disturbances in the balance of the four bodily humours (blood, phlegm, black bile, and yellow bile), and was the generally accepted paradigm of ancient and medieval medical

[13] See Simon Kemp, *Medieval Psychology* (New York: Greenwood Press, 1990) p. 114; and Angel González de Pablo, 'The Medicine of the Soul: The Origin and Development of Thought on the Soul, Diseases of the Soul and Their Treatment, in Medieval and Renaissance Medicine', *History of Psychiatry*, V (1994), 483–516. See also Richard Neugebauer, 'Medieval and Early Modern Theories of Mental Illness', *Archives of General Psychiatry*, 36 (1979), 477–83; and Jerome Kroll and Bernard Bachrach, 'Visions and Psychopathology in the Middle Ages', *The Journal of Nervous and Mental Disease*, 170 (1982), 41–9.
[14] Stephen Medcalf, 'Inner and outer', in *The Later Middle Ages*, ed. Stephen Medcalf (London: Methuen, 1981), pp. 108–71 (p. 109).
[15] Ibid., p. 117.
[16] Medieval medical writers disagreed on the significance of Aristotelian notions of sex difference: some saw male / female as opposite, others as the same but arranged differently. See Joan Cadden, *Meanings of Sex Difference in the Middle Ages: Medicine, Science and Culture* (Cambridge: Cambridge University Press, 1993), pp. 177–83.
[17] On thirteenth-century theological debates about human pain and suffering see Donald Mowbray, *Pain and Suffering in Medieval Theology: Academic Debates at the University of Paris in the Thirteenth Century* (Woodbridge: Boydell Press, 2009), pp. 13–42.

thinkers. Galen (b. c. 129) in particular linked the qualities of hot, cold, dry, and moist with their humoral counterparts, and these combinations became the permitted models for a balanced body: blood was hot and moist, yellow bile was hot and dry, black bile was cold and dry, and phlegm was cold and moist. The Galenic system of temperaments associated the predominant humour in the body with supposed character traits; the sanguine temperament was dominated by blood, the choleric by yellow bile, the phlegmatic by phlegm, and the melancholic by black bile.[18] There was thus an inherent concomitance between a melancholic 'complexion' and one's temperament.[19] Crucially, there was also an ancient connection between the four bodily humours, the four ages of man, and the four seasons, which linked the process of ageing to black bile and melancholia, a notion which remained unchanged throughout the medieval and Renaissance periods.[20] The symbiosis of life stage and physiological constitution in medieval medicine is intrinsic to my suggestion of Margery Kempe's melancholic disposition and accompanying affective receptivity, especially since this book focuses largely on her spiritual journey from the point of her conversion at around the age of thirty-six, through her middle to old age.[21]

Medieval writers developed Galen's theory, reviving ancient doctrine in the light of Christian theology. The humours are described in a Middle English translation of Gilbertus Anglicus's widely disseminated *Compendium medicinae* (c. 1240) as connected to the four elements of the universe – fire, air, water, and earth:

> Ryt so as þer ben iiij elementus, so þer be iiij humours in euery leuyng body, as j be-fore seyd, wyche humours han gret licnesse to þe iiij elementes be-fore namyd. Þese ben þe iiij humours: colere, blood, fleme, and malencolye. Colre js hoot and drye, of nature liȝt, scharp, and sotyl. Blood js hoot and moist, of nature lyȝt, soft, and rysyng vpward. Fleume js coold and moyst, of nature wete, and heuy of kynde. Malencholie is coold and dry, of nature gret, and wonder heuy. But where in eny body eny of þese iiij humours haþe more of on þan of an-oþer, þat body takyth name of þat humour.[22]

[18] OED s.v. melancholy: Etymology: Ancient Greek μελαγχολία condition of having black bile. See Jennifer Radden, *The Nature of Melancholy: From Aristotle to Kristeva* (Oxford: Oxford University Press, 2000), pp. 61–8.

[19] On the history of melancholia, see Raymond Klibansky, Erwin Panofsky and Fritz Saxl, *Saturn and Melancholy: Studies in the History of Natural Philosophy, Religion and Art* (London: Nelson, 1964).

[20] Klibansky et al., *Saturn and Melancholy*, pp. 10–11. For a more recent study see Kathleen Woodward, *Ageing and Its Discontents: Freud and Other Fictions* (Bloomington and Indianapolis: Indiana University Press, 1991).

[21] Kempe's conversion can be dated to c. 1409 when Christ ravishes her spirit, assures her of forgiveness, and tells her to give up eating meat. This is narrated in Chapter 5 then recounted in Chapter 26. See Windeatt, *BMK*, p. 71, n. 510.

[22] Gilbertus Anglicus, *Compendium of Mediaeval Medicine*, in *System of Physic* (GUL MS Hunter 509, ff. 1r–167v): A Compendium of Mediaeval Medicine Including the Middle English Gilbertus Anglicus, ed. Laura Esteban-Segura (Bern: Peter Lang, 2012), p. 39. Hereafter, *System of Physic*.

Although not the most desirable, a melancholic constitution was not intrinsically unhealthy. Some natural black bile was essential for life in keeping the blood at its correct level and removing superfluities. As Bartholomaeus Anglicus (fl. 1230–50) attested, 'Som melencolye is kyndeliche and som vnkindeclich'. The 'kyndeliche' melancholy makes the blood 'apt and couenable' and is needed for 'clensinge of al þe body and for fedynge of þe splene', which helps to control superfluity.[23] But medieval scholasticism also held that melancholia was one of the four main brain diseases, and by 1300 it was common to equate melancholia with madness.[24] In the tenth century the Arabic physician Ibn Sīnā (980–1037; Avicenna), whose writings were translated into Latin and circulated very widely in the West, connected melancholics with 'sleeplessness, obsessions' and 'senseless thoughts'. In considering disorders of the psyche, he notes that those with melancholic disease are subject to 'Suspicion, corrupted thoughts and fear'. If the disease progresses to mania, 'its sign is madness and beastly behaviour', or if it develops to psychosis the individual is dominated by fear and 'frightening darkness'; to remain in a melancholic state of 'depression and sadness' will 'finally turn to mania'.

Strikingly, the medieval understanding of the connection between the heart and brain results in Avicenna's assertion that 'the source of the disease usually originates in the heart'.[25] The Middle English *Cyrurgie of Guy de Chauliac* (translated anonymously in the mid-fifteenth century from Guy de Chauliac's Chirugia magna of 1363) illustrates the longevity of such ideas by suggesting that 'The natural melancholye is þe drastes of good blood and the trowblynesse, grete in substaunce, declynyng in colour to a manere blaknesse, in sauour to sournesse and bitternesse.'[26] Hildegard of Bingen (1098–1179), the mystic, theologian, and medical writer, also regarded the 'disease' of melancholy to cause wickedness and cognitive disorder, but in *Causae et curae* she connects it to the state of the human soul through a connection to Original Sin, and thus asserts its universal significance:

> There are other people who are sad, timid, and vague in their minds, so in them is no right constitution or state. They are like a strong wind, which is harmful to all plants and fruits. Whence phlegm grows in them, which is neither damp nor thick, but lukewarm. It is like *livor* and it is tenacious, stretching out in length, like gum resin. It brings about melancholy, which arose from the serpent's breath in the first birth from the seed of Adam, since Adam followed the serpent's advice about food.

---

[23] *On the Properties of Things: John Trevisa's translation of Bartholomaeus Anglicus De proprietatibus rerum*, 2 vols, vol. 1 (Oxford: Oxford University Press, 1975), pp. 159–62.

[24] Fernando Salmón, 'From Patient to Text? Narratives of Pain and Madness in Medieval Scholasticism', in *Between Text and Patient: The Medical Enterprise in Medieval and Early Modern Europe* (Firenze: Sismel, 2011), pp. 373–95 (p. 389).

[25] Avicenna, *The Canon of Medicine (al-Qānūn fi'l-tibb)*, 5 vols, vol. 3, trans. Peyman Adeli Sardo, ed. Laleh Bakhtiar (Chicago: Kazi Publications, 2014), Part I, pp. 33, 120, 126–7 and 131 respectively.

[26] *The Cyrurgie of Guy de Chauliac*, ed. Margaret S. Ogden, EETS o.s. 265 (London: Oxford University Press, 1971), p. 123.

[Sunt vero alii homines, qui tristes ac timidi ac vagi in mentibus suis sunt, ita quod nulla recta constitutio et status in eis est. Sed sunt ut validus ventus, qui omnibus herbis et fructibus inutilis est. Unde in his crescit flegma, quod nec humidum nec spissum est, sed tepidum, et quod est ut livor, qui tenax est, et qui se ut gummi in longum protrahit, et qui parat melancoliam, quae in primo ortu semine Adae orta est de flatu serpentis, quoniam Adam consilium illius in cibo perfecit.][27]

As well as viewing melancholia as part of the human condition, Hildegard observes that certain melancholic women lose much menstrual blood and therefore develop debilitated, fragile wombs ('quis debilem et fragilem matricem habent'). Because these women then cannot receive or retain the male seed, they are healthier ('saniores'), stronger ('fortiores'), and more joyful ('laetiores') *without* a husband, because marriage – and by default, reproduction – makes them sick and weakened ('debiles').[28] In presenting as dominated by the melancholic humour through her irrepressible lamentations, Margery Kempe might thus be regarded as constitutionally unfit for conjugal activity since sexual abstinence would have health benefits, an idea that I consider in the next chapter.

The interaction of love, desire, and melancholia was also noted by the Arabic medical writer Ibn al-Jazzar (b. c. 895), whose treatise *Zād al-Musāfir* was translated into Latin by Constantine the African (d. 1087). Constantine, a converted Christian monk as well as a medical translator, thus produced the famous *Viaticum*, which circulated very widely in Europe. Here, a correlation between the black bile of melancholy and the dyscrasia of lovesickness is established:

The love that is also called 'eros' is a disease touching the brain … Sometimes the cause of this love is an intense natural need to expel a great excess of humours … Since this illness has more serious consequences for the soul, that is, excessive thoughts, their eyes always become hollow [and] move quickly because of the soul's thoughts [and] worries to find and possess what they desire.

[Amor qui et eros dicitur morbus est cerebro contiguus … Aliquando huius amoris necessitas nimia est nature necessitas in multa humorum superfluitate expellenda … Cum hec infirmitas forciora anime subsequentia habeat, id est cogitationes nimias, fiunt eorum oculi semper concaui, cito mobiles propter anime cogitationes, sollicitudines ad inuendienda et habenda ea que desiderant.][29]

---

[27] *Hildegardis: Causae et curae*, ed. Paul Kaiser (Liepzig: In aedibus B.G. Teubneri, 1903), Liber II, p. 38. Translation from Hildegard of Bingen, *Causes and Cures: The Complete English Translation of Hildegardis Causea et Curae Libre VI*, trans. Priscilla Throop (Charlotte: Medieval IMS, 2008), p. 32.

[28] *Causae et curae*, ed. Kaiser, p. 89.

[29] Constantine the African, *Viaticum* I.20, in *Lovesickness in the Middle Ages: The* Viaticum *and Its Commentaries*, ed. and trans. Mary Frances Wack (Philadelphia: University of Pennsylvania Press, 1990), pp. 187–93.

Extreme desire, caused by an excess of humours, is pathologised in this example of psychosomatic fluidity, illustrated by the relationship between the humours, emotions, intellect, and physiology: the hollowed eyes – assumedly dark, or black ('melano') – are physical manifestations of this 'love disorder'.[30] Comparably, the treatise *De medicina animae*, which was formally attributed to Hugh of Saint-Victor (d. 1141) but probably written by Hugo of Folieto (d. c. 1174), interpreted black bile allegorically in its association with immorality and the desire for a nexus with Christ, and with a distinct emphasis on vision. Black bile:

> *issues from the eyes.* Its quantity increases in autumn ... By black bile we may, as we have said elsewhere, mean grief, which we should feel for our evil actions. But one may also speak of a different sort of grief, when the spirit is tormented by the longing to be united with the Lord.

> habet per oculos. Crescit in autumno ... In colera nigra, sicut alibi diximus, intelligi potest tristitia, ut pro his quæ male gessimus tristes simus. Sed et alia species tristitiae dicitur esse, dum mens transeundi ad Deum desiderio cruciatur.][31]

The darkness of sin and the light of vision are apparent in the Gospel of Matthew, which rules that 'The light of thy body is the eye. If thy eye be single, thy whole body shall be lightsome. But if thy eye be evil thy whole body shall be darksome. If then the light that is in thee, be darkness: the darkness itself how great it shall be!'[32] Augustine commented that:

> For so Adam in Paradise sinned, and hid himself from the face of God. As long, then, as he had the sound heart of a pure conscience, he rejoiced at the presence of God; when that eye was wounded by sin, he began to dread the divine light, he fled back into the darkness, and the thick covert of trees, flying from the truth, and anxious for the shade.

> [Nam et in paradiso peccavit Adam, et abscondit se a facie Dei. Cum haberet ergo cor sanum puræ conscientiæ, gaudebat ad præsentiam Dei: postquam peccato oculus ille sauciatus est, cœpit lucem formidare divinam, refugit in tenebras atque in densa lignorum, veritatem fugiens, umbras appetens.][33]

---

[30] OED s.v. melano: Related to the senses 'dark coloured' and 'of relating to melanin'. 'dark-coloured' and 'of or relating to melanin'. From the ancient Greek μέλας: black.

[31] My emphasis. Hugo de Folieto, *De medicina animae*. PL 177, col. 1190. Translation from Klibansky et al., *Saturn and Melancholy*, p. 108.

[32] Matthew 6:22–3.

[33] PL 38. Augustine, *Sermones Ad Populum*: Sermo LXXXVIII, Cap. VI, Col. 542 (Paris, 1841). Translation from 'On the words of the Gospel, Matt. xx. 30, about the two blind men sitting by the way side, and crying out, "Lord, have mercy on us, Thou Son of David"', in *A Select Library of the Nicene and Post-Nicene Fathers of the Christian Church*, vol. 6, ed. Philip Schaff <http://www.ccel.org/ccel/schaff/npnf106.i.html> [accessed 22nd February 2017].

For Augustine, that sin is a cause of blindness and darkness introduces a powerful subtext of the blackness of melancholy, brought on by a lost relationship with the divine.[34]

Later, Aquinas not only connected the loss of an object of desire to fear – the cognitive dissonance of the object as 'difficult for [anyone] who is unable to resist [it]' ('difficile cui resisti non potest') – but also stated that all fear arises from love, and that 'the greatest fear of all is that which has the danger of death for its object' ('Sed timor praecipuus est periculorum mortis').[35] Aquinas also linked emotion to physiological change, because he considered an individual's exterior actions to be *initiated* by the soul, and *enacted* by the 'instruments' of the bodily members. Fear hinders action as the outward members are deprived, through fear, of their heat ('propter defectum caloris qui ex timore accidit in exterioribus membris'). And if the fear of loss is intense enough to disturb the reason, it hinders action, even on the part of the soul ('Si vero timor tantum increscat quod rationem perturbet, impedit operationem etiam ex parte animae').[36] The paralysing fear of losing a beloved is thus quite literally soul-destroying, and physiologically disabling.

Gerard of Berry, who wrote the earliest surviving commentary on Constantine's *Viaticum* in the last decades of the twelfth century, elaborated on the notion of a sufferer's fixation:

> Moreover, the imaginative faculty is *fixated on it* [the object] on account of the imbalanced complexion, cold and dry, that is in its organ, for the *spiritus* and innate heat are drawn to the middle ventricle [of the brain], where the estimative faculty functions intensely. The first ventricle therefore grows cold and dries out, so that there remains a melancholic disposition and worry.

> [Ymaginatiua autem uirtus figitur circa illud propter malam complexionem frigidam et siccam que est in suo organo, quia ad mediam concauitatem ubi est estimatiua trahuntur spiritus et calor innatus ubi estimatiua fortiter operatur. Unde prior concauitas infrigidatur et desiccator, unde remanet dispositio melancolia et sollicitudo.][37]

The fixation on an object of desire to which Gerard points is both a cause *of* and reason *for* melancholia. The subject becomes fixated because of a humoral imbalance, which then causes further cooling and drying in the brain, and a melancholic disposition 'remains' (remanet). That it 'remains' evidences Gerard's understanding of melancholia as simultaneously constitutional and self-fulfilling: emotions such as intense desire trigger physiological modifications, which then perpetuate the disorder.

---

[34] See *The Five Senses in Medieval and Early Modern England*, ed. Annette Kern-Stähler, Beatrix Busse, and Wietse de Boer (Leiden: Koninklijke Brill, 2016).

[35] Thomas Aquinas, *Summa Theologiae*, I-II, 41.2 and II-II, 125.2. Translation at <http://www.newadvent.org/summa/index.html> [accessed 22nd February 2017].

[36] *Summa Theologiae*, I-II, 44.4.

[37] My emphasis. Gerard of Berry, *Glosule Super Viaticum*, in *Lovesickness in the Middle Ages*, ed. and trans. Wack, pp. 194–205 (pp. 200–1).

Robert Burton's encyclopaedic *The Anatomy of Melancholy* of 1621 draws on both ancient and medieval sources and illustrates the longevity of those theories of melancholia in the broader historical reach. The chapter entitled 'Symptoms of Maids', Nuns', and Widows' Melancholy' establishes female melancholia as proceeding from the 'vicious vapours' that come from menstrual blood. Such vapours cause inflammation:

> the whole malady proceeds from that inflammation, putridity, black smoky vapours, etc.; from thence comes care, sorrow, and anxiety, obfuscation of spirits, agony, desperation, and the like, which are intended or remitted, *si amatorius accesserit ardor* [should the amatory passion be aroused], or any other violent object or perturbation of the mind. This melancholy may happen to widows, with much care and sorrow, as frequently as it doth, by reason of a sudden alteration of their accustomed course of life, etc.; to such as lie in child-bed, *ob suppressam purgationem* [that suppresses purgation]; but to nuns and more ancient maids, and some barren women, for the causes abovesaid.[38]

Burton omits the social category of married women, since they are able to expel superfluous humours through regular intercourse and menstruation, but relegates most other women to the putrid vapours of inflammation and melancholia. Moreover, the sorrowful emotions that ensue will increase or relinquish (*intend* or *remit*) depending on the existence of an 'amatory passion' or 'violent object'.[39] Such grief results in 'much solitariness, *weeping*, distraction, etc.'[40] Again, the corporeal innateness of melancholia is perpetuated, or fulfilled, by the presence or denial of an object of powerful desire, an object whose loss – to return to the Freudian hypothesis with which this chapter began – symbolises a trauma which, in the melancholic, cannot be eased. In this way, I contend that Margery Kempe's own melancholic temperament and self-fulfilment operate via a similar desire–loss hermeneutic, through which her unremitting integration with the lost and crucified body of Christ is symptomatic of a self-consciously effected totalisation.

The Pathology of Weeping

Before developing the notion of Margery Kempe's melancholic and integrative identity, I first wish to consider the public reactions to her demonstrations of unrestrained affect, particularly in light of the medieval understanding that emotional response was understood to cause, or to create, physiological change. It is something of an inevitability that wit-

---

[38] Robert Burton, *The Anatomy of Melancholy*, ed. Holbrook Jackson (New York: New York Review of Books, 2001), pp. 414–15.
[39] OED s.v. intend: To stretch out, extend, expand, increase, intensify; s.v: remit: To give up, resign, or surrender (a right, claim, possession, etc.); to relinquish.
[40] My emphasis. Burton, *Melancholy*, p. 415.

nesses of Kempe's boisterous devotion medicalised her 'symptoms'. Indeed, the unusual collapsing and 'bursting' of her pained body in public and sacred spaces almost forces her onlookers to pathologise her explosive articulations of grief, interpreting them as sickness or disorder.[41] During her pilgrimage to Rome, for example, Wenslawe, a German priest from the Church of St John Lateran, is mystically enabled to override linguistic impediments and gifted with the capacity to comprehend Kempe, and vice versa. She falls to the ground with visible emotion:[42]

> sche fel down þerwyth & myth not beryn it. Þan sche wept bittyrly, sche sobbyd boistowsly & cryed ful lowde & horybly Þat þe pepil was oftyn-tymes aferd & gretly astoyned, demyng sche had ben vexyd wyth sum euyl spirit er a sodeyn sekenes, not leuyng it was þe werk of God but raþar sum euyl spirit er a sodeyn sekenes, er ellys symulacyon & ypocrisy falsly feyned of hir owyn self (83).

The 'pepil' – Kempe's fellow pilgrims from England and other worshippers in Rome – deny the authenticity of her emotions, disbelieving of any 'werk of God', and instead 'diagnose' diabolism, a 'sodeyn sekenes', or fraud. Such is their contempt that her countrymen forsake her, unable to reconcile themselves to her displays of otherness, and convinced that her *boystows* demonstrations of affect emanate monstrously from disorder or disfunction.[43] They are 'aferd' and 'gretly astoyned', inverting the 'affliction' of Kempe's emotive collapse into their own fear and shock.[44] Their discomfort at witnessing her anguished sobbing, however, underlies an exclusion paradigm predicated on Kempe's demonstration of a mystical esotericism that the onlookers cannot share. To these witnesses, the very excess of her response indicates the peculiar or privileged, but while they perceive something potentially harmful, Kempe is in fact *grateful* for her tears, embracing their paradoxically gratifying pain.

Kempe is informed by God that she is a mirror to humankind, a holy reflection of others' sins, for which she strives to weep and to sorrow. In functioning as a model of devotion and repentance within the parish, Kempe's tears thus become symbols of the failure of the congregation, liquid signifiers

[41] While unusual in England, Kempe's version of spirituality is closer in character to the Continental holy women about whom she learned via her acroamatic *syllabi* and pilgrimages to Europe. See, for example, *Prophets Abroad*, ed. Voaden.
[42] This church, built next to the Lateran Palace in Rome, may have added significance for Kempe because Bridget of Sweden was said to have been seen in 'levitation' there. Since Kempe would have undoubtedly been aware of these events, the efficacy of her own mystical experience in the same church would have held extra potency. See *BMK*, p. 300, n. 82/10.
[43] MED s.v. boistous: 1(a) crudeness, an unpolished art. 1(b) noisy, loud. 2. strong and powerful. 5. In physiology: dominated by the element 'earth': gross, coarse, opaque; 'thick' blood.
[44] MED s.v. astoined: 1. of persons: stupified, stunned; insensate, unconscious. 2. upset, bewildered; dumfounded; perplexed, embarrassed.

of the mass salvation that she is pledged to effect, and a reason for that congregation's antipathy:[45]

> Dowtyr, þu hast a good ȝele of charite in þat þu woldist alle men were sauyd, & so wolde I. & þei seyn þat so wolde þei, but þu maist wel se þat þei wol not hem-self be sauyd, for alle þei wil sumtyme heryn þe word of God, but þei wil not alwey don þeraftyr, & þei wil not sorwyn hem-self for her synnys, ne þei wil suffyr non oþer to suffir for hem. Neuyr-þe-lesse, dowtyr, I haue ordeynd þe to be a *merowr* a-mongys hem for to han gret sorwe þat þei xulde takyn exampil by þe for to haue sum litil sorwe in her hertys for her synnys þat þei myth þerthorw be sauyd, but þei louyn not to heryn of sorwe ne of contricyon (186).

That Kempe is a mirror of weeping contrition not only noisily reflects back her onlookers' religious shortcomings, but also makes that weeping intrusive, both audibly and visually seeping into others like an uninvited message. Jeffrey Cohen suggests that 'Kempe's sobs and screams carried her out of herself, into the bodies of her auditors and into the wideness of the world', and so Kempe's voice, in its non-verbal, liquid form, becomes the authorised and invasive voice of God on earth.[46] 'Þe Myrour Off Chastite', in the late fourteenth-century religious handbook *The Pore Caitif*, which was intended for lay use, establishes itself as a 'myrour of maidens [who should] loke þee þerinne, as folower of þe mekest maide, mairie goddis modir of heuene'.[47] Similarly, the author of the early fifteenth-century *Myroure of Oure Ladye*, written for the sisters of Syon Abbey, also explains the purpose of its title as designed to emphasise how its readers 'shulde se her [the Virgin] therin as in a myrouore, and so be styred the more deuoutly to prayse her, & to knowe where ye fayle in her praysinges, and to amende: tyll ye may come there ye may se her face to face wythouten eny myrroure'.[48] Margery Kempe is therefore designated the highest honour by Christ, as a *merowr* of sorrow upon whom others should gaze as an example, comparable even to the Virgin Mary whose infinite mourning is immortalised in the ubiquitous iconography of

---

[45] Kempe's sorrow and contrition do also have a sanctifying effect on many of those with whom she communes. After meeting Kempe several times Thomas Marshall, a man from Newcastle, weeps tears of contrition and compunction both night and day. Marshall is recorded as collapsing in a manner similar to Kempe: 'he fel down & myth not beryn it' (108). Likewise, when in Rome, the 'good women' have compassion for Kempe's sorrow, '& gretly meruelyng of hir wepyng & of hir crying, meche þe mor þei louyd hir' (99).

[46] Jeffrey J. Cohen, *Medieval Identity Machines* (Minneapolis: University of Minnesota Press, 2003), p. 156.

[47] 'The Pore Caitif, edited from MS Harley 2336 with Introduction and Notes', M.T. Brady (unpublished PhD thesis, Fordham University, 1954), p. 176. There exist in the region of forty-four known MSS of complete or partial texts, demonstrating the widespread popularity of the work.

[48] Thomas Gascoigne, 'Lyfe of Seynt Birgette', in *The Myroure of Our Ladye*, ed. John H. Blunt, EETS e.s. 19 (London: Trüber, 1873), p. 4. While the author of *The Myroure of Our Ladye* is unknown the text is regularly attributed to Thomas Gascoigne. See *The Myroure*, pp. viii–ix. Also see Brady, *The Pore Caitif*, p. cxxxii.

Mary at the Foot of the Cross. It is little wonder, then, that Kempe's parish 'audience' sometimes recoil at her weeping, as her privileged devotion is reflected back to them in illumination of where they themselves might 'fayle in her praysinges'.

Similar discomfort is exemplified by the esteemed grey friar who comes to Lynn to be in convent and who is warned of Kempe's outbursts by the parish priest. Despite her attempts to remain silent in church she is unable to bear the anguish of thinking on Christ's Passion: 'Sche kept hir fro crying as long as sche myth, and þan at þe last sche *brast owte* wyth a gret cry & cryid wondyr sor' (149); on the second occasion of her explosive response, she is evicted from the church. Recalling the psychophysical melding of inner and outer in Medcalf's analysis, Kempe's sorrow is uncontainable, resisting somatic restriction and diffusing amongst the 'pepil' in an eruption of her inner self, turning inside out. Yet, just as medieval culture conceived the body–soul dynamic as fluid, so, in the forceful projection of Kempe's cries and screams into the ears and consciousness of her spectators, the absolute division between the individual and her pathologising inspectorate is softened. Through the noisy bursting and invading of others' cognition, she explodes the ontological separation of the individual from the other, disorientating onlookers and afflicting – or infecting – them with her own agonising grief. A version of this operation is seen by George Lakoff and Mark Johnson as an 'imaginative projection', generated by the ability of the sentient human to empathise, thus triggering the transcending of bodily containment:

> A major function of the embodied mind is empathic. From birth, we have the capacity to imitate others, to vividly imagine being another person, doing what that person does, experiencing what that person experiences. The capacity for imaginative projection is a vital cognitive facility. Experientially, it is a form of 'transcendence'. Through it, one can experience something akin to 'getting out of our bodies' – yet it is very much a bodily capacity.[49]

Kempe's affective and empathic response to her visions of the Passion, for instance, illustrate exactly this transcendent 'getting out of the body', at the same time as she acts out such responses in an insistently kinetic, somatic manner. Furthermore, that she is a divinely appointed 'merowr' for the people makes such empathetic imagining more manifold since she reflects back, to astonished reception, her visionary insights. Indeed, the onlookers' discomfort at her paroxysms of crying highlights that her tears are 'themselves language', in Dhira Mahoney's words; they are 'a sign of her power, her link with the Other'.[50] Not only do Kempe's spectators recoil from the sight and sound

---

[49] George Lakoff and Mark Johnson, *Philosophy in the Flesh: The Embodied Mind and Its Challenge to Western Thought* (New York: Basic Books, 1999), p. 565.
[50] Dhira B. Mahoney, 'Margery Kempe's Tears and the Power over Language', in *Margery Kempe: A Book of Essays*, ed. Sandra J. McEntire (New York and London: Garland, 1992), pp. 37–50 (pp. 40–1).

41

of her lamentation, but their simultaneous exclusion from her revelations results also in a conflicted interplay of aversion and desire. Such witness could be edifying, however. According to Carolyn Muessig, 'performers' of Christ's Passion, such as Elizabeth of Spalbeek (fl. 1246–1304) and Margaret of Cortona (c. 1247–1297), 'acted as a conduit between God and the Christian community', transforming their audiences with their demonstrations of suffering and altering their watchers' 'interior disposition'; Kempe's reflected weeping passion could work in the same way.[51]

The Grey Friar declares, 'I wolde þis woman wer owte of þe chirche; sche noyith þe pepil' (149). Not only does she annoy the parishioners, who 'turnyd a-ȝen hir', but the even priests who intervene beg the friar to 'suffyr hir paciently' as 'oþer good men had suffyrd hir be-fore' – something of a veiled insult calling for a reluctant tolerance, a *suffering* of her diffusive sorrow, rather than an admiration of her piety (150). The friar also regards Kempe as ill – 'he leuyd it was a cardiakyl er sum oþer sekenesse' – proffering a psychosomatic explanation based on a 'cardiakyl', or heart, disease caused by superfluous humours around the heart. In fact, Avicenna stated that a weak heart is caused by an excess of black bile (the humour of melancholia), which moves through the brain 'and from the arteries to the heart and stimulates abnormal beating of the heart … decreases the heart's strength and leads to sadness, depression, and bad thoughts in a person'; this suggests that the friar's diagnosis was not completely medically spurious.[52] The heart was also connected to cognitive function in the writings of Richard Rolle, who experienced a fire of love in his breast that he perceived as altering his mind: 'My heart grew hot within me, and fire shall burn in my thinking.'[53] Kempe's own collapsing fervour is eventually addressed by the friar's attempt at diagnostic negotiation. If she will admit a 'kendly [natural] seknes' – a medical false confession of sorts – he will tolerate her crying, since pathologising her tears as products of infirmity and the frailty and failure of the female body is safer territory than investigating her mystical giftedness and potential heterodoxy. As the friar may have known, treatments for disorders of black bile did exist, and included access to light and gardens; calm and rest; purges and laxatives; inhalations and warm baths with moistening plants such as nenuphar; a diet of lamb, lettuce, and eggs; and phlebotomy.

Margery Kempe's refusal to accept this diagnosis is unrelenting. She emphasises the power of her own authentic experience: 'be *reuelacyon* & be *experiens of werkyng* it was no sekenes', and suffers 'gret peyne' at her exclusion

---

[51] Carolyn Muessig, 'Performance of the Passion: The Enactment of Devotion in the later Middle Ages', in *Visualising Medieval Performance: Perspectives, Histories, Contexts*, ed. Elina Gertsman (Abingdon and New York: Routledge, 2016), pp. 129–42.
[52] Avicenna, *The Canon of Medicine*, vol. 3, ed. Bakhtiar, p. 509.
[53] *Richard Rolle: The English Writings*, trans. and ed. Rosamund S. Allen (New York: Paulist Press, 1988), p. 43.

from sermons and social ostracisation (151).[54] Here, the multiplicity of 'peyne' signification in Kempe's perception is evident. It emanates not from physical affliction, or the melancholic diathesis that I argue gives rise to her weeping and sorrowing, but in the psychological and spiritual distress caused by the ecclesiastical men who expel her from the Christian ceremonies that sustain her very soul. Doubly marginalised, then, by exclusion from liturgical rite and by her categorisation as dysfunctional, made abject by her female embodiment, Kempe prays that her intrusive weeping be quelled during the Mass:

> take þes cryingys fro me in þe tyme of sermownys þat I cry not at þin holy prechyng & late me hauyn hem be my-self alone so þat I be not putt fro heryng of þin holy wordys, for *grettar peyn may I not suffyr* in þis worlde þan be put fro þi holy worde heryng. And, ȝyf I wer in preson, *my most peyn* xulde be þe forberyng of þin holy wordys & of þin holy sermownys (181–2).

In begging that her tears become private, she acknowledges their affront to the friar and many members of the congregation. But given the proliferation of medical texts from the thirteenth century that gave religious clerics and friars (and, by infiltration, their parishioners) access to medical knowledge, it is unsurprising that Kempe's social milieu interprets her explosive weeping as a product of the dysfunctional female body.[55]

In the *Timaeus*, Plato (b. 427 BC) had compared the womb to a living creature – an animal.[56] Hippocrates (b. c. 460 BC) discussed the condition of uterine displacement, which was also referred to as the 'hysterical bolus'. This theory of the 'suffocated womb', based on Galenic and Aristotelian writings, held that certain imbalances of the body or temperature could cause the womb to be drawn upward, causing physical symptoms. Such ideas circulated in the West from the central Middle Ages, especially through the *De mulierum affectibus*.[57] *The Knowing of Woman's Kind in Childing* describes the extreme visibility of the painful condition of 'suffocation', which caused swooning and would thus easily be confused with Kempe's collapsing:

---

[54] Even Kempe's priestly amanuensis turned his back on her after the friar's declaration. It is only after reading Mary of Oignies' (1177–1213) *Vita*, which was authenticated via male redaction (Jacques de Vitry, her confessor, wrote two books of her life), that Kempe's scribe returns to her with contrition.

[55] Monica Green has shown how female healthcare moved almost entirely into the male domain in the later Middle Ages. Her handlist of owners of *Trotula* manuscripts in the vernacular in England in the Middle Ages shows that most owners were noblemen or men of religious orders. See Green, *Making Women's Medicine Masculine*, pp. 325–31. Many medieval scholars of medicine were clergymen since they mostly attended the medieval universities of northern and western Europe. However, Kempe's priest scribe reads *The Prykke of Lofe* by pseudo-Bonaventure, the life of Elizabeth of Hungary, and Richard Rolle's *Incendium Amoris*, as well as the Bible, St Bridget's *Revelations*, and Hilton's writings, which, in contrast, support the tradition of pious weeping (143; 153–4).

[56] Danielle Jacquart and Claude Thomasset, *Sexuality and Medicine in the Middle Ages*, trans. Matthew Adamson (Cambridge: Polity Press, 1988), p. 173.

[57] Jacquart and Thomasset, p. 174.

> Suffocacion of þe maryce ys an angvych þat doth women to suell at þe poynt of here herte & makyth hem to *sovnde & to fall dovne*, þer tethe yonyde to-gedyre with-owt dravynge ore schevynge of breth, & but they be holpe þe sonere in suche case hit ys wondure & euere they releue.[58]

The medieval medical and theological connection between the uterus and heart is illustrated in this passage by the heart swelling in direct response to a uterine problem. Symptoms of *sounding* and falling down are reminiscent of Kempe's lamentatory collapse, as is the impaired breathing which causes 'þe body' to be 'as dede. & þat ys cause þat women oþer-whyll *ly a-s'v'ovnynge as þey were dede*'.[59] Similarly, 'The 'Book on the Conditions of Women', one of the *Trotula* texts, states:

> Sometimes the woman is contracted so that the head is joined to the knees, and she lacks vision, and she loses the function of the voice, the nose is distorted, the lips are contracted and she grits her teeth, and the chest is elevated upward beyond what is normal.

> [Quandoque mulier contrahitur ita quod capud iungitur genibus, et uisu caret, et uocis officium amittit, nasus distorquetur, labia contrahuntur, et dentes strin-git, et pectus sursum preter solitum eleuatur.][60]

Again, these symptomatic bodily contortions call to mind the muffled noises and flailing exhibited by Kempe in church.

The 'anguysch' of suffocation is predominantly caused by the cold sinews of the uterus seeking heat from other internal organs, moving around the body as if it were an animated and self-governed being of its own:

> The ij anguysch ys suffocacyon of matrice, þat is whan þe matrice rysyth out of hys ryȝht plase & goyth ouer-hy, & þe cause þer-of I schall schev yow by resonne. I have tolde yow here be-fore þat þe matryce is made of synow & eche synov be kynde ys colde & eche þing þat ys colde sekyth hete, & þer-fore þe matrice þat ys cold of hym-selfe, yf hit be not holp with oþer thyngis, hit sekyth hete & so sume tymme hit goyth vp to þe most hottest place of þe body of woman, þat ys þe hert, þe lyuyre, þe mylte & þe longys, þe wyche cleue to gedyre a-boute þe stomack. And be-cause þat all þe breth þat we draw comyth by contynuall clappynge of þe longis & whan þe matrice, þat ys full of synovs, tochyth þe longis, hit pressyth hem & comburth hem þat þey may not meve ne clappe for-to drav brethe & whan þe breth may not in ne ovt, þe body ys as dede. & þat ys cause þat women oþer-whyll ly a-s'v'ovnynge as þey were dede.[61]

The manifestation of uterine suffocation also depended on the woman's pre-vailing humour. A dominance of the black bile of melancholy could cause

---

[58] My emphasis. *The Knowing of Woman's Kind in Childing*, p. 46.
[59] My emphasis. *The Knowing of Woman's Kind in Childing*, p. 50.
[60] 'Book on the Conditions of Women', in *The Trotula*, pp. 84–5.
[61] *The Knowing of Woman's Kind in Childing*, p. 50.

disturbances in vision and the apparent signs of madness.[62] Hippocrates, in *The Sacred Disease*, had noted how patients with an excess of bile were noisier and more restless.[63]

In the twelfth century the complex of melancholia was connected by Hildegard of Bingen to a spiritual crisis, suggesting that a domination of black bile caused evil thoughts that could have lethal consequence:

> Those who have an excess of bile are not insane, but they are assailed by many wicked thoughts in denial of God, and they think of this state of mind as a great affliction and even a sickness unto death. Thus they put the devil to flight. People think, however, that they are possessed although they are not. If they persevere under this heavy affliction, they become martyrs.

> [Qui autem in melancolia abundant, non insaniunt, sed multe maligne cogitationes Deum contradicentes sepe ad eos currunt, et has quasi pro molestia et prop grauedine mortis habent. Ideoque diabolus ab eis fugit, sed homines dicunt, quod obsessi sint et non sunt, et si in hac molestia perseuerauerint, martyres sunt.][64]

For Hildegard, not only does the individual with a surplus of black bile have the affliction of 'wicked thoughts', but to endure this 'sickness' is sanctifying to the extent that they become martyrs. This dissonance of constitutional affliction and holy advantage holds equivalence with the melancholic predisposition to affective receptivity that this chapter explores. For the medieval doctor, however, suffocation of the womb was caused fundamentally by the retention of 'seed' in virgins and widows (a point that is developed in Chapter 2). Such retained matter could lead to madness, spasm and fainting, and apparent death.[65]

As *The Knowing of Woman's Kind in Childing* attests, other uterine disorders, such as precipitation, were known to 'trovbelyth þe braynne', and Kempe's weeping is indeed often so great that it is 'as sche xulde a deyid þerwyth' (139).[66] Given the atmosphere of such ideas, the people of Lynn 'concludyn þat sche had a deuyl wythinne hir which cawsyd þat crying. & so þey seyden pleynly & meche mor euyl' (105). Other 'amateur physicians' diagnosed her

[62] Jacques Despars' late medieval commentary on Avicenna's *Canon* discusses the *conversio* of suffocation into individual outcomes. See Jacquart and Thomasset, p. 175.

[63] See Simon Kemp, *Medieval Psychology* (New York and London: Greenwood Press, 1990), p. 115.

[64] Hildegard of Bingen, *Epistolarivm: Pars Tertia CCLI-CCCX*, ed. L. Van Acker and M. Klaes-Hachmöller (Turnhout: Brepols, 2001), Epist. CCLXXXVII, 'Hildegardis ad quondam sacerdotem', pp. 40–1. Translation from *The Letters of Hildegard of Bingen*, vol. 3, ed. Joseph L. Baird and Radd K. Ehrman (New York and Oxford: Oxford University Press, 2004), Letter 287, pp. 83–4.

[65] See Jacquart and Thomasset, p. 175.

[66] *The Knowing of Woman's Kind in Childing*, p. 52. A failure to control one's passions is seen in Galenic terms as a cause of madness, 'and that ungoverned passion might increase to the point of becoming an incurable disease of the soul'. See Kemp, *Medieval Psychology*, p. 115.

with the 'falling evil', owing to the 'horrowr' of her writhing, wailing, and the blackening of her complexion:

> Sum seyde þat sche had þe fallyng euyl, for sche wyth þe crying wrestyd hir body turning fro þe o side in-to þe oþer & wex al blew & al blo as it had ben colowr of leed. & þan folke spitted at hir for horrowr of þe sekenes, & sum scornyd hir and seyd þat sche howlyd as it [had] ben a dogge & bannyd hir & cursyd hir & seyd þat sche dede meche harm a-mong þe pepyl (105).

In fact, the 'falling evil' (modern-day epilepsy) was often confused with uterine suffocation at this time.[67] Certainly, the spasmodic twisting from side to side, change of pallor from blue to ashen, and atavistic howls described here could reasonably indicate a physical affliction to her discombobulated spectators. But the 'pepyl' fail to comprehend the spiritual ecstasy of Kempe's cries. While she writhes in quasi-masochistic lamentation, she both resists the socially prescribed containment of her female flesh and retains a powerful union with her beloved, Christ. Indeed, this is something that Elizabeth Robertson sees as her attempt to overthrow judgements about female bodies by medical, clerical, and patriarchal authorities, arguing that 'The very excess of her writing, her extremes of tears and sensual expressiveness, suggest a destabilization of those assumptions', and thus take medical theories to 'their logical extreme'.[68] Her kinaesthetic bouts of crying are not, then, the 'horrowr of ... sekenes', but rather a means of self-medication that productively perpetuates her melancholic lamentation so that she might *feel* God's privileged 'habundawns of lofe'.

Weeping and mourning therefore form the symptomatic language of another text which runs parallel to Kempe's own: the unsanctioned narrative of somatic disorder that is the preferred interpretation of many of her onlookers. Others – even the 'red ink annotator' of the manuscript, who engages in approving, extra-narrative marginalia in a dialectic with the descriptions of her weeping – recognise the gift of those tears.[69] However, she is concomitantly helpless in their profusion or absence – that 'sche myth nowt chesyn, but þat wolde þei not belevyn' (83–4) evidences how she cannot choose to cry. This powerlessness is an affliction itself, yet it is one of divine genesis and one for which she desires no cure or relief. When the Archbishop of York *boystowsly* asks her 'Why wepist þu so, woman?', Kempe replies with vehement one-upmanship: 'Syr, ʒe xal welyn sum day þat ʒe had wept as sor as I' (125). In asserting a spiritually superior position over the ecclesiast who seeks to silence and fetter her as a heretic, she not only displays formidable courage,

---

[67] Jacquart and Thomasset, p. 175.
[68] Elizabeth Robertson, 'Medieval Medical Views of Women and Female Spirituality in the *Ancrene Wisse* and Julian of Norwich's *Showings*', in *Feminist Approaches to the Body in Medieval Literature*, ed. Linda Lomperis and Sarah Stanbury (New York and London: University of Pennsylvania Press, 1993), p. 158.
[69] Johanne Paquette, 'Male Approbation in the Extant Glosses to the *Book of Margery Kempe*', in *Women and the Divine in Literature before 1700*, ed. Kerby-Fulton, pp. 153–69.

but also reclaims her endangered body by asserting the edifying quality of her tears as free-flowing matter that resists manacling or confinement. While Kempe's violent sobbing affronts those spectators who pathologise her 'symptoms', that same aetiology is, for her, a desired state of mystical rapture and a means of remaining spiritually fruitful. As she sobs and swoons during Mass, reliving the trauma of Christ's Passion and reopening the wounds of his bleeding body, she enacts the self-fulfilment of the melancholic state to which she is painfully, and ecstatically, inclined.

'… difficile cui resisti non potest': Affective Receptivity and Medicalised Spirituality

The dominance of black bile in the body has been regarded historically as a productive facilitator of affective receptivity. Melancholics have long been accorded an ontological connection with creative energy or brilliance and cognitive and emotional intelligence – a dichotomy of disorder and giftedness and a physiological predisposition to mystical experience that is paradoxically advantageous. Aristotle first asked:

> Why is it that all those men who have become extraordinary in philosophy, politics, poetry, or the arts are obviously melancholic, and some to such an extent that they are seized by the illnesses that come from black bile, as is said in connection with the stories about Heracles among heroes?[70]

Other ancient writers, like Theophrastus in his book on melancholy, examined the interplay between melancholia and frenzied creativity, and so 'the dark source of genius – already implicit in the word "melancholy" – was uncovered'.[71] In the second century AD Rufus of Ephesus had claimed that melancholics had the gift of prophecy.[72]

The Iberian philosopher and medical writer Ibn Rushd (1126–98), whose name is Latinised to Averroës, linked enhanced psychic faculties to melancholic types, regarding their cold, dry constitutions as a necessary foundation for superior imaginative experience. This was due to the imagination requiring images that can be sustained and well defined: a cold and dry constitution delays motion and helps the image to persist. Since the 'vapours' of black bile also encourage sleep, melancholics, he writes, have more frequent and 'truer' dreams, often perceiving in waking what others dream when they are asleep.[73]

---

[70] Aristotle, *Problems: Books 20–38, Rhetoric to Alexander*, vol. 2, ed. and trans. Robert Mayhew and David C. Mirhady (Cambridge, Mass. and London: Harvard University Press, 2011), Book XXX, i, p. 277.

[71] Klibansky et al., p. 41.

[72] Ibid., p. 50.

[73] Averroës, *Epitome of Parva Naturalia*, trans. Harry Blumberg (Cambridge, Mass: Medieval Academy of America, 1961), pp. 50–1.

Such notions endured and are evidenced in Burton's work, which further suggested that melancholic inner sensory perception is potentially painful and linked to a 'terrible object', in striking resonance with the object-fixation of the yearning melancholic considered above:

> Phantasy, or imagination, which some call estimative, or cogitative … is an inner sense which doth more fully examine the species perceived by common sense, of things present or absent, and keeps them longer, recalling them to mind again, or making new of his own … In melancholy men this faculty is most powerful and strong, *and often hurts*, producing many monstrous and prodigious things, especially if it be stirred up by some terrible object, presented to it from common sense or memory.[74]

Not only is the faculty of imaginative cognition stronger in the melancholic here, but that it 'often hurts' by drawing on memories of 'terrible object[s]' forges a connection between mystical perception, melancholia, and pain that Kempe's experiences illustrate. Indeed, Dyan Elliott notes how 'complexions, sound or unsound, inform a person's spiritual aptitude', and that 'the humours act as a conduit for the passions which, in turn, have a major impact on the imagination'.[75] In considering the 'ideal types' of medieval complexion, she sees the efficacious potential of the female melancholic: 'another, and more promising, possibility for the female disposition was melancholic, as the dominant humour, black bile, was associated with earth (cold and dry)'.[76] A woman who was naturally melancholic (as I suggest Margery Kempe to be, and as Hildegard of Bingen implies that she herself was) would have a 'physical predisposition to mystical rapture'.[77]

The phenomenon of Kempe's craved weeping is also cyclical. Her melancholia is perpetuated by her perception, internalisation, and mourning of the 'terrible object' that is the crucified Christ, in a multipliable, self-fulfilling paradigm, spiralling infinitely. Amy Hollywood considers the fixations of Beatrice of Nazareth and Margaret Ebner in a similar way, in that 'the idealized other they incorporate is idealized precisely in his suffering and death. Melancholia here feeds melancholia rather than allaying it – the death of the other leads to the idealization of and desire for one's own death'.[78] For Kempe, this is only partly true: her ambivalence towards her own pain and death is

---

[74] My emphasis. Burton, p. 159.

[75] Dyan Elliott, 'The Physiology of Rapture', in *Medieval Theology and the Natural Body*, ed. Biller and Minnis, p. 149. See also Elliott, *Proving Woman: Female Spirituality and Inquisitional Culture in the Later Middle Ages* (Princeton and Oxford: Princeton University Press, 2004), pp. 205–8.

[76] Elliott, 'The Physiology of Rapture', p. 157.

[77] Ibid., p. 159. On the gendering of melancholia, see Lynn Enterline, *The Tears of Narcissus: Melancholia and Masculinity in Early-Modern Writing* (Stanford: Stanford University Press, 1995) and Julia Schiesari, *The Gendering of Melancholia: Feminism, Psychoanalysis and the Symbolics of Loss in Renaissance Literature* (Ithaca, NY: Cornell University Press, 1992).

[78] Hollywood, 'Acute Melancholia', p. 402.

an ongoing theme in this book. But while her tears function as boisterous intrusions to her community at large, they also signify a melancholic woman who is simultaneously reliant on and distraught at the most devastating image of Christian narrative, unable to accept or relinquish it and so forced, like an 'open wound', to bleed her tears of lamentation.

Bleeding Tears

If we free ourselves by confession of the sins that sadden us we are purified by tears … Through blood thou hadst the sweetness of love-now, through black bile or 'melancholia', hast thou grief for sin.

[Ab his enim vitiis, pro quibus tristes efficimur, si per confessionem ejecta fuerint, per lacrymus purgamur … Habuisti per sanguinem dulcedinem charitatis. Habes nunc per choleram nigram, sue melancholiam, tristiam pro peccatis.][79]

Margery Kempe's tears – as plenitudinous within scholarly debate as in their own existence – are, as I have argued, not arbitrary expressions of mystical experience, but rather signifiers of a melancholic complexion, liquid articulations of her constitutional receptivity. The melancholic has a natural predisposition to rapture, and Kempe, for the same reasons, is predisposed to weeping. As she develops in spiritual maturity and realises the productive value of this weeping as a means of achieving a privileged dialogue with Christ, she also recognises their conventionality in the experience of contemplation.[80] When she hears her priest read of how 'owr Lord wept' in Jerusalem, as he anticipated the 'myscheuys & sorwys' that would ensue, Kempe weeps 'sor' and cries 'lowde' (143), at once grieving for and identifying with the Christ whose lost body signifies the wounds for which she will infinitely weep. The cold, dry melancholic complexion is, I suggest, exacerbated by her copious crying, dehydrating her further and sustaining her melancholia in a hermeneutic of mournful self-fulfilment.[81] Such 'bleeding tears', inspired by the envisioned wounds of Christ, offer Kempe the pseudo-stigmatic opportunity to partake in a Christ-like dissonance of salvation and disease.

---

[79] Hugo de Folieto, *De medicina animae*. PL 177, col. 1191. Translation from Klibansky et al., p. 109.

[80] Kempe's amenuensis trusts in her weeping much more after reading of the crying of Marie of Oignies and Elizabeth of Hungary. See *BMK* pp. 152–3. Kempe may have been influenced by the ideas of St Jerome and St John Climacus, which inspired Walter Hilton's *Scale of Perfection* and which was read to Kempe over a number of years. Angela of Foligno and Marie of Oignies also caused disruption in church by their crying. See Santha Bhattacharji, *God is an Earthquake: The Spirituality of Margery Kempe* (London: Darton, Longman and Todd, 1997), pp. 44–50.

[81] The gendering of this idea is emphasised by the first commentator of *De secretis mulierum*, who asserts that 'women cry a great deal because they have much humidity that their body must expel'. *De secretis mulierum*, trans. Lemay, p. 130.

Gregory of Nyssa (c. 330–395), bishop and rhetorician, called tears 'the blood in the wounds of the soul'.[82] The tenth-century German monk Grimlaïcus of Metz advised the male recluses to whom his Rule was addressed to cause 'the blood of the confessing soul [to] flow out through tears' (*sanguis animae confitentis per lacrymas profluat*).[83] And similarly, the author of *The Prickyng of Love* perceives that his 'yʒen were filled ful of his [Christ's] blod'.[84] Indeed, Liz Herbert McAvoy has noted how blood flow and tears were 'constantly allied' in the Middle Ages, tending to be associated with feminine piety because of their association with the suffering of the Virgin as *mater dolorosa* as she beholds the wounds of Christ at the foot of the cross.[85] The Middle English translation of Philip of Clairvaux's *Vita* of Elizabeth of Spalbeek describes her experiencing a stigmata of the eyes: 'Also y and my felawes, booth abbots and monkes, ate mydnyghte and sum othere oures also, sawe blode comynge oute at hir eyen and dropped doune and dyed the linnyn garment that sche was cladde with ouerest'.[86] As well as from her eyes, Spalbeek bleeds from wounds in her hands, feet, and sides. Philip emphasises the stigmatic nature of the blood, stating 'Wee sawe blode, not allynges rede but as it were mengyd with water, rennynge oute thorowe an hool of hir coot made aboute the pappe.'[87] In describing the blood in the same manner as Christ's blood is depicted in the Bible, Philip shows Elizabeth to engender an *imitatio Christi* since her blood is identified precisely with Christ's blood, a recognisable motif given the popularity of blood piety in medieval society.[88] The cultural coalescence of blood and tears, made explicit through stigmatic weeping, thus offers Elizabeth an opportunity for the internalisation and re-enactment of trauma described by Hollywood; her tears are recognised, symbolic articulations of

---

[82] Gregory of Nyssa, *Oratio funebris de Placilla* (PG 46.880C). Cited from Mary Carruthers, 'On Affliction and Reading, Weeping and Argument: Chaucer's Lachrymose Troilus in Context', *Representations*, 93, No. 1, 2006, 1–21 (p. 7).

[83] From Liz Herbert McAvoy, *Medieval Anchoritisms: Gender, Space and the Solitary Life* (Cambridge: D.S. Brewer, 2011), p. 35.

[84] From Vincent Gillespie, 'Strange Images of Death: The Passion in Later Medieval English Devotional and Mystical Writing', *Analecta Cartusiana*, 117 (1987), 110–59 (p. 129).

[85] McAvoy, *Medieval Anchoritisms*, p. 35.

[86] 'The Middle English Life of Elizabeth of Spalbeek', in *Three Women of Liège: A Critical Edition of and Commentary on the Middle English Lives of Elizabeth of Spalbeek, Christina Mirabilis, and Marie D'Oignies*, ed. Jennifer N. Brown (Turnhout: Brepols, 2008), pp. 27–50 (p. 41).

[87] Ibid. That the blood runs from Elizabeth's 'pappe' is significant in its allusion to the medieval connection between blood and breast milk. This idea is considered in Chapter 3.

[88] John 19:34: 'But one of the soldiers with a spear opened his side, and immediately there came out blood and water'. There is a physiological reason for Christ's spilling of water as well as blood. Extreme blood loss causes shock to the body (now termed 'hypovolemic shock'). Symptoms include extreme thirst (as Christ was said to experience: see John 19:28) and the accumulation of fluid around the heart and lungs (now termed 'pericardial effusion' and 'pleural effusion').

her own weeping wounds.[89] This same motif can be seen in a Marian lyric which describes how the Virgin's 'blody terys fro my herte roote rebowne', the 'bloody tears' originating in Mary's heart and springing ('rebowne') up to her eyes, emphasising the connection between blood and its fluid transference as a material (and maternal) conduit of emotion.[90]

In concord, Margery Kempe's tears are symbolic of the wounding that she experiences at Calvary, when her crying first becomes loud and causes her somatic collapse and dismantling. After her conversion and before her pilgrimage to the Holy Land, she weeps soft 'plentyouws teerys of contricyon' (2). But it is the experience of visiting the place of Christ's execution and the friars' graphic descriptions of each stage of his suffering that prompt Kempe to envision the Passion with forceful affective devotion:

> & the forseyd creatur wept & sobbyd so plentyvowsly as þow sche had seyn owyr Lord wyth hir bodyly ey sufferyng hys Passyon at þat tyme. Befor hir in hyr sowle sche saw hym verily be contemplacyon, & þat cawsyd hir to haue compassyon. &, whan þei cam vp on-to þe Mownt of Caluarye, sche fel down þat sche mygth not stondyn ne knelyn but walwyd & wrestyd wyth hir body, spredyng hir armys a-brode, & cryed wyth a lowde voys as þow hir hert xulde a brostyn a-sundyr, for in þe cite of hir sowle sche saw verily & freschly how owyr Lord was crucified. Beforn hir face sche herd and saw in hir gostly sygth þe mornyng of owyr Lady, of Sen Iohn & Mary Mawdelyn, and of many oþer þat louyd owyr Lord. & sche had so gret compassyon & so gret peyn to se owyr Lordys peyn þat sche myt not kepe hir-self fro kryng & roryng þow sche xuld a be ded þerfor. And þis was þe fyrst cry þat euyr sche cryed in any contemplacyon (68).

The verisimilitude with which Kempe recounts this episode is illustrated by the very physical way in which the trauma unfolds.[91] She sees Christ in temporal immediacy, as if it were with her 'bodyly ey' in the present moment

[89] On female stigmata, see Caroline Walker Bynum, *Holy Feast and Holy Fast: The Religious Significance of Food to Medieval Women* (Berkeley, Los Angeles and London: University of California Press, 1987). On the development of stigmatic experience see Carolyn Muessig, 'Signs of Salvation: The Evolution of Stigmatic Spirituality Before Francis of Assisi', *Church History*, 82 (2013), 40–68. On the connection between stigmata, pain and illness, see Gábor Klaniczay, 'Illness, Self-Inflicted Body Pain and Supernatural Stigmata: Three Ways of Identification with the Suffering Body of Christ', in *Infirmity in Antiquity and the Middle Ages: Social and Cultural Approaches to Health, Weakness and Care*, ed. Christian Krötzl, Katariina Mustakallio, and Jenni Kuuliala (Farnham and Burlington: Ashgate, 2015), pp. 119–36.
[90] IMEV 3692, 'Mary at the Foot of the Cross', no. 40, l. 3, in *Middle English Marian Lyrics*, ed. Karen Saupe (Kalamazoo: Medieval Institute Publications, 1997), TEAMS online edition <http://d.lib.rochester.edu/teams/publication/saupe-middle-english-marian-lyrics>. MED s.v. reboune: To recoil from an impact or a force; be driven back forcibly; spring back, return.
[91] On the connection between image, vision and the body, see Cordelia Warr, 'Re-reading the Relationship between Devotional Images, Visions, and the Body: Clare of Montefalco and Margaret of Città di Castello', *Viator*, 38 (2007), 217–49.

('at þat tyme'), as opposed to retrieving the image through memory or imagination. This cognition enables Kempe to experience two realities in simultaneity, echoing scientific theories of the melancholic's heightened receptivity and imposing a *truth* on the contemplation as she sees Christ 'verily', in her soul. On Calvary she collapses in corporeal failure, her weeping a symptom of heartbreak – of lovesickness – for the lost object of her desire ('hir hert xulde a brostyn a-sundyr'), her cries in 'lowde voys' the thundering articulation of loss, threatening the annihilation of her physical self as she presumes the conclusion to be her own death ('þow sche xuld a be ded þerfor'). Such co-suffering evidences the internalisation of Christ's crucifixion within her own body, and the interiorisation of Jerusalem inside her soul such that 'in the cite of hir sowle sche saw veryly'. In fact, Kempe tells Christ that if she might 'wepyn [in hell] & mornyn for þi lofe as I do her, Helle xuld not noyin me, but it xulde be a maner of Heuyn' (215). To incorporate, and to thus perceive, the event of the Passion, Kempe shows us how the wounds of Christ are her own, their painful internalisation revealed outwardly by her cries of grief. It is a grief that is, though, agonisingly necessary.

This vociferous weeping lasts for ten years, climaxing at Easter time when it causes her physical weakness: 'And euery Good Friday in alle þe forseyd ȝerys sche was wepyng & sobbyng v er vj owrys to-gedyr & þerwyth cryed ful lowde many tymes so þat sche myth not restreyn hir þerfro, which madyn hir ful febyl & weke in hir bodily mytys' (140).[92] Despite mental and physical exhaustion, Kempe seeks out the discomfort, fearing its loss and the subsequent obstruction of Christ's grace: 'And þerfor, Lord, I schal not sesyn, whan I may wepyn, for to wepyn for hem plentyuowsly, spede ȝyf I may. And, ȝyf þu wylt, Lord, þat I sese of wepyng, I prey þe take me owt of þis world' (142). The fear of losing her gift of tears is so acute that it is a reason for mortal departure, as those tears are the very representation of Christ's presence in her soul. Indeed, biblical texts indicate the generative value of female weeping, such as this passage from Jeremiah:

> Consider ye, and call for the mourning women, and let them come: and send to them that are wise women, and let them make haste: Let them hasten and take up a lamentation for us: let our eyes shed tears, and our eyelids run down with waters. For a voice of wailing is heard out of Sion.[93]

As Santha Bhattachaji suggests, Kempe's tears represent 'an intense joy', arising from 'a paradoxical sense of the almost unbearable presence of Christ'.[94] Their absence, in contrast, suggests a spiritual dryness, or *acedia*, a state which

---

[92] Kempe's boisterous crying 'enduryd þe terme of x ȝer' (p. 140).
[93] Jeremiah 9:17–20.
[94] Santha Bhattachaji, 'Tears and Screaming: Weeping in the Spirituality of Margery Kempe', in *Holy Tears: Weeping in the Religious Imagination*, ed. Kimberly C. Patton and John Stratton Hawley (Princeton and Oxford: Princeton University Press, 2005), pp. 229–41 (p. 229).

Mary Carruthers notes can be remedied by weeping: 'Tears' effect upon a barren soul is life-giving' because they are 'moist and hot', balancing and softening the cold and hard constitution of the spiritually bereft individual.[95] As Evagrius Ponticus (345–99) wrote, 'Pray first for the gift of tears so that by means of sorrow you may soften your native rudeness.'[96] And when Julian of Norwich experienced great sickness and pain she described herself 'as baren and as drye as [she] had never had comfort but litille'.[97] Kempe's tears are therefore an embodiment of grace, of which she desires limitless quantities: 'I wolde I had a welle of teerys' (140–1). That well of tears is coexistent with the open wounds for which she weeps, constructing an infinite process of mourning and melancholia which has the paradoxical benefit of retaining the lost Christic figure, signifying the antithesis of spiritual dryness. As Carruthers illustrates, medieval writers saw weeping as the rebalancing of a cold and hard constitution by making it moist, since tears signify spiritual fecundity and provide multipliable nourishment. Further to this theological understanding, Margery Kempe's tears might be viewed as *reanimating* the melancholic state by purging moisture and drying her further, according to medical theory. Nevertheless, their fecundity is tangible. Christ informs Kempe that God, Mary, and all the saints in heaven are sustained by her tears: 'þu hast ȝouyn hem drynkyn ful many tymes wyth teers of thyn eyne' (52). Her tears are the drink of angels, too, and medicinally potent: they are 'very pyment to hem' (161).[98] Conversely, as Julian of Norwich tells Kempe during her visit to her cell in Norwich, tears are torturous to the diabolic: 'for Ierom seyth þat terys turmentyn mor þe Devylle þan don þe peynes of Helle' (43), a sentiment that is enforced when Kempe envisions St Jerome in Rome and is told that her tears are a 'synguler & a specyal ȝyft' (99). Spiritually fruitful in their holy signification, therefore, Kempe's tears simultaneously perpetuate the psychosomatic template of melancholia and her mystical perceptivity in powerful repetition.

That same spiritual fecundity vanishes, however, when Kempe becomes temporarily barren of tears:

> sche was sumtyme so bareyn fro teerys a day er sumtyme half a day & had so gret peyne for desyr þat sche had of hem þat sche wold a ȝouyn al þis worlde, ȝyf it had ben hir, for a fewe teerys, er a suffyrd ryth gret bodily peyne for to a gotyn hem wyth (199).

Her 'gret peyne for desyr' reveals a lovesickness for which she would sacrifice the earth, while the incorporation of the term 'bareyn' further symbolises the

---

[95] Carruthers, 'On Affliction', p. 7.
[96] Ibid., p. 8.
[97] Julian of Norwich, 'A Revelation of Love', in *The Writings of Julian of Norwich*, ed. Watson and Jenkins, p. 331.
[98] MED s.v. piment: A sweetened, spiced wine used for refreshment and in medical recipes.

status of her tears as indicators of spiritually fertile potential.[99] Not only is her very desire for crying painful, but she is prepared to suffer '*gret* bodily peyne' to regain her tears. The indefinite boundaries between the somatic and the spiritual, the internal and external, and the ascetic function of pain, here conflate. When Jesus removes for a time Kempe's 'lowde' crying, substituting it with a more 'stille' sorrow 'as God wolde mesur it hys-selfe' (155), public accusations of hypocrisy initiate bodily pain and spiritual progress: '& so slawndir & bodily angwisch fel to hir on euery syde, & al *was encresyng of hir gostly comfort*' (156). Moreover, this episode reveals a potent enactment of the tradition of *Christus medicus* (Christ the Physician), a ubiquitous notion in the Christian Middle Ages that originated from the biblical conceit of Christ as a healer of body and soul.[100] In this episode, Christ increases and decreases Kempe's weeping in a pseudo-medical action, replaying the tenets of humoral theory by rebalancing her capacity for crying in order to max-imise her spiritual health. Her own powerlessness to control the measure of her tears is also evident during a vision received on a Good Friday when the sight of the crucifixion engenders such traumatic perception that Kempe's quasi-suicidal cry is cause for her physical removal to the prior's cloister:

> [The liturgical re-enactment of Christ's death drew] hir mende al holy in-to þe Passyon of owr Lord Crist Ihesu, whom sche beheld wyth hir *gostly eye* in þe sight of hir sowle as verily as þei sche had seyn hys precyows body betyn, scorgyd, & crucified wyth hir *bodily eye*, which syght & gostly beheldyng wrowt be grace so feruently in hir mende, wowndyng hir wyth pite & compassyon, þat sche sobbyd, roryd, & cryed, and, spredyng hir armys a-brood, seyd wyth lowde voys, 'I dey, I dey', þat many man on hir wonderyd & merueyled what hir eyled. And þe more sche besijd hir to kepyn fro crying, þe lowdar sche cryed, for it was not in hir powyr to take it ne leuyn it but as God wolde send it. Than a preyst toke hir in hys armys & bar hir in-to þe Priowrys Cloistyr for to latyn hir takyn þe eyr, supposyng sche schulde not ellys han enduryd, hir *labowr* was so greet (140).

As Margery Kempe attempts to quieten and cease weeping, her cries only become 'lowdar', since it is 'not in hir powyr' to stop what God controls. Crying is thus an intimately experienced phenomenon outside her autonomy and a product of divine will to which she must submit. The dramatic oscilla-tion between ghostly and bodily perception in this episode reveals a complex consciousness that resists straightforward categorisation, yet it also illustrates her authentic understanding. In aligning her two 'eyes' as one, the painful reality of Christ's tortured flesh, perceived through her ghostly eye, is as immediate and acute as her bodily eye would have it, making 'real' the event

---

[99] MED s.v. barein: 1a) Barren (woman); sterile (woman or man). 2) Unproductive, non-bearing, fruitless. 4) Intellectually or morally sterile.
[100] See Naoë Kukita Yoshikawa, 'Introduction', in *Medicine, Religion and Gender in Medieval Culture*, ed. Yoshikawa, pp. 1–24. The tradition of *Christus medicus* is explored further in Chapter 4 of this study.

and dissolving the distinctions between worldly and spiritual experience. The real-time portrayal of Christ's mutilation is animated through the echoing of rhetorical triads: Christ is 'betyn, scorgyd, & crucifyed', whilst Kempe 'sobbyd, roryd, & cryed'. Similarly, the present-tense leap through time in the climactic cry 'I dey, I dey' engenders an urgent immediacy and final articulation of pain, as her mourning of the lost Christ is so intense that the inevitable outcome must be her death. The potency of this vision, as Kempe hovers in a liminal zone somewhere between earthly and ephemeral realities, causes her to be literally 'wownd[ed]' by compassion, the tangible flesh and blood of the scene emphasising real bodily damage, witnessed 'verily', and the endless outpouring of blood and tears.[101] And, as does the lamentation of Mary, whose role in the scene is diminished by Kempe's own performance, the portrayal of a great 'labowr' reminds us that it is the pain and love of Christ – the spiritual fecundity of woundedness – with which Kempe is now identified.[102] Indeed, metaphors of spiritual birthing are seen elsewhere in the *Book* – 'sumtyme sche was al on a watyr wyth þe labowr of þe crying' (185), for example – and suggest a drenching in fluid like the nourishing generation of amniotic water. Kempe joins a well-established tradition of 'ghostly labowr', as Karma Lochrie has shown, citing the Dominican theologian Felix Fabri (1438–1502), who documented how female visitors to Jerusalem often 'cried out, roared, and wept, as though giving birth'.[103] Kempe is now able, in agonising temporality, to substitute Christ's sacrifice for her own.

The *realness*, or truth, of Kempe's grief is illuminated in Chapter 60, when a priest criticises her tears at the sight of a Pietà in Norwich:

'Damsel, Ihesu is ded long sithyn'. Whan hir crying was cesyd, sche seyd to þe preste, 'Sir, hys deth is as fresch to me as he had deyd þis same day, & so me thynkyth it awt to be to ȝow & to alle Cristen pepil. We awt euyr to han mende of hys kendnes & euyr thynkyn of þe dolful deth þat he deyd for vs' (148).

Not only is Christ's death perpetually 'fresch' in Kempe's perception, but she regards the ongoing contemplation of his 'dolful deth' to be the duty of the good Christian, who should '*euyr*' have mind of his kindness. In foregrounding the *euyr*-ness – the *eternity* of mournful meditation – she reasserts herself not only as a model, or *merowr*, of devotion, in rebuking the priest, but also as a mourner in perpetuity.[104] At St Stephen's Church she falls to the ground and roars at the graveside of the previous vicar, generating such 'holy thowtys & so holy mendys þat sche *myth not mesuryn* hir wepyng ne hir crying' (147). Such

---

[101] MED s.v. verreili: 1 (a) In accordance with the facts, truly; honestly; truthfully.
[102] MED s.v. labour: 1. Work, esp. hard work. 2. Pains taken. 4(b) Pain, sickness, disease, also, the active phase of an intermittent disease; of birth.
[103] Lochrie, *Margery Kempe and Translations of the Flesh*, p. 192.
[104] On this episode and Kempe's multitemporality, see Carolyn Dinshaw, 'Margery Kempe', in *The Cambridge Companion to Medieval Women's Writing* (Cambridge: Cambridge University Press, 2003), pp. 222–39, esp. 231–2.

an incalculable capacity for psychological pain evokes the advice of Julian of Norwich, who writes that '[God] makyth vs to askyn & preyn wyth mornynggys & wepyngys so plentyvowsly þat þe terys may not be nowmeryd' (43), and of Chaucer's Man in Black, whose mourning bears infinite pain: 'This ys my peyne wythoute red [remedy], / Alway deynge and be not ded'.[105]

These boundless tears, the teleological outpouring of melancholia, is exemplified by Kempe's uncontrollable crying on Palm Sundays. Her feelings are so great during one episode that 'sche myth not *beryn* it', again beholding Christ in her 'gostly syght as verily as he had ben a-forn hir in hir bodily syght' (184–5). The homogeneity of interior and exterior cognizance compels her to articulate mystical experience outwardly: 'sche *must nedys* wepyn, cryin, & sobbyn whan sche be-held hir Sauyowr suffyr so gret peynys for hir lofe' (185). In this way, her crying is not the hysterical language of a woman religious, an idea proposed by several scholars, so much as an interiorised necessity; it is the reversal of that expression, the emanation of what is already there.[106] As a melancholic Kempe's phenomenological experience *must* emanate through weeping, as she 'melt[s] al in-to teerys' (124). This uncontrollable expulsion of emotion is illustrated when the Palm Sunday sermon causes her to burst outwards. She could 'no lengar kepyn þe fir of lofe clos wyth-inne hir brest, but, *wheþyr sche wolde er not*, it wolde aperyn wyth-owte-forth swech as was closyd wyth-inne-forth' (185). That 'sche xulde a *brostyn* for pite' depicts Kempe's conflation of her tears with her death. In imagining that her very body will explode with the pressure of her suffering she evidences what Jeffrey Cohen sees as her 'emptying herself from her own body'.[107] As Vincent Gillespie has argued, in order to be open to change, one must undertake a process of 'kenosis', or 'self-emptying', an act of courage and letting-go in order to achieve God's grace.[108] Kempe's dependence on weeping for her identification and very existence – that she must bleed the tears of Christ – indicates a difficult passage ahead and a helpless route towards annihilation.

[105] Geoffrey Chaucer, *The Book of the Duchess*, in *The Riverside Chaucer*, ed. Larry D. Benson (Oxford: Oxford University Press, 1987), ll. 587–8, p. 337.
[106] See Hope Phyllis Weissman, '*Hysterica Compassio* in the Late Middle Ages'; David Knowles, who argues that there is a 'large hysterical element in Margery's personality' in *The English Mystical Tradition*, p. 146; Wolfgang Riehle, who regards Kempe as having a 'sick, neurotic psyche' in *The Middle English Mystics*, p. 96; and Julia Long, who suggests that Kempe 'experiences … "ghostly labours" at Calvary resembling an hysterical childbirth', in 'Mysticism and Hysteria: The Histories of Margery Kempe and Anna O.', in *Feminist Readings in Middle English Literature: The Wife of Bath and All Her Sect*, ed. Ruth Evans and Lesley Johnson (London and New York: Routledge, 1994), pp. 88–111; and William B. Ober, who sees Kempe's experiences as symptomatic of 'both hysteria and mysticism', in 'Margery Kempe: Hysteria and Mysticism Reconciled', *Literature and Medicine*, 4 (1985), 24–40 (p. 39).
[107] Jeffrey J. Cohen, *Medieval Identity Machines* (Minneapolis: University of Minnesota Press, 2003), p. 173.
[108] Vincent Gillespie, 'Dead Still / Still Dead', *The Mediaeval Journal*, 1 (2011), 53–78 (pp. 60–3).

However, although Amy Hollywood suggests that female mystics idealise and desire their own death in identification with Christ, Kempe's conceptualisation of her own death is more ambivalent.[109] While her desire for contemplative pain persists, she reveals a fear of physical pain and dying that emphasises the importance of melancholic weeping over corporeal pain for her construction of self. Kempe imagines 'what deth sche mygth deyn for Crystys sake', however, the nature of the death must be 'soft' as it is punctuated by an underlying fear:

> Hyr þow[t] sche wold a be slayn for Goddys lofe, but dred for þe poynt of deth, & þerfor sche ymagyned hyr-self þe most soft deth, as hir thowt, for dred of inpacyens, þat was to be bowndyn hyr hed & hir fet to a stokke & hir hed to be smet of wyth a scharp ex for Goddys lofe (30).

God is pleased with Margery's willingness to die in his name, although her choice of a quick and 'soft' death jars with Christ's own embracing of pain: 'it lykyn me wel þe peynes þat I haue sufferyd for þe' (30). The pain exchange is neither literal nor reciprocal, as Kempe's earthly reluctance to succumb to extremes of bodily anguish marks a devotional impasse of sorts: Christ's endurance of corporeal pain is a model for which she willingly suffers spiritually, but which she is unwilling to mirror physically. Her fear of death frequently occurs during periods of sickness, for example, during her pilgrimage in Venice when 'owyr Lord mad hir so seke þat sche *wend to be ded*, & sythyn sodeynly he mad hir hool a-ȝen' (66); similarly, on her return to Lynn she falls 'in gret sekenes in so mech þat sche was anoyntyd for dowt of deth' (104).[110] Kempe's sense of spiritual incompletion is revealed when she then asks God to allow her to travel to the shrine of St James at Santiago de Compostela before she dies. Though she is informed that she will not die yet, her mortal anxiety is paralysing. Like the crying that threatens to split apart her bodily frame, her pain is such that to remain existent seems impossible: 'owr Lord Ihesu Crist seyd to hir in hir sowle þat sche xuld [not] dey ȝet, and sche wend hir-selfe þat sche xulde not a leuyd for hir peyn was so gret' (104). The slipperiness of Kempe's response to suffering is, in fact, synonymous with her equally paradoxical desire for infinite tears of grief. While their source is reliant on the wounded and *difficile* Christic body, it is that very object, and the longing and mourning upon which it insists, which *resisti non potest*. Like Chaucer's Man in Black, she is 'Alway deynge and be not ded'.

Tears are thus the liquid manifestation of Kempe's disintegration. Unlike the female ascetics who seek out bodily anguish in their desire for Christic imitation, Kempe dismantles herself in a sacrificial offering via a complex outpouring of melancholy, a grief which she cannot control, and from which

---

[109] Hollywood, 'Acute Melancholia', p. 402.

[110] MED s.v. doute: 1(a) A feeling of uncertainty, doubt, or perplexity. 3(a) Anxiety; fear, fright; for fear of (death, etc.). That Kempe is given extreme unction indicates the severity of her illness.

she cannot escape.[111] When secreted in the prior's cloister, she cries 'as ȝyf hir sowle & hir body xulde a partyd a-sundyr' (138). On the verge of rupture and fragmentation, it is a woundedness of self that signals Kempe's own version of the violent *imitatio* of her contemporaries. Though she does not desire death in the form of accident or illness, it is her only option in the event of the terminal drying up of her tears: 'And, ȝyf þu wylt, Lord, þat I sese of wepyng, I prey þe take me owt of þis world' (142). It is this unyielding boundedness to tearful mourning that preserves her infinite union with Christ, yet which also inspires the scepticism of her *even cristen*, who are as divided in their diagnoses as Kempe is in her burst and fractured body.

This is the woundedness of melancholia: a boundless state in which Kempe is immersed and with which her identity is inextricably bound up. For if her tears cease to exist then so must she, and so must the Christ whose own wounded body she retains through her weeping. For Kempe, therefore, to relinquish productivity in crying for the world's sins as a sorrowing intercessor, to dry up the 'open wounds' – in Freud's words – that weep for the lost Christ, is to be annihilated. Without tears, she is nothing but mutilated flesh: 'ȝyf if wer thy wille, Lord, I wolde for þi lofe & for magnifying of þi name ben hewyn as small as flesch to þe potte' (142).[112] In crying her infinitely bleeding tears of lamentation she fulfils the trajectory of her existence by retaining that 'violent object' of Burton's imagining through a cycle of traumatic repetition. It is thus safe to contend that Kempe's melancholia and the way in which it engenders affective receptivity are central features of her route towards union with Christ, and provide a powerful way of reading mystical experience. Her weeping allows us to read the *Book* not as the embodiment of pathological disorder, but as a teleology of Margery Kempe herself – the way in which, in tearful understanding, she was ordained, and how she must always be.

[111] See Sarah Macmillan, 'Mortifying the Mind: Asceticism, Mysticism and Oxford, Bodleian Library, MS Douce 114', in *The Medieval Mystical Tradition in England: Exeter Symposium VIII*, ed. E.A. Jones (Cambridge: D.S. Brewer, 2013), pp. 109–24.

[112] It is notable that similar lexis is employed by the man whom Kempe propositions in Chapter 4 of the book in order to show disgust and corporeal annihilation: 'And he sayd he ne wold for al þe good in þis world; he had leuar ben hewyn as small as flesch to þe potte' (15).

2

'Þe mukke' of Marriage and the Sexual Paradox

The wife hath not power of her own body, but the husband. And in like manner the husband also hath not power of his own body, but the wife.

I Corinthians 7:4

… þe dette of matrimony was so abhominabyl to hir þat sche had leuar, hir thowt, etyn or drynkyn þe wose, *þe mukke* in þe chanel, þan to consentyn to any fleschly comownyng saf only for obedyens.

BMK, 11–12

At around the age of thirty-six or thirty-seven Margery Kempe, whilst lying in bed with her husband John, hears 'a sownd of melodye so swet & delectable, hir þowt, as sche had ben in Paradyse' (11).[1] So sublime is the music that upon hearing any subsequent melody or auditory 'myrth' she crumbles to plenteous weeping and sighing since she is now conscious of the meaning of heaven, perceiving its sensory *truth*. As she begins to share this revelation with her acquaintances, disclosing how 'It is ful mery in Hevyn', she is met with wrath, as the people challenge the audacity of a woman who claims to know about a place to which she has not been: 'Why speke ȝe so of þe myrth þat is in Heuyn; ȝe haue not be þer no mor þan we' (11). In attempting to articulate, in the earthly world, her knowledge and experience of the divine, Kempe reveals both her experiential polarisation from the parishioners in Lynn, and her mystical receptivity: a receptivity which bridges the divide between heaven and earth, which dissolves the borders of body and soul, and which evidences the fluid porousness of her 'gostly' and 'bodyly' vision, as we saw in Chapter 1. This new understanding of the cosmos gives Kempe claim to a metaphysical wisdom that will mark the transference of all her desires to a heavenly trajectory: 'sche desyryd no-thyng so mech as Heuyn' (13). In her cognition, therefore, she *has* 'be þer'.

---

[1] My estimation of Kempe's age is based upon Hope Emily Allen's calculation that Margery and John Kempe's vow of chastity occurs in June 1413, when Margery Kempe is about forty years old. The book tells us in Chapter 3 that she asks John to live chaste after perceiving this heavenly music, and that he agrees 'iij or iiij ȝer aftyr' (12). This places the episode around the year 1399 or 1400.

It is perhaps unsurprising, then, that Kempe juxtaposes this moment of ecstatic, heavenly discernment with the concomitant revulsion that ensues when she is faced with the prospect of a sexual encounter with John: it is 'aftyr þis tyme' that she cannot bear the prospect of 'fleschly comownyng' with him (11–12). This abhorrence of sexual intercourse is described through imagery of ingesting glutinous, oozing, and dirty matter; the 'wose' and 'mukke' – the mud and sewage of the channel – represent base, contaminatory substances, and in Middle English 'wose' also has connotations of digestive juices.[2] The foulness of the consumption and digestion of 'mukke' thus confirms Kempe's post-conversion misogamy; regarding sexual contact as polluting and repulsive, she would rather be violated by poison than by the sinful contagion of her husband's body. As Caroline Walker Bynum has comprehensively shown, ingestion is imbued with a particular significance for medieval religious women, since curing and healing with food is a form of *imitatio Christi*. In 'merg[ing] their own humiliating and painful flesh with that flesh whose agony, espoused by choice, was salvation', women such as Angela of Foligno 'found the taste of pus "as sweet as communion"'.[3] As I shall argue in this chapter, Kempe's assertion that she would prefer to ingest 'mukke' illustrates a strategy of pain substitution that declares not only her revulsion from sexual obligation but also the intensification of her physical connection to Christ's body, whose suffering flesh she seeks, instead, to interiorise.

Following this revelatory moment in the year 1399 or 1400, John continues to enforce his entitlement to marital 'obedyens' and 'wold haue hys wylle, & sche obeyd wyth *greet wepyng* & sorwyng for þat sche myght not levyn chast' (12).[4] Kempe's distress is articulated by 'greet wepyng' that neither relieves her suffering nor spares her from John's 'vsyng' via the marriage contract. We are told, 'in al þis tyme sche had no lust to comown wyth hir husbond, [as] it was very peynful & horrybyl vn-to hir' (14). Even when she is in spatial and doctrinal safety – in the marriage bed – she cannot endure sexual intercourse with him: 'Sche lay be hir husbond, & for to comown wyth hym it was so abhomynabyl on-to hir þat sche mygth not duren it, & ȝet was it leful on-to hir in leful tyme yf sche had wold' (15).[5] She accepts that sexual activity would be permissible at this 'tyme' in the Christian calendar, but the doctrinal legitimacy of the potential encounter does not negate its repugnancy, and she is unable to 'duren' the possibility.[6] Furthermore, Kempe will also have

---

[2] MED s.v. wose n. 2: 3(a). The substance produced by the action of digestive juices on food, the product of the first stage of digestion.

[3] Bynum, *Holy Feast and Holy Fast*, p. 246.

[4] There were strict codes applicable to the sex lives of married couples. See Georges Duby, *The Knight, the Lady and the Priest: The Making of Modern Marriage in Medieval France*, trans. Barbara Bray (Middlesex: Penguin Books, 1983), esp. pp. 57–74.

[5] MED s.v. lefful: 1(a) permissible, allowed (b) permitted by civil law, legal (c) permitted or *sanctioned by religious law*.

[6] Medieval penitentials forbade marital sex on fast days, feast days, before communion, and after receiving the sacrament, during Lent, Advent, and Whitsuntide, on certain days of

had seventeen years of childbearing by this point, initiated by a traumatic first birth that is recounted, tellingly, early in the *Book* and which – perhaps paradoxically – signifies the moment of her epiphanic spiritual conversion.

Though Jerome had established three grades of chastity – virginity, widowhood, and marriage – that placed marriage at the bottom, Kempe was probably aware of the lives of married saints like Hedwig of Silesia (c. 1174–1243), Dauphine of Puimichel (1283–1360), Dorothy of Montau (1347–94), Angela of Foligno (c. 1248–1309), Marie of Oignies (1177–1213), and Elizabeth of Hungary (1207–31), who were praised for the purity of their marriages which were based not upon lust but 'faith, fertility, and sacrament'.[7] Bridget of Sweden, whom Kempe certainly emulates, was known to have had a pious marriage and developed the ascetic practices of prayer, fasting, and sleep-deprivation over its duration.[8] *The Pore Caitif*, which is likely to have been in the reading milieu of Kempe's priestly confessors, tell us that the Virgin Mary 'dispise[s] lusti filþes', and that St Lucy, 'spouse of crist … hatid filþis of þis world', sentiments that add to a culture which elevated female chastity while simultaneously enforcing the doctrine of marriage.[9] The inescapable pain of Kempe's sexual marriage thus perpetuates in an abject cycle of pseudo-masochism: her desire for *Heuyn*, though ultimately rewarding, has an agonisingly high cost on earth.[10]

---

each week, during menstruation, pregnancy, and lactation. The primary purpose of these prohibitions was to avoid ritual pollution. See James Brundage, '"Allas! That evere love was synne": Sex and Medieval Canon Law', *The Catholic Historical Review*, 72 (1986), 1–13 (p. 10). See also Dyan Elliott, *Spiritual Marriage: Sexual Abstinence in Medieval Wedlock* (Princeton: Princeton University Press, 1993), pp. 150–1.

7 See Connor McCarthy, *Marriage in Medieval England: Law, Literature and Practice* (Cambridge: Boydell and Brewer, 2004), pp. 107–25 (p. 108); and Clarissa Atkinson, *Mystic and Pilgrim*, pp. 157–94. See also Michael Goodich, 'Sexuality, Family, and the Supernatural in the Fourteenth Century', in *Medieval Families: Perspectives on Marriage, Household, and Children*, ed. Carol Neel (Toronto and London: University of Toronto Press, 2004), pp. 302–28. Kempe may have known the *Vita* of Dorothy of Montau, although she does not mention her by name. David Wallace has connected the revived cult of Dorothea in the 1930s with the discovery of Kempe's *Book* in *Strong Women: Life, Text, and Territory, 1347–1645* (Oxford: Oxford University Press, 2011), p. 61. See also Ute Stargardt, 'The Beguines of Belgium, the Dominican Nuns of Germany, and Margery Kempe', in *The Popular Literature of Medieval England*, Tennessee Studies in Literature, 28, ed. Thomas J. Heffernan (Knoxville: University of Tennessee Press, 1985), pp. 277–313. On Kempe's literary and religious influences, see Wolfgang Riehle, *The Secret Within*, pp. 246–81. See also Alexandra Barratt, 'Margery Kempe and the King's Daughter of Hungary', in *Margery Kempe: A Book of Essays*, ed. McEntire, pp. 189–201; Alexandra Barratt, 'Continental Women Mystics and English Readers', in *The Cambridge Companion to Medieval Women's Writing*, ed. Dinshaw and Wallace, pp. 240–55; and Susan Dickman, 'Margery Kempe and the Continental Tradition', in *The Medieval Mystical Tradition in England: Papers Read at Dartington Hall, July 1984*, ed. Marion Glasscoe (Cambridge: D.S. Brewer, 1984), pp. 150–68.

8 Bridget Morris, *St Birgitta of Sweden* (Woodbridge: Boydell and Brewer, 1999), pp. 42–63.

9 *The Pore Caitif*, p. 178 and p. 193 respectively.

10 On female virginity in late antiquity see Elizabeth Castelli, 'Virginity and Its Meaning for Women's Sexuality in Early Christianity', *Journal of Feminist Studies in Religion*, 2 (1986), 61–88.

The pain imperative of marriage is intensified by the ubiquity of medical texts which, paradoxically, establish sexual *abstinence* as detrimental to health, causing pain and affliction in the female body. 'On Treatments for Women', one of the *Trotula* texts, asserts that celibate women who wish to engage in sexual activity, but do not, become seriously ill: 'These [women], when they have desire to copulate and do not do so, incur grave illness' (que cum uoluntatem habeant coeundi et non coeunt, grauem incurrunt egritudinem).[11] Thus, despite the potential advantage of a quest for marital chastity and a concomitantly fruitful end to her reproductive capacity – a potential quasi-menopause, of sorts – there is a tension in what I term the *pain paradox* of marriage, which is the basis for this chapter. Scholarly attention has been paid to the theological difficulties inherent in chaste marriage, but no work has been conducted on the inherent conflict between theological and medical advice which constructs a paradigm through which it is impossible to manoeuvre painlessly.[12] Medieval medical theory, in its proposition of celibacy as physically damaging, stands in opposition to the doctrine that upholds virginity as the highest state, thus creating a pain imperative from which Kempe is ultimately unable to escape. She is, then, trapped within an imprisoning hermeneutic, faced with the discomforting choice of spiritual or physical suffering in a never-ending paradox of pain.[13] This chapter therefore explores a series of entangled dichotomies. It begins with an exploration of Margery Kempe's first, traumatic episode of childbirth as an acute spiritual crisis which, I contend, obfuscates her subsequent identity as a mystic-wife-mother. In turning to Kempe's growing desire for a 'curative' vow of chastity, the chapter then examines the 'pain paradox' of celibacy: the medical texts that warn of the physical dangers of chastity to the female body, and the opposing spiritual pain that Kempe experiences in maintaining a sexual marriage. Progressing thereafter to Kempe's innovative strategies for relief, through the substitutional operations of ascetic activity and the multiple fortifications with which she surrounds her 'dangerous' female body, finally achieving a vow of chastity with John, the chapter ultimately assesses her eventual marriage to the Godhead as the antithesis of marital 'mukke', brought about by her progress towards wholeness and purification. Like the slurry that she is prepared to endure having thrown at her naked body for

---

[11] 'On Treatments for Women', in *The Trotula*, pp. 120–1.

[12] See Jo Ann McNamara, 'Chaste Marriage and Clerical Celibacy' in *Sexual Practices in the Medieval Church*, ed. Vern L. Bullough and James A. Brundage (New York: Prometheus, 1982), pp. 22–33; Penny S. Gold, 'The Marriage of Mary and Joseph in the Twelfth-Century Ideology of Marriage', in *Sexual Practices in the Medieval Church*, pp. 102–17; and Elizabeth M. Makowski, 'The conjugal debt and medieval canon law', *Journal of Medieval History*, 3:2 (1977), 99–114.

[13] On gendered pain in scholastic thought, especially Eve's legacy, see Mowbray, *Pain and Suffering in Medieval Theology*, pp. 43–60. Mowbray suggests that theologians like Aquinas saw women as experiencing three types of suffering: carrying the foetus and giving birth, hardship and suffering in conception (due to the sin of sexual pleasure), and subjection to male hegemony.

God's love, Kempe selects alternative metamorphoses of 'muck', yet I ask, lastly, if divine union does provide a satisfactory analgesic to the problem of earthly marriage.

The Birth of Fear and Loathing: The Remaking of Margery Kempe

It is not by chance that the *Book* opens with an account of Margery Kempe's first childbirth. The postpartum trauma, described in visceral detail at the very start of Chapter 1, occurs soon after she turns twenty, after she is married, and signals a deliberate narrative fashioning which situates that personal trauma as a foundational event for the later, mystical traumas that she will experience and relive. In enduring the abject event of near-annihilation in childbirth, Kempe undergoes a dichotomous loss of self, brought about by her new status as a young, wounded mother, and by her temporary exclusion from the Christian rite of confession when she is abandoned and liminal, blocked from absolution and from cure. That it is the appearance of a 'most bewtyuows' Christ, whose blessed 'chere' (8) triggers her instant stabilisation and 'wholeness', teaches Kempe two important lessons. First, that she is henceforth the privileged child of God, with direct access to Christ and mystically authorised to circumvent clerical mediation. And second, that since Christ signifies cure, the loss of the Christic-object will forevermore signify a concomitant loss of self, and of existence. Through her near-annihilation and woundedness, and through the dramatic movement of her exclusion from and reunion with Christ, Kempe's melancholic diathesis is tested to the extreme. As Liz Herbert McAvoy has argued, there exists an association of 'the curative properties of the blood-bath with a maternal blood sacrifice', and further still with *Christus medicus*, who washes the sins of the world with his own bleeding wounds.[14] In turning here to the conception of Kempe's understanding of trauma, of those sacrificial wounds which will weep throughout her life in anamnestic empathy and devotion, deadly childbirth is shown to converge with the birth of the *Book*. By uncovering the painful genesis of Kempe's adult life, which paradoxically gestates into a recognition of Christ's curative power, she is synchronically unmade and remade.

In her short life so far, the course of Kempe's social, familial, and working journey has taken a conventional path. The *Book* presents her passing through the phases of life as to be expected: 'sche *was* maryed' at twenty, '*was* wyth chylde wyth-in schort tyme, *as kynde wolde*' (6). The simple narrative progression of this passage, *as nature would have it*, illustrates the unremarkable inevitability of Kempe's transition from maidenhood to wifehood and motherhood and marks a measured foreshadowing of the violent illness which follows.

---

[14] Liz Herbert McAvoy, 'Bathing in Blood: The Medicinal Cures of Anchoritic Devotion', in *Medicine, Religion and Gender in Medieval Culture*, ed. Yoshikawa, pp. 85–102 (p. 98).

Kempe would have been expected to engage in household tasks during her teenage years, and her marriage would have been considered a promising link between two prominent families: the Brunhams of Lynn, a wealthy elite family (John Brunham was one of the most eminent and active Lynn burgesses of the later fourteenth century), and the Kempes, who were prosperous merchants and jurats.[15] Her marriage thus occurred at a usual age and stage. Whilst her identity would have undergone a rapid shift during this period, the transition is a recognisable one rooted in cultural norms and societal expectations.[16] Kempe's sense of self is thus socially objectified and signified through a process of familiar symbols, marked indeed by a pride in her newly married status: the *Book* makes clear that John is a '*worschepful* burgeys', and even after her conversion she vaingloriously dresses in fancy clothing, driven by an acute recognition of her 'worthy kenred' (6, 9).

Scholars have frequently interpreted the childbirth episode in the terms of modern psychiatry, as an example of postpartum psychosis.[17] Although such retrospective applications provide interesting methodological possibilities, I prefer to consider the episode in the terms of a pivotal spiritual crisis brought about by a near-death experience, manifested as diabolically life-threatening. Indeed, the event is predicated on the acceleration and braking of narrative temporality, from a brisk and linear traverse through the socio-religious rituals of marriage and childbirth, to an aborted confession which interrupts Kempe's trajectory via a sharp turn into the realm of subjectivity and despair. At this point of disruption, of traumatic synchronicity, Kempe painstakingly reveals to her readers the source of her own wounds and the lessons that she learns in discovering their panacea. Her postpartum trauma is a critical example of the fragmentation and deconstruction of bodily integrity, significant not only because of its childbirth context, but also because of its near-death context. Running in parallel to the narrative of psychosomatic injury is thus the narrative of spiritual injury – two traumas in one – both of import for Kempe's evolving identity. The episode further offers explication of her

---

[15] See Kim M. Phillips, 'Margery Kempe and the Ages of Women', in *A Companion to 'The Book of Margery Kempe'*, ed. Arnold and Lewis, pp. 21 and 24. See also Susan Maddock, 'Margery Kempe's Home Town and Worthy Kin', in *Encountering The Book of Margery Kempe*, ed. Kalas and Varnam (forthcoming); and Goodman, pp. 48–55 and pp. 65–6.

[16] On the normalcy of this age of marriage see Goodman, p. 66. On Kempe's downplaying of her social experience, see Janel M. Mueller, 'Autobiography of a New 'Creatur': Female Spirituality, Selfhood, and Authorship in *The Book of Margery Kempe*', in *Women in the Middle Ages and Renaissance*, ed. Rose, pp. 155–71. For the opposing view that Kempe's domesticity is a vital component of her spiritual journey, see Sandra McEntire, 'The Journey into Selfhood: Margery Kempe and Feminine Spirituality', in *Margery Kempe: A Book of Essays*, pp. 54–5.

[17] Richard Lawes, for example, argues that Kempe's symptoms equate with 'a depressive psychosis in the puerperium, the most common of the post-natal psychoses'. See Lawes, 'The Madness of Margery Kempe', in *The Medieval Mystical Tradition, VI*, ed. Glasscoe, pp. 147–68.

frequent, mournful claims throughout the *Book* that she is 'brostyn a–sundyr' (68) and 'brostyn for pite' (185). In reiterating these feelings of *undoing*, she draws upon and relives the trauma of her first childbirth, when Christ's eventual appearance reconfigures her wholeness. That medicinal Christ, therefore, whose presence Kempe experiences 'verily' in mystical contemplation, must be retained in melancholic fixation to heal her 'open wounds'.

Kempe's first experience of motherhood at a little over twenty years of age puts her in mortal danger. We are told that 'sche was labowrd wyth grett accessys tyl þe child was born, & þan, what for labowr sche had in chyldyng & for sekenesse goyng beforn, sche dyspered of hyr lyfe, wenyng sche myght not leuyn' (6). That she fears for her life in the final stages of labour is unsurprising after a problematic pregnancy characterised by great *accessys* and *sekenesse*.[18] The multiplicity of maternal pain is generally situated as inevitable in medieval medical texts. *De secretis mulierum*, for example, claims an instantaneous correlation of human generation and pain: 'If a woman feels cold and has pain in her legs immediately after coitus with a man, this is a sign that she has conceived' (Si enim mulier quando fuerit in coitu cum viro, post coitum sentit frigus, & dolorem in cruribus, signum est quod concepit).[19] The writer of *The Knowing of Woman's Kind in Childing* considers the link so intrinsic that s/he rather unsympathetically advises abstinence if pain is to be avoided altogether: 'But sche þat wol haue no travyll in chyldynge, let kepe here fro þe recevynge of sede of man &, oon my parell, sche schall nevyre drede þe travelynge of chylde.'[20] And *The Cyrurgie of Guy de Chauliac* emphasises the perilous surgical procedures required in cases of difficult childbirths, stillbirths, and maternal death.[21] Pain, and the 'drede', or fear, of pain, are therefore an unavoidable paradigm for the woman of reproductive age.

Margery Kempe's association of reproduction and pain thus begins during the months of gravidity and culminates in a difficult birth. With no prior term of reference or mode of codification for this pain and fear other than the despair that it causes, the only imaginable trajectory at this moment is death; she is left 'wenyng sche myght not leuyn'. She sends 'for hyr gostly fadyr' to be relieved of the 'thyng in conscyens which sche had neuyr schewyd' (6). This specific sin, the 'thing in conscyens', that hastens her call for the confessor, has been suggested by several critics to be of a sexual nature, with which I concur, particularly in the light of her apparent shame in not naming it and the persistent and compulsive sexual thoughts that plague her throughout the *Book*.[22] The sin, however, is never fully confessed: the confessor 'was a lytyl to

---

[18] MED s.v. acces(se): 1(a) An attack of illness characterised by fever; 1(d) Attack or seizure of any disease.

[19] *De secretis mulierum*, trans. Lemay, p. 120. Albertus Magnus, *De secretis mulierum*, p. 100.

[20] *The Knowing of Woman's Kind in Childing*, p. 50.

[21] *The Cyrurgie of Guy de Chauliac*, pp. 530–1.

[22] See McAvoy, *Authority*, p. 34; and Weissman, '*Hysterica Compassio*', in *Acts of Interpretation*, ed. Carruthers and Kirk, pp. 207–8. Conversely, Stephen Medcalf argues that Kempe's sin is not sexual but heretical, as she heeds the words of her parish priest,

hastye & gan scharply to vndernemyn hir er þan sche had fully seyd hir entent' (7). The intolerance of the male cleric, who rebukes her before she has finished instead of administering the remedial rite, initiates a profound fear in Kempe which replays that which she has just experienced in labour. The excruciating physical pain of childbirth is now compounded with an ineffable spiritual pain, as she is prematurely silenced by the priest's intimidations – 'sche wold no mor seyn for nowt he myght do' (7) – leaving her once again trapped in a liminal site of uncertainty and dread, 'for dreed she had of dampnacyon on þe to side & hys scharp repreuyng on þat oþer syde' (7). That Kempe aligns the confessor's reproving comments with an eternity of damnation illustrates the deep fear and 'dreed' which he instils in her, an understandable concern given that in some medieval parishes women who died in childbirth in their postlapsarian state were often refused burial in holy ground.[23] Those who died 'badly', without the correct sequence of rituals and absolution, were thought to be not only sinful, 'pestilent dead', but also a danger to the community, which might be infected by the contagion of the corpse that was 'sin incarnate'.[24] While the physical presence and moral authority of the 'gostly fadyr' reinforce her hidden understanding of the significance of her sin, the threat of his chastisement on the one hand and the threat of hell on the other ensnare her in a damnation that she can escape only by leaving her*self* instead of the birthing room.

Kempe's intense shame about her sin has already caused prior distress. Integrated within the description of the childbirth trauma are recollections of the previous, diabolic persuasions of 'hyr enmy', who convinced her not to confess, so that instead she undertook 'penawns be hir-self a-loone', fasting and performing other 'dedys of almes' (7). Such internal secreting of this shame is antithetic to the *modus operandi* of the confession rite, which exists to external-ise and articulate the Christian's sin for the efficacious purpose of absolution.[25]

William Sawtre, who was burned for heresy in 1401. See *The Later Middle Ages*, ed. Medcalf, pp. 116–17. For examples of Kempe's sexual preoccupation in the *Book* see *BMK*, I, ch. 4, when she is tempted by lechery and agrees to a sexual encounter with a fellow parishioner, only to discover the request was a test. See also Ch. 59 when she temporarily loses God's grace and envisions 'mennys membrys', and also the instances when she fears rape and defilement when travelling on pilgrimage, for example, Book II, Ch. 6.

[23] See Gail McMurray Gibson, 'Blessing from Sun and Moon: Churching as Women's Theatre', in *Bodies and Disciplines: Intersections of Literature and History in Fifteenth-Century England*, ed. Barbara Hanawalt and David Wallace (Minneapolis and London: University of Minnesota Press, 1996), pp. 139–54.

[24] Stephen Gordon, 'Disease, Sin, and the Walking Dead in Medieval England c. 1100–1350: A Note on the Documentary and Archaeological Evidence', in *Medicine, Healing and Performance*, ed. Effie Gemi-Iordanou, Stephen Gordon, Robert Matthew, Ellen McInnes, and Rhiannon Petitt (Oxford: Oxbow Books, 2014), pp. 124–58. See also Katharine Park, 'Birth and Death', in *A Cultural History of the Human Body in the Medieval Age*, ed. Linda Kalof (London: Bloomsbury, 2010), pp. 17–38 (p. 35).

[25] An important decree of the Fourth Lateran Council in 1215 was *Omnis utriusque sexus*, demanding annual confession and communion. See R.N. Swanson, *Religion and Devotion in Europe, c. 1215–1515* (Cambridge: Cambridge University Press, 1995),

Kempe's inner accumulation of guilt provides a striking parallel with a passage from *The Knowing of Woman's Kind in Childing*, which posits that shame is a central cause of difficulty in childbirth: 'Now wol I tell yow what may lette a woman with chylde of ryȝht delyuerance. Sche may be dystrovbelyd yf sche be angury or *prowde* or *shamfull*, or ellysþat hit be here fyrst chylde.'[26] The *Sickness of Women* similarly proposes that the afflictions of the female body are a source of shame: 'ther bien many wymmen that han many diuers maladies and sikenessis nygh to the deth and they also bien shameful to shewen'.[27] These examples throw into sharp perspective the symbiosis of medical and theological ideologies, where the sins of pride and shame engender physical effects on the body and thus adversely affect the physical processes of labour.

Given that Kempe also struggles with pride and materialistic greed after her conversion ('sche wold not leeuyn hir pride ne hir pompows aray' [9]), and that this is indeed her first experience of childbirth, she fits most of the hindrances to labour laid out in the first passage, making her unconfessed sin a plausible cause of the near-annihilation of her body and soul. *De secretis mulierum* warns against 'irregular' sexual intercourse ('inordinatus coitus') because the foetus will not be produced in the proper manner and will therefore be at risk of deformity and monstrosity.[28] That sin is understood in this treatise to relate to the laws of religion and nature reinforces the possibility that Kempe's confessor, perhaps learned of similar texts, was 'to hastye' as a result of his anxiousness to castigate her sinful *irregularity* of nature and to assert his ecclesiastical role as moral warden.[29] Now polarised from the aspirational model of the Virgin Mary, her secret sin, the collective female punishment of Original Sin, and the concomitant medieval distaste for the fleshy, unruly female body render her trapped in abject transgression.

Margery Kempe therefore goes 'owt of hir mende & [is] wondyrlye vexid & labowryd wyth spyrytys half ȝer viij wekys & odde days' (7) in a spiritual trauma that emerges from the mortal danger of childbirth and a crisis of self. The ensuing period of derangement and distraction of 'half ȝer viij wekys & odde days' (7) mirrors the approximate length of a pregnancy, illustrating

---

pp. 25–30. The language of the 21st Constitution of the Fourth Lateran Council takes a noticeably medical flavour: 'The priest shall be discerning and prudent, so that like a skilled doctor he may pour wine and oil over the wounds of the injured one. Let him carefully inquire about the circumstances of both the sinner and the sin, so that he may prudently discern what sort of advice he ought to give and what remedy to apply, using various means to heal the sick person'. From The Fourth General Council of the Lateran, 1215 AD. 21: 'On yearly confessions to one's own priest, yearly communion, the confessional seal', in *Papal Encyclicals Online* <http://www.papalencyclicals.net> [accessed 15 February 2016].

26 *The Knowing of Woman's Kind in Childing*, pp. 60–2.
27 *The Sickness of Women*, p. 485.
28 Albertus Magnus, *De secretis mulierum*, p. 93. *De secretis mulierum*, trans. Lemay, p. 114.
29 Monica Green, 'From "Diseases of Women" to "Secrets of Women": The Transformation of Gynaecological Literature in the Later Middle Ages', *Journal of Medieval and Early Modern Studies*, 30 (2000), 5–39.

what McAvoy sees as 'an apt "punishment" to fit a perceived "sin" of concupiscence', but also mirrors the period of human gestation, gesturing towards this life episode as a crucial process of rebirth.[30] She is thus subject to two labours of physical and spiritual rupture. With the confessional rite aborted, Kempe is *unmade* and subject to diabolical 'steryngys' – visions antithetic to mystical rapture yet redolent of her melancholic propensity to imaginative perception, to 'truer dreams'.[31] She is nearly destroyed by the frenzied illness, imagining violent episodes with diabolic figures who taunt her and torture her, embodying the very punishment that she believes necessary for her damaged soul:

> And in þis tyme sche sey, as hir thowt, deuelys opyn her mowthys al inflaumyd wyth brenny[n]g lowys of fyr as þei schuld a swalwyd hyr in, sum-tyme *rampyng* at hyr, sum-tyme thretyng her, sum-tym *pullyng* hyr & *halyng* hir boþe nygth & day duryng þe forseyd tyme (7).

The devils' threats with their hungry mouths of fire not only signify traditional depictions of the burning mouth of hell and eternal pain and punishment, but also foreshadow the many threats of burning that she will suffer during the course of her holy journey.[32] Furthermore, that she fears that they might have 'swalwyd hyr in' evokes another version of captivity: to be ingested into the devils' bodies as the literal embodiment of evil. In this hallucinatory episode Kempe perceives the *spyrites* 'sum-tyme rampyng at hyr, sum-tyme thretyng her, sum-tyme pullyng hyr & haling hir boþe nygth & day' (7). To be pawed and threatened and pulled and dragged is to be physically mauled and wounded, a phenomenological muddying of body and soul marked by relentless torture. The author of *The Pore Caitif* warns of such darkness, born of sin: when one is tempted by 'dilectacioun' and loses 'vertu of [one's] heeris, aliens shulen take him, þat ben vnclene spiritis, and þey shulen *bynde* him with *boondis* of dyuerse desiris, & þey shulen *blynde* þe iȝen of his *herte, þat he se not liȝt*'.[33] Such is the hold of the 'deuelys' – a bondage that will soon be physically re-enacted – that Kempe denounces her faith, her family and her friends, replaying the diabolic and torturous machinations on her own body in frenzied self-mortification, blind to the light of God and of divine vision:

---

[30] McAvoy, *Authority and the Female Body*, p. 36.

[31] Some medical texts acceded to the possibility of demonic causes for mental disturbance. See Catherine Rider, 'Demons and Mental Disorder in Late Medieval Medicine', in *Mental (Dis)Order in Later Medieval Europe*, ed. Sari Katajala-Peltomaa and Susanna Niiranen (Leiden and Boston: Brill, 2014), pp. 47–69.

[32] In Canterbury, for example, Kempe is accused of Lollardy by the monks at the monastery, who, when she leaves, cry after her, 'Þow xalt be brent, fals lollare. Her is a cartful of thornys redy for þe & a tonne to bren þe wyth' (28).

[33] My emphasis. *The Pore Caitif*, p. 184. MED s.v. herre, pl. herris: 2(a) One of the four cardinal points of the heavens or the earth; (b) one of the celestial poles; (c) a matter of cardinal importance.

Sche wold a fordon hir-self many a tym at her steryngys & ben damnyd wyth hem in Helle, & in-to wytnesse þerof sche bot hir owen hand so violently þat it was seen al hir lyfe aftyr. And also sche roof hir skyn on hir body a-ȝen hir hert wyth hir nayles spetowsly, for sche had noon oþer instrumentys, & wers sche wold a don saf sche was bowndyn & kept wyth strength boþe day & nyȝth þat sche myȝth not haue hir wylle (8).

Kempe craves self-destruction – to 'fordon' herself – a suicidal wish to annihilate the body that harbours her sin and the pain of torture by the 'spy-rites'.[34] Unable to verbally articulate her suffering she self-mutilates, wounding her guilty body and tearing open fissures and wounds in a non-verbal articulation of undoing: an attempt to literally *carve out* an escape from the torturous locus of the self. In pseudo-stigmatic *imitatio* she bites her hand with such violence that she is permanently scarred 'al hir lyfe aftyr'. This stigmata, however, is not born from the desire to experience Christ's pain on the cross, but rather to wound the body that is *separated* from him and bound instead to her diabolical imprisoners.[35] Like Scarry's notion of pain-utterances as a form of proto-language, because pain 'actively destroys' language, Margery Kempe's articulation is also destroyed. Attempts to voice her confession have gone unheard, replaced instead by submersion in a postpartum trauma of non-verbal frenzy.[36]

The 'spetows' *roofing*, or riving (tearing apart), of her skin with her own fingernails, notably around her heart – the violent act of scarification – is not only the non-verbal crescendo of the event, however, but also a way of regaining self-possession. In this way Kempe scripts her rebirth in torturous reply, rewriting it onto her body and regaining agency in an embodiment of the birth-moment of language to which Scarry points. The carving of marks into her flesh, the *making* of open wounds, signals her returning voice as she transforms, once more, into the editor of her text, the warden of her own enclosure. Kempe's riving around her heart is, though, an inversion of the medieval devotion to the Sacred Heart made popular by twelfth-century Cistercians, especially Bernard of Clairvaux (1090–1153) and later writers such as Gertrude of Helfta (1256–c. 1302), who employ imagery of feeding and refuge and situate the heart as connected to Christ's wounds as a primary symbol of God's love.[37] The heart is also likened to the uterus in medieval culture since conversion to Christianity is assimilated with the conception and birth of Christ in one's heart. Some holy women, such as Clare of Montefalco, were documented as literally harbouring

---

[34] MED s.v. fordon.

[35] On stigmata in the Middle Ages see Giles Constable, *Three Studies in Medieval Religious and Social Thought: The Interpretation of Mary and Martha, The Ideal of the Imitation of Christ, The Orders of Society* (Cambridge: Cambridge University Press, 1995).

[36] Scarry, *The Body in Pain*, pp. 4–6.

[37] On the Sacred Heart see Caroline Bynum Walker, *Jesus as Mother: Studies in the Spirituality of the High Middle Ages* (Berkley, Los Angeles and London: University of California Press, 1982), pp. 192–3. The German Dominican priest Henry Suso (1295–1363) is depicted in iconography inscribing the IHS Christogram onto his chest.

relics within their hearts, a discovery made during the post-mortems conducted for the purposes of canonisation.[38] This was a metaphor that was developed by thirteenth- and fourteenth-century writers who saw Mary's pain at the foot of the cross as like a second childbirth, and her swooning and need of support as identifiable with a labouring woman's need of a midwife.[39] Certainly, Simeon's prophecy to Mary at the Temple of Jerusalem that 'a sword will pierce your heart', only days after her purification, heightens the association of Christ's birth with his loss, located in the heart-womb.[40] While Kempe's stigmatic tearing at the flesh around her heart so soon after childbirth creates open wounds that connect with Christ's, its destructive despair reveals how she has not yet been purged of the sin that remains, instead of Christ, inside her soul.

Accordingly, she continues to flail and rive and *labowr* (a Middle English term with connotations of hard, painful work as well as birthing), observed by a silent body of 'kepars' who restrain and bind her to prevent further injury: '& wers sche wold a don saf sche was bowndyn & kept wyth strength boþe day & nygth þat sche mygth not haue hir wylle' (8).[41] The injuries that she inflicts on her anguished postpartum body are, then, limited by the physical force of her 'kepars' and the cords and ties that bind her, preventing the actualisation of her suicide threat. Such binding was advised by medical writers such as Bartholomaeus Anglicus, who suggests that signs of 'frensey' include 'raginge', 'castinge of hondes', and a patient who 'bitiþ gladliche and rendiþ [tears at] his wardeyne and his leche'. The text advises that such patients should 'be wel iholde oþir ibounde in a derk place'. A 'parafrenesis' can also, pertinently, be caused by 'a posteme of þe stomake oþir þe modir [uterus]'.[42] Binding is also recommended for postpartum bleeding in *The Knowing of Woman's Kind in Childing*, which advises practitioners to 'let here be bovnde with wympyls or with othyre softe thyngis'.[43] But while soft and soothing treatments are suggested for physical postpartum injuries, stiff bonds are employed by Kempe's custodians: she is 'kept wyth *strength*' in order to restrict and enclose her flailing body-in-pain. The male attendants, who are also assumedly her binders, survey her agonised performance as terminal; her actions are such 'þat *men* wend sche schuld neuyr *a skapyd ne levyd*' (8).[44] Like

[38] See Katherine Park, 'Relics of a Fertile Heart: The Autopsy of Clare of Montefalco', in *The Material Culture of Sex, Procreation, and Marriage in Premodern Europe*, ed. Anne L. McClanan and Karen Rosoff Encarnación (New York: Palgrave, 2002), pp. 115–33.
[39] On the medieval connection of the heart and uterus see Katherine Park, *Secrets of Women: Gender, Generation, and the Origins of Human Dissection* (Brooklyn: Zone Books, 2006), pp. 60–7.
[40] Luke 2:35.
[41] MED s.v. labour: 1. Work, esp. hard work. 2. Pains taken. 4. Pain, sickness and disease; *laboure of birthe*.
[42] *On the Properties of Thinigs*, pp. 348–9.
[43] *The Knowing of Woman's Kind in Childing*, p. 104.
[44] Although the usage of the noun 'men' here might signify 'men' in the sense of mankind, the later distinction between 'hyr maydens & hir kepars' (8) during the episode implies the denotation of 'men' and 'kepars' as male.

her earlier self-diagnosis that such pain must signal impending death, these anonymous men regard her condition as a captivity from which she will be unable to escape or even continue to live. The men's presence also signifies a violation of the highly gendered childbirth room in contravention of the strict codes of lying-in practices which meant that women were confined for the forty days prior to their purification in the Churching ceremony.[45]

Just as Kempe's previous entrapment between the threat of hell 'on þe to side' and her confessor's chastisement on 'þat oþer syde' represents a punitive ensnarement, so the ensuing *labowr* of diabolic vision is one from which, her onlookers perceive, she will not be freed. Along with Kempe's enclosure in the birthing room and the bindings which now contain and constrict her desperate body from effecting its own annihilation, these multivalent forms of bondage intensify the trauma to the point that Kempe must evacuate her*self* – go 'owt of hir mende' – in order to escape the incarceration of unconfessed sin and pain. The trauma of this episode is thus the antithesis of the private birthing experience and traditional lying-in period, when mothers were attended extensively by midwives and other women.[46] Women of reasonable status were often bestowed with brooches, pendants, and books depicting icons of healing saints, as well as jewelled girdles from statues of female saints, in order to ease their confinement.[47] Some birthing rooms contained prayer rolls and amulets which utilised the healing power of the written word.[48] In addition to her abjection in childbirth, Kempe is therefore excluded from many of the religious and comforting tokens of a 'good birth', instead manacled and quashed by her keepers and treated as a threatening locus

---

[45] See Gail McMurray Gibson, 'Scene and Obscene: Seeing and Performing Late Medieval Childbirth', *The Journal of Medieval and Early Modern Studies*, 29 (1999), 7–24; and Joanne M. Pierce, '"Green Women" and Blood Pollution: Some Medieval Rituals for the Churching of Women after Childbirth', *Studia Liturgica*, 29:2 (1999), 191–215. On Kempe's childbirth see Jennifer Wynne Hellwarth, *The Reproductive Unconscious in Medieval and Early Modern England* (New York and London: Routledge, 2002), pp. 43–60.

[46] On male and female roles in birthing practices see Monica Green, 'Women's Medical Practice and Health Care in Medieval Europe', in *Women's Healthcare in the Medieval West* (Aldershot: Ashgate, 2000), I, pp. 39–78. See also Angela Florschuetz, 'Women's Secrets: Childbirth, Pollution, and Purification in Northern Octavian', *Studies in the Age of Chaucer*, 30 (2008), 235–68. Florschuetz argues that the intrusion of male presence in the lying-in room was a defilement of female secrets and boundaries.

[47] Archaeological excavations in King's Lynn have unearthed pilgrim badges depicting the Virgin's girdle. Kempe was likely familiar with birth girdles and their apotropaic power. See Mary Morse, '"This moche more ys oure lady mary longe": Takamiya 56 and the English Birth Girdle Tradition', in *Middle English Texts in Transition: A Festschrift Dedicated to Toshiyuki Takamiya on His 70th birthday*, ed. Simon Horobin and Linne R. Mooney (York: York Medieval Press, 2014), pp. 199–219.

[48] See Carole Rawcliffe, 'Women, Childbirth, and Religion in Later Medieval England', in *Women and Religion in Medieval England*, ed. Diana Wood (Oxford: Oxbow Books, 2003), pp. 91–117.

of disorder.[49] Her treatment literalises the medico–philosophical notion of the post-labour woman as an extension of her unruly and wandering womb, as 'On Treatments for Women' exemplifies: 'The womb, as though it were a wild beast of the forest, because of the sudden evacuation falls this way and that, as if it were wandering. Whence vehement pain is caused' ('Matrix namque tamquam fera siluestris propter subitam euacuationem huc et illic quasi uagando declinat. Vnde uehemens dolor efficitur').[50] That her namesake is Saint Margaret, the patron saint of childbirth, renders this early–adult experience, then, as multivalently aberrant.

Cure is eventually delivered when Kempe envisions Christ in the likeness of a man 'wyth so blyssyd a chere þat sche was strengthyd in alle hir spyritys'; now she is 'stabelyd in hir wyttys & in hir reson as wel as euyr sche was beforn' (8). The beauty of Christ's visage instantly transmogrifies her to a state of stability and wholeness, while the verisimilitude of the vision bears witness to her melancholic receptivity, as she perceives the very air through which Christ is revealed and then concealed: 'sche saw *veryly* how þe eyr openyd as brygth as ony levyn [lightning], & he stey up in-to þe eyr, not rygth hastyli & qwykly, but fayr & esly þat sche mygth wel be-holdyn hym in þe eyr tyl it was closyd a–geyn' (8).[51] This is a spiritual medicine in perpetuity. The torn and ruptured skin across her heart is replaced by a hair-shirt which Christ ordains inside it: 'I schal ȝiue þe an hayr in þin hert' (17). The eating of meat is replaced with Christ's flesh and blood in the Eucharist, prescribed 'euery Sonday' as salvific blood to transform the sullied blood of her wounds (17). And the dismissive confessor is replaced by Christ himself, to whom she is told she will have the freedom to 'sey what [she] wyld' at six o'clock each day (17). This is a divine medicine through which she is reintegrated to the Christian liturgy and rites from which she was previously excluded. Through the invasion of the private birthing space Kempe's womanly *secretys* were exposed and she humiliated, shackled, reduced to animal, and then remade. Only when 'sche lay a-loone and hir kepars wer fro hir' (8) does that same space become receptive to Christ's presence in a privileged vision which purifies her lost childbearing sanctuary and gives Kempe a new 'secret'. Now, since Christ signifies the cure for her ruptured and wounded body – for her very identification – the loss of that divine-object will equate to Kempe's own loss of existence, reopening the bleeding wounds of trauma.

By the end of her reproductive life, Kempe has given birth to 'xiiij childeryn' (115), spending the greater part of twenty years in pregnancy.[52] The visuality

---

[49] On the 'good birth' see Park, 'Birth and Death', *A Cultural History of the Human Body in the Medieval Age*, ed. Kalof, pp. 22–7.

[50] 'On Treatments for Women', *The Trotula*, pp. 118–21.

[51] MED s.v. leven.

[52] Laura L. Howes calculates that Kempe would have been pregnant for a total of 126 months out of 240 months, 'or just over half of the time between her twentieth and fortieth birthdays'. See 'On the Birth of Margery Kempe's Last Child', *Modern Philology*, 90 (1992), 220 – 225 (p. 224).

of this pregnant body publicly identifies her as a mother, associated with earthly domesticity and generation. Moreover, 'þe drawt of owyr Lord' has become symbiotic with postpartum illness and pain, explaining perhaps her special place of devotion at the Gesine (childbed) Chapel in her parish church at Lynn.[53] The memory of this first childbirth thus impresses an indelible mark upon her soul, but it is a mark that is possible to edit out through the almost-complete redaction of child-narratives in the *Book*. The trauma thus symbolises a transition not only into adulthood – from young wife to mother – but into mystical experience, too. Unmade by clerical exclusion and injured by sin and bodily abjection, she is remade as Christ's privileged disciple. It is also an event that functions as the centre from which her future spiritual development will emanate, as a perpetual reminder of the threat of annihilation when her physician, Christ, is lost. The stigmatic wounding of her hand and heart as externalisations of her legitimacy as an apprentice holy woman are imprints of the sins for which she weeps. And those sins, particularly of her past concupiscence, will besiege her beyond the door of the childbirth room and serve as a powerful motivation for her quest for a chaste marriage. But in beholding and receiving Christ in all his 'blyssyd … chere', Margery Kempe receives a salve for her melancholic woundedness, paving the way for the rest of her spiritual passage.

The Pain Paradox of Celibacy

In þe tyme þat þis creatur had reuelacyons, owyr Lord seyd to hir, 'Dowtyr, þow art wyth childe.' Sche seyd a-ȝen, 'A, Lord, how xal I þan do for kepyng of my chylde?' Owir Lord seyd, 'Dowtyr, drede þe not, I xal ordeyn for an kepar'. 'Lord, I am not worthy to heryn þe spekyn & þus to comown wyth myn husbond. Ner-þe-lesse *it is to me gret peyn & gret dysese*' (48).

It is little wonder that when God discloses to Kempe that she is again pregnant, she describes it as a 'gret peyn & gret dysese'. Her suffering in marriage, the pain of the conjugal debt, which grieves her, and the physical pains of childbirth which will continually resound as a piercing subtext signify an aberrant mothering hermeneutic that impedes her devotional advancement. That we are told that this pregnancy occurs during 'þe tyme þat þis creatur had reuelacyons' and thus in the throes of her spiritual flourishing explains her rumination on the inconvenience of caring for, or 'kepyng', the child. It is, in short, a 'gret dysese' – a diathesis of motherhood as sickness, scripturally inscribed as a collective womanly cross to bear.[54]

---

[53] See Gail McMurray Gibson, *The Theatre of Devotion*, p. 64.
[54] Genesis 3:16: 'To the woman also he said: I will multiply thy sorrows, and thy conceptions: in sorrow shalt thou bring forth children, and thou shalt be under thy husband's power, and he shall have dominion over thee'.

Indeed, St Paul's sanction, quoted at the beginning of this chapter, dictates the loss of corporeal autonomy in marriage through the Christian tradition of conjugal debt, which posed a strategic problem for holy married women who sought a spiritual life. This echo of Genesis, when 'a man shall leave father and mother, and shall cleave to his wife: and they shall be two in one flesh' (2:24), served to emphasise the clear somatic role of the marriage institution as a site of concession where sexual activity could take place (albeit preferably for the purpose of reproduction) in a less sinful context.[55] However, where the marriage institution liberated spouses in this respect, it simultaneously constrained them, as payment for sexual license required the relinquishing of one's own corporeal agency. A similar dichotomy of spirit and flesh, and the internal battle which is thus generated, was also acknowledged by St Paul: 'the flesh lusteth against the spirit; and the spirit against the flesh. For these are contrary one to another; so that you do not the things that you would' (Galatians 5:17). Furthermore, that the Church Fathers identified Original Sin as the first sexually transmitted disease illustrates an early association with female transgression and somatic malady and establishes an inescapable synthesis of spirit and body that renders female spiritual progression as inherently problematic.[56]

The possibility that chaste marriage, which became popular from the time of the early Church, might provide a remedy, however, was similarly fraught; Dyan Elliott regards it as 'somewhat of an anomaly because it occasions a blurring of what were widely perceived as two discrete groups: the continent and the married'.[57] But the retrieval of bodily autonomy via chaste marriage could be justified through a claim to a higher spiritual force than biblical doctrine alone – the claim to a superior piety – something that is, I suggest, most easily accessed through mystical privilege. Female mystics' esoteric spirituality and direct communion with Christ constitutes such 'superior piety'. Furthermore, the manner in which chastity in marriage could transcend gender distinctions had the effect of female empowerment with the distinct possibility of disrupting the hegemonic equilibrium.[58] Indeed, what Elliott terms as the 'reproductive imperative' of marriage is necessarily immobilised after a vow of

---

[55] On the varying levels of the sinfulness of sex in different contexts, set out by medieval canon lawyers such as Peter Lombard, see Pierre J. Payer, *The Bridling of Desire: Views of Sex in the Later Middle Ages* (Toronto: University of Toronto Press, 1993).

[56] This was discussed by Norman Powell Williams in the 1920s; work which was to be followed by the emergence of feminist scholarship that sought to challenge the 'inevitability' of such social constructions for medieval religious women. See Norman Powell Williams, *The Ideas of the Fall and of Original Sin: A Historical and Critical Study* (London: Longmans, 1927), pp. 226–31.

[57] Elliott, *Spiritual Marriage*, p. 17. After the imposition of celibacy upon the clergy in the late eleventh and early twelfth centuries the support for chaste marriage dwindled and it was thereafter discouraged among the laity. See Jo Ann McNamara, 'Chaste Marriage and Clerical Celibacy', in *Sexual Practices*, ed. Bullough and Brundage, pp. 22–33.

[58] See Rosemary Radford Ruether, 'Misogyny and Virginal Feminism in the Fathers of the Church' in *Religion and Sexism: Images of Women in the Jewish and Christian Traditions*, ed. Rosemary Radford Ruether (New York: Wipf and Stock, 1974), pp. 150–83.

chastity has taken place, and such a quasi-menopause, as I see it, is an important socio-somatic juncture in Kempe's life-course. The linguistic flexibility within the medieval terminologies of chastity and virginity, which could be interchangeable, opened up new interpretative possibilities for the religious women who sought out their own version of the inimitable Virgin Mary. The terms *castitas* and *virginitas* might refer to physical intactness, to a commitment to a celibate life, or even to sexual faithfulness in a monogamous marriage.[59] Aquinas had described Christ's relationship to humanity as 'a kind of spiritual marriage' ('matrimonium quoddam spirituale'), further evidencing spiritual marriage's fluid, and achievable, potential.[60] The attainment of Kempe's chaste marriage will therefore mark a critical turning point for her movement towards a spiritual life in enabling a version of virginity, a concomitant closeness to Mary and to Christ, and a symbolic relinquishment of childbearing.

In the theological and medical texts of the Middle Ages, celibacy is constructed as inescapably painful, through the 'pain paradox' that I here explicate. To procreate in marriage, for example, elevates marriage and motherhood in St Paul's doctrine: 'Yet she shall be saved through childbearing; if she continue in faith and love and sanctification with sobriety' (1 Timothy 2:15). Yet this tenet marks a curious re-evaluation of Eve's curse and its universal application to women who are told that 'in *sorrow* shalt thou bring forth children' (Genesis 3:16; my emphasis). Despite the undeniably gendered nature of the transgression,[61] this same 'sorrowful' childbearing facilitates salvation, albeit with the conditional obedience and sober modification required by Christian motherhood.[62] If, in the biblical tradition, motherhood is construed as an edifying route for female salvation, then the notion of chaste marriage and its inherent denial of procreative functionality is inherently problematic. In response, the impossible model of the spiritual marriage of Mary and Joseph became a vehicle through which canonists could separate lay and theological ideals of marriage, and the emergence of pastoral manuals and canonistic sources thus sought to emphasise what Elliott posits as 'the dramatic reassertion of the centrality of sexual intercourse in marriage'.[63] But as the writer of *The Pore Caitif* advised,

[59] See *Menacing Virgins: Representing Virginity in the Middle Ages and Renaissance*, ed. Kathleen Coyne Kelly and Marina Leslie (London: Associated University Presses, 1999), pp. 15–25. On the different interpretations of medieval virginity see Sarah Salih, *Versions of Virginity in Late Medieval Europe* (Cambridge: D.S. Brewer, 2001).

[60] Thomas Aquinas, *Summa Theologiae*, I[a] q. 95 a. 1 arg. 5. Translation from Thomas Aquinas, *Summa Theologiae: A Concise Translation*, ed. Timothy McDermott (Allen, Texas: Christian Classics, 1989), vol. 51:30.1, p. 516.

[61] 'And Adam was not seduced; but the woman being seduced, was in the transgression' (1 Timothy 2:14).

[62] On Holy Kinship and the salvific possibilities for married women and mothers, see Pamela Sheingorn, 'Appropriating the Holy Kinship: Gender and Family History', in *Medieval Families*, ed. Neel, pp. 273–301.

[63] See Elliott, *Spiritual Marriage*, pp. 25–6 and pp. 140–2; and Penny S. Gold, 'The Marriage of Mary and Joseph in the Twelfth-Century Ideology of Marriage', in *Sexual Practices*, ed. Bullough and Brundage, pp. 102–17.

although in marrying 'þou hast not synned', to remain 'vnweddid & maiden' is a superior state since it causes a woman to 'þenthiþ þilke þingis þat ben of þe lord', rather than busy herself with the worldly concerns of pleasing her husband.[64]

However, in the central paradox of this chapter, the contemporary explosion of medical and scientific texts which underscored women's pronounced sexual appetite and established sexual abstinence as physically damaging and painful constructed an all-encompassing hermeneutic that maintained chastity in marriage as inadvisable. Even the linguistic term for the womb, 'moder', in some Middle English treatises, illustrates the utter collapsing into one of women's biological and social functions in the medieval imaginary.[65] Kempe's growing fervour for a vow of chastity is therefore deeply entangled in dichotomies of pollution and pain, scripture and science, domesticity and biology, and serves to complicate her trajectory towards a religious life. The *Trotula* text 'On Treatments for Women' establishes the notion of celibacy as a physical problem causing pain:

> There are some women to whom carnal intercourse is not permitted, sometimes because they are bound by a vow, sometimes because they are bound by religion, sometimes because they are widows, because to some women it is not permitted to take fruitful vows. These women, when they have desire to copulate and do not do so, incur grave illness.

> [Sunt autem quedam mulieres quibus non committitur carnale commercium, tum quia uoto, tum quia religione tenentur, tum quia uidue sunt, quia quibusdam mulieribus non licet ad fecunda uota transire, que cum uoluntatem habeant coeundi et non coeunt, grauem incurrunt egritudinem.][66]

The author of this passage accepts unquestioningly the necessity of celibacy for some women. It also accepts the accompanying pain as a given, homologising theological and physiological 'truths' and reinforcing the pain imperative of chastity. An indomitable female sexual appetite is assumed ('que cum uoluntatem habeant coeundi' – *when* they have desire to copulate), despite the obvious fact that such women have clearly chosen – with the exception of the widow – to live celibate. The suggested remedy is a cotton plug, soaked in oil and placed into the vagina, underlining a tension between physical and spiritual health where the female body, imprisoned by its scriptural and reproductive functions, should simply be soothed and controlled: '[it] dissipates the desire and dulls the pain' ('castigat luxuriam et dolorem sedat').[67] The inevitability of female suffering is inherent in the author's suggestion of the symbolic 'packing' and pacifying of the woman with the plug, rendering the treatment of symptoms subordinate to the immutable reality of the pain.

---

[64] *The Pore Caitif*, p. 187.
[65] The term 'moder' is employed, for example, in the Middle English Gilbertus Anglicus' *Compendium medicinae*. See *System of Physic*, p. 260.
[66] 'On Treatments for Women', in *The Trotula*, pp. 120–1.
[67] Ibid.

The phenomenology of pain as gendered is evident through its rootedness in sexual activity and, by extension, potential reproductive capacity. The 'Book on the Conditions of Women' states that:

> Galen says that women who have narrow vaginas and constricted wombs ought not to have sexual relations with men lest they conceive and die. But all such women are not able to abstain, and so they need our assistance.

> [Galyenus dicit mulieres que habent uuluas angustas et matrices strictas non debent uiris uti, ne concipiant et moriantur. Sed omnes tales non possunt abstinere, et ideo nostro indigent auxilio].[68]

Despite the marriage debt being imbued with potential mortal danger, the pain imperative remains unquestioned in this example. The writer not only acknowledges that one should *expect* to become pregnant if engaging in sexual activity, and that abstinence prevents the pains of childbirth, s/he concedes the apparently obvious fact that not all women are 'able' to abstain; those who do will suffer the 'grave illness' associated with celibate living. Similarly, *The Knowing of Woman's Kind in Childing* asserts that if a woman conceives 'so muste sche nedys have travill in delyuerance, for þe wyche I can no medycyne writ'.[69]

According to the French doctor and medical professor Bernard of Gordon (fl. 1283–1309), women are more damaged by sexual abstinence than men because they take less exercise.[70] The reason for their more sedentary lives is, according to Bernard, connected to a multifarious framework of inadequacy: a lack of heat to produce semen leads to a lack of energy, which in turn leads to a lack of physical activity. Joan Cadden has suggested that the failure of medieval authors to distinguish between behavioural habits as being the source of the medical condition, and the medical condition as the source of the behaviour, 'is an indication of the extent to which medical and scientific ideas about sex were integrated with gender constructs and also of the cultural assumption that the integration was appropriate, requiring no explanation or justification'.[71] This concomitance of medico-cultural phenomena is also applicable to medical writers' benign acceptance of the unfortunate 'fact' of pain in both celibate *and* sexual female lifestyles, a notion that is reinforced by the medieval understanding of the conflation of character and constitution. Since women are cold and moist by constitution, and thus mostly of phlegmatic or melancholic temperaments, inactive and sedentary behavioural characteristics are denoted.[72] Within this paradigm, Margery Kempe's melancholic diathesis locates her at increased physical risk of pain in a celibate life.

[68] 'The Book on the Conditions of Women', in *The Trotula*, pp. 96–7.
[69] *The Knowing of Woman's Kind in Childing*, pp. 49–50.
[70] Cadden, *Meanings of Sex Difference*, p. 172.
[71] Ibid., p. 173.
[72] Cadden, *Meanings of Sex Difference*, p. 184. See also *Galen on the Usefulness of the Parts of the Body*, ed. M.T. May, 2 vols, vol. 2 (Ithaca: Cornell University Press, 1968), p. 630; and Klibansky et al., *Saturn and Melancholy*, p. 379.

This risk of pain is similarly heightened by the tendency for celibate women who were once sexually active to experience a suffocation of the womb.[73] The 'Book on the Conditions of Women' makes clear that this is a disease of the celibate: 'This happens to those women who do not use men, especially to widows who were accustomed to carnal commerce' ('Contingit autem hoc eis que uiris non utuntur, maxime uiduis que consueuerunt uti carnali commercio').[74] The writer's synthesis of medical disorder and the 'carnal commerce' of the marriage debt replays the amalgamation of social and medical ideology, a motif that reoccurs in *De secretis mulierum*, which states that 'This sickness [suffocation] happens in women because they are full of corrupt and poisonous menses' ('Hæc enim ægritudo contingit in mulieribus ex eo quod abundat in eis menstruum corruptum & venenosum'). The first commentator then focuses on the susceptibility of newly chaste women:

This affliction happens most often to widows, women whose husbands are no longer with them, and so their menses become corrupted in the womb and thick humours are generated, which in turn produce weakness in the heart. Coitus is exceedingly beneficial to these women.

[Illa passio maxime accidit viduis quæ prius habuerunt viros, & jam non habent, unde menstruaearum corrumpunter in matrice, & generantur grossi humores, qui in corde debilitates generant, & ideo ipsis multum valet coitus.][75]

Retained menses, where 'corrupt' menstrual matter is left to fester in the womb when the heat of the male is not used to draw it out, is often connected to uterine suffocation in medieval medical texts. Moreover, *The Knowing of Woman's Kind in Childing* notes how religious women especially might experience amenorrhoea (absent menses): 'tho þat syngvn & wake mekyll, as do þes religios, for of her wakynge & travelynge in syngynge here blode wastyth & defyet well here repast'.[76] The increased expenditure of energy required for the religious activities of waking early and labouring in singing is here responsible for menstrual retention that, in turn, causes uterine suffocation. This is amplified by the linguistic fecundity of the term *travelynge*, which, in Middle English, also denotes the labour of childbirth and thus interweaves the notions of religious practice, sexuality, reproduction, and pain with which this chapter is concerned.[77] Indeed, the interrelation of Kempe's melancholia and risk of uterine suffocation due to menstrual retention and religious praxes

---

[73] The symptoms of uterine suffocation are described in Chapter 1, pp. 43–6.
[74] 'The Book on the Conditions of Women', in *The Trotula*, pp. 84–5.
[75] *De secretis mulierum*, trans. Lemay, p. 132. Albertus Magnus, *De secretis mulierum*, pp. 111–12 and p. 113.
[76] *The Knowing of Woman's Kind in Childing*, p. 48.
[77] MED s.v. travailen, *ppl.* travailinge: 1(b) to perform hard physical labour, toil; 1(c) to labour in the service of God; work for divine approval; 4(a) To suffer pain or physical torments; undergo maltreatment or punishment; (b) to suffer from disease or injury, be afflicted with an illness or debilitating condition, be or become unwell; (e) to suffer the pain of childbearing, be in labour, give birth.

creates a concoction of physical (or *bodyly*) pain to equal the spiritual (or *gostly*) pain experienced in rendering the marriage debt. But just as the medical texts evidenced here intrinsically synthesise female physiology and behaviour, so the moist and 'liquid' medieval female body may be alternatively regarded as porous and 'naturally' adaptive, capable of modification, development, and transformation. Indeed, Karmen MacKendrick has argued for medieval bodies as being inherently multiple: 'the premodern sense of the spirited body is … far less unified, orderly, singular or stable [than the modern]'.[78] Given the dramatic shift in the social structure of Margery Kempe's life after her negotiated vow of chastity, new corporealities are made possible. As will emerge, the discourses of medicine and theology facilitate a female body which continues to exist within a pain imperative, but which opens up a new *modus operandi* where Kempe can engender a transformed mode of embodied existence.

Ascetic Pain Substitution

In her quest for a vow of chastity, Margery Kempe adopts a transformational strategy of pain substitution that transposes, or even replaces, the sin (and therefore the pain) of marital sex onto individual acts of bodily penance. As she is hasty to inform her readers early in the *Book*: 'sche dred no devylle in Helle, for sche dede so gret bodyly penawnce' (13). Such a strategy – a form of self-medication – where pain is relieved through its production, is another variation of the pain paradox that I argue to be a central concern, and a means of negating the Church Fathers' view that Original Sin was a sexually transmitted disease. Indeed, her attempts to persuade John centre around the notion of abstinence as a form of punishment in itself: that in resisting bodily lust they will in effect be chastised, offering reparations to God whom they had 'dysplesyd'. Kempe decides that 'now it wer good þat þei schuld be her boþins wylle & consentyng of hem bothyn punschyn & chastysyn hem-self wilfully be absteynyng fro her lust of her bodys' (12), thus establishing her willingness to substitute one form of pain for another. As her husband is unprepared as yet to forgo the conjugal debt, Kempe 'dede gret bodyly penawnce' in a manner strikingly similar to the religious activities described in *The Knowing of Woman's Kind in Childing* above: 'Sche was schreuyn sum-tyme twyes or thryes on þe day … Sche ʒaf hir to gret fastyng & to gret wakyng; sche roos at ij or iij of þe clok & went to cherch & was þer in hir prayers on-to tyme of noon and also al þe aftyrnoon' (12). The self-imposed discomfort of sleep deprivation and fasting illustrates Kempe's determination to be punished corporeally for the similarly physical defilement that she perceives in sexual activity. Like her preparedness to ingest 'mukke', the opposite penance of

---

[78] Karmen MacKendrick, 'The Multipliable Body', *Postmedieval: A Journal of Medieval Cultural Studies*, 1 (2010), 108–14 (p. 109).

fasting not only denotes the use of food, or the absence of food, to control the self, but also represents a method of gaining power through an asceticism that harnesses particular religious and cultural meanings; as Bynum puts it, 'The point was pain because the pain was Christ's'. Fasting holy women were admired by their medieval hagiographers because their bodies ceased to excrete, thus avoiding the messy subtext of human embodiment.[79]

Such acts of fasting are intensified through Kempe's wearing of a hair-shirt, which she thereafter wears daily as a continual reminder of sin, and as a symbol of marital division and pain substitution. For while John remains unaware of his wife's uncomfortable attire, and Kempe even bears children in that time, the hair-shirt symbolises a remove between them (and that 'chylderyn' is pluralised denotes the length of time that this particular act of penance lasted). Though their sexual marriage continues, Kempe's hidden hair cloth is a confidential pact, like her private discernment of God's words, which punishes the body that continues, against her will, in its biologically reproductive function:

> Þan sche gat hir an hayr of a kylne swech as men dryen on malt & leyd it in hir kyrtylle as sotyllych & preuylich as sche mygth þat hir husbond xuld not aspye it, ne no mor he dede, & ȝet sche lay be hym euery nygth in his bedde, & weryd þe hayr euery day, & bar chylderyn in þe tyme (12).

In distancing her body from her husband, symbolically at least, Kempe becomes closer to God. Through the private and intimate pain caused by the constant discomfort of wearing coarse fibres against her skin, in sharp opposition to the enforced intimacy of her marital encounters, her intimacy with Christ supersedes that with John.[80] That this form of penance is a hidden one also gives Kempe privileged access to God through a private pain substitution that only she can decipher. Imprisoned within the 'carnal commerce' of the marriage union, Kempe therefore engineers a self-imposed enclosure, the haircloth an anchoritic interpretation signifying isolation from the world on her route towards God. Unable yet to live chastely, she instead punishes the body that continues in its reproductive efficacy. The wearing of a hair-shirt was, in fact, a common practice amongst holy ascetics. After the death of her husband, for example, Bridget of Sweden 'weer nere next hir bare skyn a corde of hempe with many knottes harde bounden to hir & in lyke wyse about euery of hir legges vnder hir knees'.[81] Certainly, that Kempe does not wait until she is a widow to don such a shirt evidences the urgency of her wish to hasten towards her hagiographical role models and to accelerate beyond wifely repro-normativity. The strategies of enclosure of Gertrude

---

[79] Caroline Walker Bynum has identified how food formed the social context of women's world and was thus an apt ascetic tool for women who used fasting to control bodily functions. See Bynum, *Holy Feast and Holy Fast*, pp. 211–14.

[80] MED s.v. privelie; also privileche: 2(a) intimately.

[81] Thomas Gascoigne, 'Lyfe of seynt Birgette', in *The Myroure of oure Ladye*, p. lii.

of Helfta, who utilised her sickness to achieve isolation, leads Alexandra Barratt to conclude that true enclosure was 'a state of mind'.[82] Conversely, Liz Herbert McAvoy has argued for Kempe's more literal undertaking of anchoritic performances – the *Book*'s 'insistent discourses of enclosure' – and the way in which she moves innovatively towards Pepwell's description of her as a 'deuote ancres of Lynne'.[83] But I want to suggest, beyond this, that the societal and domestic restrictions placed upon Margery Kempe – not least her role as a wife and mother – significantly *limit* her ability to commit entirely to a life of asceticism. By wearing the haircloth secretly, she erects a shielding barrier which encloses her in a private pact with God, but which simultaneously acknowledges her inability to declare such a re-identification publicly. Nonetheless, in both punishing and protecting the generative potentiality of the hidden womb, she reclaims the 'secrets' of the birthing room of her first traumatic childbirth – violated and intruded upon by her 'kepars', as we have seen – and transforms that same oppressive maternity into spiritual fruit.

The efficacy of this interiorised penance is divinely acknowledged by Christ, who endows Kempe with a metaphorical haircloth in her heart: 'And, dowtyr, þu hast an hayr vp-on þi bakke. I wyl þu do it a-way, & I schal ȝiue þe an hayr in þin hert þat schal lyke me mych bettyr þan alle þe hayres in þe world' (17). This mystical transplantation is resonant with the equivalence of the heart and womb, a 'replacement maternity' where Jesus can gestate in Kempe's uterus-heart in perpetuity, like the mystical implantation of Christ's heart experienced by Catherine of Siena.[84] But while Christ's gift frees Kempe from the physical binds of the haircloth, she is simultaneously reincarcerated. Implicit in the heart's haircloth is Christ's validation of Kempe's need for a punishment that is permanent and internalised forever. Though she is appropriated with heavenly perspicacity, therefore, the legacy of Eve's transgression and subsequent stain on the female soul is another internal scar that she must still, apparently, suffer. Liz Herbert McAvoy regards this episode as entirely liberating for Kempe; that she 'is "reborn" to herself and to God and, in effect, emerges from her own rent and fissured body into the arms of her loving father and spouse – Christ'; I would add that this comes at a cost, as that rebirth is paradoxically dependent on the tainted maternal body within which she is painfully enclosed.[85] Indeed, Christ's offer of the redemptive, internal haircloth is echoed shortly after by the monk at Canterbury whose hegemonic anxiety over Kempe's authoritative religious discourse leads him to wish her

[82] Alexandra Barratt, 'Context: Some Reflections on Wombs and Tombs and Inclusive Language', in *Anchorites, Wombs and Tombs: Intersections of Gender and Enclosure in the Middle Ages*, ed. Liz Herbert McAvoy and Mari Hughes-Edwards (Cardiff: University of Wales Press, 2005), pp. 27–40 (p. 36).
[83] Liz Herbert McAvoy, '"Closyd in an hows of ston": Discourses of Anchoritism and *The Book of Margery Kempe*', in *Anchorites, Wombs and Tombs*, pp. 182–94 (p. 192).
[84] See *The Life of St Catherine of Siena: Blessed Raymond of Capua, Confessor to the Saint*, trans. George Lamb (Charlotte: Tan Books, 2011 reprint), pp. 144–5.
[85] McAvoy, *Authority and the Female Body*, p. 40.

to be entirely contained in a different way: 'I wold þow wer closyd in an hows of ston þat þer schuld no man speke wyth þe' (27).

As Dyan Elliott has shown, clerical concern over female penitential practices increased when those acts of asceticism threatened the exaction of the marriage debt. In order to preserve his authority, the husband was permitted, in medieval doctrine, to interfere with his wife's asceticism, but not vice versa.[86] Kempe's subversive acts of pain substitution, in default of her desired vow, demonstrate her resolution in following a purer channel to God, circumventing spousal authority. Despite the danger of wifely insubordination, she drives forwards in her conviction that earthly pain will facilitate an eternity of spiritual health. Such determination shows religious steadfastness but also feeds into the medieval fear of the female body as a site of danger and pollution, invested with an inherent capacity for pain which renders women powerful, and potentially deadly, agents.

Deadly Touching: Towards a Protective Vow

According to the medical corpus, pious married women who were reluctant to pay the marriage debt regularly, like Kempe, suffered from retained and 'corrupt semen' due to lack of the heat of the male. The ensuing and corrupt 'fumes' are described in *The Knowing of Woman's Kind in Childing* as 'euyll', the linguistic field of malignancy emphasising menstruation as synchronically polluting and divinely ordained:

> But nature, þat hatyth euery corrupcion & voydyth afthyre hys povere all þynge þat is [noyant] to body of man, enforsyth euery monyth onys to purge & *clense þe body of euyll humorys* & corrupte. And so þis *purgacyon ys ordende* to women & ys clepid menstrual be-cause hit commyth euery monyth onys.[87]

Women are thus perceived as *naturally* contaminated, their intrinsic 'euyll' requiring 'ordende' purgation. The tension between the binary curse of Eve and the purity of the Virgin Mary posed problems for medieval interpretations of the female body and resulted in the fusion of scientific and religious doctrine where moral codes were inscribed on a dyscrasic female body.[88] Cultural anxieties about even pious touching posed a dilemma for religious women in the Middle Ages; the sense of touch, as Fernando Salmón argues, is imbricated not only in a history of sexuality but also in definitions of 'the self and its boundaries', where 'touch left the self in a territory that only existed through the practice of relating to other beings

---

[86] Elliott, *Spiritual Marriage*, p. 154 and p. 187.
[87] My emphasis. *The Knowing of Woman's Kind in Childing*, p. 54.
[88] See Charles T. Wood, 'The Doctor's Dilemma: Sin, Salvation, and the Menstrual Cycle in Medieval Thought', *Speculum*, 56 (1981), 710–27.

and objects'.[89] The touch of the 'contaminated' female was therefore a loaded one, both for the toucher and the touched, as the meaning was located precisely in the moment of physical connection between subject and object: as some medieval writers would have it, the dangerous female and her prey.[90] *The Pore Caitif*, for instance, elucidates female touch as the very cause of the Fall of Man, as, in beholding what was forbidden, 'eue [would] hadde not touched þe forbodun tre'.[91] But the story of the *un*touched virgin martyr St Agnes was 'prescribed' by the 'hooli doctour' St Ambrose for the 'edificacioun of maidens'. When led to a brothel, naked, to be 'spuylid' for her faith, the 'iustice' who would rape Agnes 'feldoun to his face: & was stranglid of þe deuel', '*bifore he shulde touche hir*'.[92] Conversely, the unclean Delilah is held to be the cause of Samson's downfall, with her 'wanton & vnchastisid fals fleish, þat in a fewe daies shal be stynkinge erþe & filþe'.[93] Here, the female body is understood to be possessed of a powerful contaminatory force that can cause harm by both actualised and suspended touch. Margery Kempe, I want to suggest, utilises and exploits the haptic semiosis of the dangerous female body in her quest for a chaste marriage.

The polluting threat of female touch is generally focused upon the risk to the 'object' – that is, the male, or the unborn child. Menstrual blood in particular was considered contaminative, thought to produce leprosy, elephantiasis, and epilepsy in the newborn infant. *De secretis mulierum* explains the female body's toxicity in terms of an airborne latency:

> This [poison] is caused in menstruating women by the flow itself, for the humours first infect the eyes, that move through the whole body, then the eyes infect the air, which infects the child.

> [Causa hujus in mulieribus apparet quibus menstrua fluunt, quiaipse fluxus feu humores qui moventur per totum corpus, primo inficiunt oculos, & oculis infectis aër inficitur, & tunc aër ille inficit puerum.][94]

Women's 'corrupt' humours are regarded by this writer as imbued with the power to transmit atmospherically; her 'venom' is able to infect and injure.

---

[89] Fernando Salmón, 'A Medieval Territory for Touch', in *Sexuality and Culture in Medieval and Renaissance Europe*, ed. Philip M. Soergel (New York: AMS Press, 2005), pp. 59–81 (p. 60 and p. 68). Caroline Walker Bynum discusses holy women such as Bridget of Sweden, Clare of Montefalco and Douceline of Marseilles, whose reticence towards 'touch' indicates a reflection of ancient notions about the polluted female. Lutgard of Aywières 'panicked at an abbot's insistence on giving her the kiss of peace'. See Bynum, *Holy Feast*, pp. 212–13.

[90] For a full-length study of the anthropology of pollution and contamination see Mary Douglas, *Collected Works Volume II: Purity and Danger: An Analysis of Concepts of Purity and Danger* (London and New York: Routledge, 1966; 2003 reprint).

[91] My emphasis. *The Pore Caitif*, p. 179.

[92] My emphasis. *The Pore Caitif*, pp. 192–3.

[93] *The Pore Caitif*, p. 183.

[94] *De secretis mulierum*, trans. Lemay, p. 129. Albertus Magnus, *De secretis mulierum*, p. 109.

By attributing the female body with imperceptible, airborne potency, the example evidences the masculine fear of those bodies as powerful and eso-teric, themselves products of the moral diathesis which they are said to infect in others. Whilst many medical writers emphasised the positive function of menstruation through its purgative effects, Joan Cadden notes how 'the misogynistic possibilities of menstruation did not go unexploited'.[95] Centuries earlier, naturalists like Isidore of Seville (c. 560–636) saw women of childbear-ing age as possessing a supernatural, alchemical quality whilst menstruating, which could affect nature: 'crops do not germinate, wine sours, grass dies, trees lose their fruit, and iron rusts'.[96] Such sentiments recur throughout the medical texts of the Middle Ages, where those dangers are capable of being transferred to the unborn child. The *Knowing of Woman's Kind in Childing* connects female sexual activity in the later stages of pregnancy with risk to the unborn child: '& þat in þat tyme *sche* entermet hyre not with no disport of [deduyt] & namly ny here tyme, for with suche puttynge þe secundynne might brek & so þe chylde be abortyffe and stroyde for euyre'.[97] More fan-tastically, the medieval understanding of the monstrous imagination, which originated in Galenic thought, held that the mother could literally *imagine* her unborn baby into a monster, a concept exploited in *De secretis mulierum* in relation to deviant female sexuality.[98] Women's bodies were therefore them-selves aetiological, their toxicity permeating the air – the very atmosphere of human existence – as a malign force which was at once inferior and powerful.

Margery Kempe thus negotiates her vow of chastity in a cultural context of conflicting discourses, her aspiration to a celibate life as a quasi-virgin bride of Christ persistently undercut by the latent subtext of the toxic body that might, potentially, turn against itself. In direct opposition to medico-theological teaching on transgressive female flesh from the central Middle Ages, later ecclesiastical directives about the marriage debt overtook previously sacro-sanct doctrine on traditional periods of abstinence.[99] Contradicting the advice of many medical treatises, the payment of the debt during menstruation or pregnancy, or after childbirth, became permissible and less sinful, even when that exaction threatened the health of the woman. However, Kempe utilises the discourse of women's dangerous corporeality and untouchability in a stra-tegic move to negotiate a vow with John – an untouchability that resonates

---

[95] Joan Cadden, *Meanings of Sex Difference*, p. 175.
[96] Ibid.
[97] My emphasis. *The Knowing of Woman's Kind in Childing*, p. 60.
[98] *De secretis mulierum*, trans. Lemay, p. 116. On this notion, see Sarah Alison Miller, *Medieval Monstrosity and the Female Body* (New York and Oxon: Routledge, 2010), p. 86; William F. MacLehose, 'Nurturing Danger: High Medieval Medicine and the Problem(s) of the Child', in *Medieval Mothering*, ed. John Carmie Parsons and Bonnie Wheeler (New York and London: Garland Publishing, 1996), pp. 3–24; and Marie-Hélène Huet, *Monstrous Imagination* (Cambridge, MA: Harvard University Press, 1993).
[99] See Elliott, *Spiritual Marriage*, p. 150; and James A. Brundage, 'Sexual Equality in Medieval Canon Law', in *Medieval Women and the Sources of Medieval History*, ed. Joel T. Rosenthal (Athens: University of Georgia Press, 1990), pp. 66–79.

with Jesus' warning to Mary Magdalene by the sepulchre to avoid touching him in his own liminal state: 'Do not touch me, for I am not yet ascended to my Father'.[100] John's disquiet over Kempe's fasting practices shows his recognition that her purified flesh is unavailable, whilst her growing alliance with God paradoxically intensifies the mortal danger that she represents to him. Eventually, she achieves a divine compact that protects her from his carnal advances:

> Anoþer tyme, as þis creatur prayd to God þat sche myt leuyn chast be leue of hir husbond, Cryst seyd to hir mende, 'Þow must fastyn þe Fryday boþen fro mete & drynke, and þow schalt haue þi desyr er Whitsonday, for I schal sodeynly sle þin husbonde'. Þan on þe Wednysday in Estern Woke, aftyr hyr husbond wold haue had knowlach of hir as he was wone be-for, & whan he gan neygh hir, sche seyd, 'Ihesus, help me', & he had no power to towche hir at þat tyme in þat wyse, ne neuyr aftyr wyth no fleschly knowyng (21).

Fasting is a powerful enough penance in this example to satisfy the Old Testament God who is willing to 'sle' John on Kempe's behalf. Her invocation of the Name of Jesus, which mysteriously prevents the husband from touching the wife forever after, perhaps renders him impotent, removing his 'power'. Medieval devotions to the Holy Name of Jesus were popular methods of piety, promoted by Anselm of Canterbury (1033–1109) and Bernard of Clairvaux. Richard Rolle was well known for such devotion, instigated by a diabolic vision that was obliterated after his prayer 'O Jesus, how precious is your blood'.[101] The invisible fortification that Kempe creates through such a call to Jesus serves to enclose her, like the secret haircloth, equipping her with a divinely sanctioned weapon and assigning her inherent complicity in God's grim plan for John. From the pain of fasting she has thus benefited twofold. First, fasting purifies and cleanses the flesh, and, as pseudo-Athanasius had asserted, 'purifies the mind, drying up bodily humours and putting impure thoughts to flight'.[102] In balancing the excess tears and moisture of her constitution, fasting thus regulates the body as well as symbolically purifying it. Second, the collegiality with God that results from this renewed cleanness accords her a mystical power that has the potential to replace, or substitute, her own penitential pain with that of her husband via his sudden annihilation.

---

[100] John 20:17.

[101] *Richard Rolle: The English Writings*, ed. Allen, p. 16 and p. 40. Kempe is familiar with Rolle's works. See Chapter 1 of this study, p. 43, n. 55. On The Name of Jesus, see R. Lutton, 'The Name of Jesus, Nicholas Love's Mirror, and Christocentric devotion in late Medieval England', in *The Pseudo-Bonaventuran Lives of Christ: Exploring the Middle English Tradition*, ed. I. Johnson and A.F. Westphall (Turnhout: Brepols, 2013), pp. 19–53. See also Denis Renevey, 'Name above Names: The Devotion to the Name of Jesus from Richard Rolle to Walter Hilton's *Scale of Perfection* I', in *The Medieval Mystical Tradition in England, Ireland and Wales, Exeter Symposium VI, Papers Read at Charney Manor, July 1991*, ed. Marion Glasscoe (Cambridge: D.S. Brewer, 1999), pp. 103–21.

[102] Bynum, *Holy Feast*, p. 216.

Kempe's willingness to sacrifice her husband is repeated shortly after, when his hypothetical question receives an unwelcome response:

> he [John] asked his wyfe þis qwestyon, 'Margery, yf her come a man wyth a swerd & wold smyte of myn hed les þan I schulde comown kindly wyth ȝow as I haue do be-for, seyth me trewth of ȝowr consciens – for ȝe sey ȝe wyl not lye – wheþer wold ȝe suffyr myn hed to be smet of er ellys suffyr me to medele wyth ȝow a-ȝen as I dede sumtyme?' 'Alas, ser,' sche seyd, 'why meue ȝe þis mater & haue we ben chast þis viij wekys?' 'For I wyl wete þe trewth of ȝowr hert'. And þan sche seyd wyth gret sorwe, 'For-soþe I had leuar se ȝow be slayn þan we schuld turne a-ȝen to owyr vnclennesse' (23).

Not only has Kempe's divine fortification proved efficacious, illustrated by these eight weeks of chaste living, but a sexualised life is for her now more debilitating than would be the death of her husband. John can, as such, no longer regard his wife as an indebted spouse, but must see her rather as a fond companion (she does, at least, wish his death with 'sorwe'!) – but one who, nevertheless, would sacrifice his life for her own salvation. His retort is heavy with the burden of social expectation – 'ȝe arn no good wyfe'. Kempe is not swayed, however, and reiterates God's promise to her that he will take John's life: 'for I teld ȝow ner iij ȝer sythen þat ȝe schuld be slayn sodeynly, & now is þe thryd ȝer, & ȝet I hope I schal han my desyr' (23). Yet the metaphysical power of John's avoidance of the marriage debt is revealed when Kempe asks him why he has not 'medelyd' with her for the past eight weeks. His answer confirms both the fear he has developed for his lethal wife, and the concurrent power of the realm of touch, whose primary function of enveloping an otherwise 'internal [medieval] body of fluid characteristics' left the authenticity of the self entirely dependent on its relationship to the Other, as Salmón notes.[103] John responds that 'he was so *made a-ferde whan he wold a towchyd hir* þat he durst no mor don'. The threat of her female body, and Christ's protection of it, is thus utilised forcefully by Kempe to engineer that body as an untouchable site of intangible power. Sarah Salih sees John as the 'virgin martyr' of the *Book* through his use of the decapitation topos.[104] Though his life has been spared thus far, the absence, now, of physical touch, and the medieval understanding of mutual contact as being requisite for existence, mark his metaphorical death and his wife's status as pseudo-pain-giver. Salmón argues that 'the loss of the *sense* of touch, was equated with the death of the individual', a cause for John's quasi-death, then, in multiple ways.[105] Margery Kempe has engineered a layering of powerful fortifications – her haircloth, her fasting, her dangerous body, her call to Jesus – that makes her ultimately untouchable.

---

[103] Salmón, 'A Medieval Territory of Touch', in *Sexuality and Culture in Medieval and Renaissance Europe*, ed. Soergel, p. 68.
[104] Sarah Salih, *Versions of Virginity*, p. 200.
[105] Salmón, 'A Medieval Territory of Touch', *Sexuality and Culture*, ed. Soergel, p. 68.

Societal and theological conventions meant that a decision by John to under-take a solemn vow of chastity was both irrevocable and potentially emasculat-ing. A solemn vow differed from a 'simple' vow, which, whilst also requiring mutual consent, was not a public and official pronouncement.[106] The solemn vow that Kempe desires would be made in front of a church official, and was thus enforceable by the Church.[107] She is clear that it is this binding agreement alone that will satisfy her: 'I pray ȝow, suffer me to make a vow of chastyte in what bysshopys hand þat God wele' (24). Her husband is acutely aware of the manifold ramifications. Socially, a wife who gained moral superiority over her husband by preceding him in chastity threatened male authority in marriage, making her a dangerous prospect.[108] Indeed, women who committed to chaste living in marriage were often referred to as widows; something of an ironic designation in the light of Margery Kempe's lingering threat of John's death and reduced status, since his wife has metaphorically signalled his social and experiential demise.[109] Doctrinally, the risk of annihilation is equally real, because, as Elliott asserts, 'One who failed to fulfil a vow of chastity was, argu-ably, committing spiritual suicide'.[110] John is thus forced to choose between the pain of damnation if he were to break a vow, or the risk of sudden death from a vengeful God. He states, 'Nay … þat wyl I not grawnt ȝow, for now may I vsyn ȝow wyth-owtyn *dedly synne* & þan myght I not so' (24). Margery Kempe has thus projected her inescapable pain onto John through a synthesis of multiple and mortal threats. In wishing to achieve a form of self-inflicted widowhood, she gains agency over her fortified body, its protection from marital touching a reclamation of her virginity that paves the way for a solemn vow.

That the 'Book on the Conditions of Women' describes conjugal debt as 'carnal commerce' marks an exchange that is echoed in religious doctrine, illustrating the broad cultural understanding that the debt is a commodity of intrinsic value.[111] As matrimonial theory was being shaped during the

---

[106] Makowski, 'The Conjugal Debt and Medieval Canon Law', pp. 109–10.
[107] Elliott, *Spiritual Marriage*, pp. 158–9.
[108] An Augustinian sermon suggested that this undermines masculine leadership. See Elliott, *Spiritual Marriage*, pp. 158–9.
[109] Gratian cites the plight of Ecdicia, 'who, associating freedom from the debt with the restoration of autonomy, began to dress like a widow and manage her property independently. Probably to ensure that other husbands do not blindly let go of the reins by vowing continence, Gratian then assures couples that mental continence and a pious rendering of the debt are perfectly acceptable, although virginity is undoubtedly superior'. Elliott, *Spiritual Marriage,* p. 158.
[110] Ibid., pp. 158–9.
[111] 'Book on the Conditions of Women', in *The Trotula*, pp. 84–5. The medieval discourse surrounding 'carnal commerce' was happening at the same time as a commercial revo-lution in medieval society, when physical commodities were being increasingly traded and the language of business and economics began to enter clerical texts and sermons. See *Mendicants and Merchants in the Medieval Mediterranean*, ed. Taryn E.L. Chubb and Emily D. Kelley (Leiden: Brill, 2014). See also Siegfried Wenzel, *Latin Sermon Collections from Later Medieval England* (Cambridge: Cambridge University Press, 2005); and *Money, Commerce and Economics in Late Medieval English Literature*, ed. Craig E.

twelfth century, sex and marriage became ideologically separated, a separation promoted by theologians such as Hugh of Saint-Victor (d. 1141). His own reference to 'carnal commerce' in the context of its legitimate absence in chaste marriage posits the greater sacrament of the compact of love as having more value than the corporeal trading of sexual debt.[112] Employing identical terminology in his medical explication of uterine suffocation, Constantine the African concludes that its cause is an absence of 'carnal commerce'.[113] It is unsurprising, therefore, that the final negotiations between Kempe and John over a formally canonised pledge of chastity take a similar bargaining pattern. In Kempe's poignant recollection of a hot summer's evening, as she walks with John, carrying beer and cake, he finally offers a transaction, despite (or because of) his wife's deadly warnings:

> Margery, grawnt me my desyr, & I schal grawnt ʒow ʒowr desyr. My fyrst desyr is þat we xal lyn stylle to-gedyr in o bed as we han do be-for; þe secunde þat ʒe schal pay my dettys er ʒe go to Iherusalem; & þe thrydde þat ʒe schal etyn & drynkyn wyth me on þe Fryday as ʒe wer wont to don (24).

But Kempe is resolute and unprepared to compromise her ascetic fasting: 'Nay ser', she retorts, 'to breke þe Fryday I wyl neuyr grawnt ʒow whyl I leue' (24). Evidently, her transition from John's wife to Christ's bride is instigated already: God's command to fast is paramount and she relinquishes her earthly marital subservience instinctively. Though she will endure 'gret peyne' in her heart through the continuation of any 'carnal commerce', it is preferable to the mortal pain of disobeying God: 'But, blyssyd Lord, þow knowyst I wyl not contraryen þi wyl, and mekyl now is my sorwe les þan I fynde comfort in þe' (24). But God, as divine mediator and marriage counsellor, releases Kempe from her commitment to fasting in order to be free of the binds of conjugal debt. As he decrees that 'I wyl no lengar þow fast, þerfor I byd þe in the name of Ihesu ete & drynk as thyn husbond doth' (24–5), domestic arrangements retain a superficial normality for the sake of John's dignity; moreover, as ultimate securer of the transaction, Christ the Physician cures the pain of Kempe's sexual imperative and the ascetic fasting practices that have been her torment.

Margery and John Kempe's vow of chastity in the presence of Philip Repyngdon, Bishop of Lincoln, thus marks the culmination of a protracted negotiation. The bishop's agreement that 'I wyl fulffyllen ʒowr desyr ʒyf ʒowr husbond wyl consentyn þerto' (34) is answered with the symbolic meeting of hands between husband, wife, and ecclesiast – a paradoxically physical touch that, through the weight of its meaning, sanctions the subsequent and total *absence* of touch, at least in the carnal sense. The private agreement of chastity between Kempe and John is thought to have occurred in June 1413, and

---

Bertolet and Robert Epstein (London and New York: Palgrave Macmillan, 2018). My thanks to Trish Skinner for these suggestions.
[112] From Elliott, *Spiritual Marriage*, pp. 137–8.
[113] From Jacquart and Thomasset, p. 174.

their meeting with the bishop shortly after.[114] This makes Margery Kempe approximately forty years old, approaching the final few years of her natural reproductive life and a point in the medieval life cycle where a progression to chastity was considered by some an almost natural step.[115] That Kempe answers the bishop and his clerks so 'redyly & pregnawntly' after the vow, during what can only be described as a clerical interrogation of her revelations, implies a linguistic fecundity that symbolically and instantaneously replaces her reproductive capacity through the relinquishment of marital conjugality.[116]

The *Book*, however, records that 'long befor þis tyme' (38) God had freed her from the constraints of childbirth.[117] Though she was in a weakened post-partum state (she was 'beryng chylder & sche was newly delyueryd of a chyld' [38]), she was instructed to go to Norwich to disclose her revelations to the vicar of St Stephens. In designating her as God's interlocutor, Jesus simultaneously relieves her of the burden of future maternity: 'owyr Lord Cryst Ihesu seyd to hir sche xuld no mor children beryn' (38). It is therefore possible that the terminus of Kempe's reproductivity was divinely sanctioned some time before Church and spouse solemnised the vow. The *Book*'s achronicity renders problematic the claim that the delivery of her last child was indeed a *long tyme* before the vow, but this alternative spiritual transaction signals another private 'pact' with God which has been to the exclusion of her husband and the Church, and thus a further fortification within which she has been protected. Sarah Salih suggests that Kempe refuses to 'make her natural motherhood relevant to her sanctity and to sanctify the identity of "mother"', and instead 'reformulat[es] the self as virginal', arguing that 'the physical loss of virginity is not insuperable ... individual efforts can remake the body'.[118] In such a way, Margery Kempe manoeuvres innovatively within the non–absolute categories of sexuality in the medieval imaginary, securing a metamorphosis of body and of self through the dynamic potentialities of spiritual marriage.

---

[114] Hope Emily Allen calculates that, owing to their marriage occurring after 1393, and the production of fourteen children, the agreement could not have been made before 1405 and would have been prior to Archbishop Arundel's death in 1414. Because the only year between 1405 and 1414 in which Midsummer Even was on a Friday was 1413, Allen surmises that the vow was most likely to have occurred on 23 June 1413. See *BMK*, p. 269. Barry Windeatt concurs. See *BMK*, ed. Windeatt, p. 104.

[115] See Elliott, *Spiritual Marriage*, p. 41. See also Peter Brown, *The Body and Society* (London and Boston: Faber and Faber, 1988), pp. 69–82, pp. 149–50 and p. 378.

[116] MED s.v. pregnaunt: (a) With child, pregnant; (b) imaginative, quick, discerning; (c) of a prophecy, vision, pageant: highly significant; having hidden meaning; (d) of evidence, an argument, etc.: cogent, convincing, compelling. Although the intention is likely to have been to emphasise Kempe's cogency in this episode, the MED illustrates how the concomitant Middle English meanings of generation, imagination and vision are in fact primary.

[117] Since we are told in Chapter 43 that the vicar of St Stephen's in Norwich was Richard of Caister, who was vicar there from 1402 until his death in 1420, Kempe must have visited him between 1402 and 1413, when the vow of chastity takes place. This visit occurs after delivering what is implied as her last child, because of God's revelation that 'sche xuld no mor children beryn' from that point. See *BMK*, p. 276, n. 38/12, and Windeatt, *BMK*, p. 113.

[118] Salih, *Versions of Virginity*, p. 232 and p. 181 respectively.

The Analgesia of Mystical Marriage

On 9 November 1414, the feast of the dedication to St John Lateran, whilst in the Church of the Apostles at Rome, Margery Kempe is married to the Godhead.[119] God discloses that 'I wil han þe weddyd to my Godhede, for I schal schewyn þe my preuyteys & my cownselys, for þu xalt wonyn wyth me wyth-owtyn ende' (86). This mystical union occurs less than eighteen months after Margery and John negotiate their vow, when Margery Kempe is approximately forty-one years old. As a spiritual zenith, it is preceded by her marriage to the Manhood, which she communicates through the wearing of a ring, commissioned on the 'byddyng of God' (78). The direct revelation of God's request to wear the ring, and its importance as a visual symbol of union following her physical *dis*unity with John after the vow, merges private discernment with a public declaration of her transfigured socio-religious status. The ring, which 'owyr Lord had comawndyd hir to do makyn whil she was at hom in Inglond', is engraved with 'Ihesus est amor meus' (78), revealing an economic as well as spiritual richness. On the occasion of the vow, Kempe also dons the customary mantle of the vowess, which signified her chastity. In adopting the ring and the mantle, therefore, Kempe proclaims her status as vowess and quasi-widow, although, as Mary Erler has indicated, 'strictly speaking, the clothing which accompanied this vow – not only the mantle and ring, but also the veil and the wimple – did not signal widowhood, or even vowed widowhood, as many commentators have suggested, but vowed chastity in a lay state'.[120] The profundity of Kempe's betrothal and cognizance of her pseudo-widowhood is nevertheless illustrated when she temporarily loses the ring later in Rome and forcefully articulates its recondite meaning to the Italian landlady, who, incredibly and notwithstanding a language divide, 'vndirstond[s] what sche ment' (78). The ring – or what it *means* – thus accords Kempe with enhanced mystical perspicacity, transcending the division between material and spiritual erudition, and paving her way towards the superior state of wife of the Godhead.

While, then, she sits in the Church of the Apostles, God reveals his pleasure in her on account of her belief in the sacraments, her faithful longevity, and, 'specialy', her belief in the 'manhode of [His] Sone & for þe gret compassion þat þu hast of hys bittyr Passyon' (86). That Kempe's meditative focus on Christ's Passion is prioritised in this list illustrates its primacy for the experien-

---

[119] Hope Emily Allen calculates the year as 1414 because of Kempe's previous record that she had left Richard, a broken-backed man, in Rome two years prior to this marriage. As this was 1417, and Kempe would have spent only one winter in Rome, Allen concludes that she must have been in Assisi on Lammas Day of 1414. See *BMK*, pp. 298–9.

[120] Mary Erler, 'Margery Kempe's White Clothes', *Medium Aevum*, 62 (1993), 78–83 (p. 78). See also Hope Emily Allen in *BMK* p. 274, n. 34/10–12; and Gunnel Cleve, 'Semantic Dimensions in Margery Kempe's "Whyght Clothys"', *Mystics Quarterly*, 12 (1986), 162–70 (p. 164).

tial pain in her life so far: its *bittyrness*, interiorisation, compassion, and conduit for union.[121] But the spiritual apotheosis of her marriage to the Godhead, while climactic, is discordant both in its analgesic effect and the extent of Kempe's own internal security. For in spite of her craving for spiritual oneness with God, its manifestation must, insistently, operate via the Christic body to which, as she confesses, she is profoundly attached: 'al hir lofe & al hir affeccyon was set in þe manhode of Crist & þerof cowde sche good skylle & sche wolde for no-thyng a partyd þerfro' (86).[122] As her meditations on the Passion indicate, she is inextricably bound to the cultural and Christocentric significance accorded to flesh and to embodiment. It is God incarnate for whom she yearns, and union must necessarily therefore be based on the very corporeality that she knows, even in its flawed and painful form.

Kempe's silence at God's declaration speaks volumes. She is so 'ful sor aferd of þe Godhed' that she 'kept sylens in hir sowle & answeryd not þerto' (86), maintaining her sealed boundaries of self and enclosure lest Christ incarnate be removed from her soul. Appropriately, it is Jesus Christ, 'þe Secunde Persone in Trinite', who mystically intervenes, his emphasis on her relative spiritual immaturity and inexperience reminiscent of the nervous young bride on her wedding day: 'Fadyr,' he says, 'haue hir excused, for sche is ȝet but ȝong & not fully lernyd how sche xulde answeryn' (87). When God '[takes] hir be þe hand in hir sowle be-fore þe Sone & þe Holy Gost & þe Modyr of Ihesu', his words echo the traditional Christian marriage ceremony and legitimise the mystical rite not only as doctrinally valid, but also as concrete as the earthly referents with which Kempe is familiar:

> I take þe, Kempe, for my weddyd wyfe, for fayrar, for fowelar, for richar, for powerar, so þat þu be buxom & bonyr to do what I byd þe do. For, dowtyr, þer was neuyr childe so buxom to þe modyr as I xal be to þe boþe in wel & in wo, – to help þe and comfort þe (87).

The use of the mother–child dynamic as a metaphor for the unconditional love that will underpin the union is made problematic by the painful significa- tion that Kempe's maternity – and the sexual activation that it symbolises – has represented thus far, despite its theological tradition.[123] Notwithstanding, her deep anxiety about feelings of insignificance is coupled with the intense *comfort* that she perceives, physically and spiritually, in the event: 'felyng ryth vnworthy to any swech grace as sche felt, for sche felt many gret com- fortys, boþe gostly comfortys & bodily comfortys' (87). As a medieval term of cultural profundity – and a primary function of the *Book* itself, which is

---

[121] MED s.v. bitter: 2(a) Of suffering; grievous, *severe*.

[122] On Margery Kempe's union with Christ incarnate as an example of the medieval devo- tional tradition of sweetness, see Laura Kalas Williams, 'The *Swetenesse* of Confection'.

[123] 'For whoever does the will of my Father in heaven is my brother and sister and mother': Matthew 12:50. On this tradition see Caroline Walker Bynum, *Jesus as Mother*, pp. 110–66.

retrospectively described as a 'schort tretys and a comfortabyl' by the Proem's scribe – the 'comfortys' she gains are strengthening and remedial, providing relief, gratification, encouragement and courage, and spiritual joy.[124]

Such joy and spiritual gratification in divine wedlock is concomitantly manifested in a heightened sensory perception as a symbolically fecund replacement of Kempe's sexual and reproductive self, following her vow of chastity and marriage to the Godhead. Immediately after the mystical union, Kempe's senses conflate the physical and heavenly:

> Sum-tyme sche *felt swet smellys* wyth hir nose; it wer swettar, hir thowt, þan euyr was ony swet erdly thyng þat sche smellyd be-forn, ne sche myth neuyr tellyn how swet it wern, for hir thowt sche myth a leuyd þerby ʒyf they wolde a lestyd. Sum-tyme sche herd wyth hir *bodily erys* sweche sowndys & melodijs þat sche myth *not wel heryn what a man seyd to hir* in þat tyme les he spoke þe lowder (87–8).

Such rapturous and synaesthetic discernments continue over a period of twenty-five years, bestowing Kempe with joy and grace and endowing her with the intensified receptiveness to visionary stimulation that was examined in Chapter 1.[125] She *feels* smells, she *tastes* them as 'swet'; her 'bodily erys' are so suffused with heavenly melody that they block out people's speech. She is also gifted other auditory 'tokenys' by the third person of the Trinity, the Holy Ghost: the sound of blowing bellows and the songs of doves and robins (90–1). She sees 'white thyngys' flying around her like motes in the sunlight, explained by God as betokening angels all around her (and symbolising a heavenly replacement of the devils whose torturous actions plagued her at the beginning of her earthly marriage and childbirth [88]). Indeed, she is told that 'þu xalt heryn þat þu neuyr herdist, & þu xalt se þat þu neuyr sey, & þu xalt felyn þat þu neuyr feltist' (89). Spiritual wedlock has, therefore, unlocked in Kempe a capacity for elevated delectation that could potentially act as a powerful analgesic in counteracting her earthly pains in illness, public scorn, and pious grief. It also serves to undermine Wolfgang Riehle's recent assessment that Kempe is lacking in joy.[126] Permitted entry into a new sensory cosmos after the removal of her earthly shackles, her melancholic perspicacity facilitates a kaleidoscopic cognizance that opens up a renewed access to the divine. The use of sensory stimulation for medical purposes was a popular treatment in the Middle Ages: treatises frequently advise, for example, olfactory fumigations as a means to thwart physiological disorder. The Hippocratic idea of uterine displacement – that the movement of the womb in an upwards

[124] MED s.v. comfort: 1(a) Encouragement; (b) courage; 2(a) A feeling of relief, consolation, or gratification; 3(a) Pleasure, delight, gratification; (b) spiritual gratification, joy.
[125] That Kempe senses such sounds and melodies every day for 'xxv ʒere when þis boke was wretyn', and that Book I was revised between 1436 and 1438, places this episode at around 1413 and thus at more or less the exact time of her vow in 1413 and mystical marriage in 1414, corroborating the chronology.
[126] Wolfgang Riehle, *Inner Lives,* p. 257 and p. 280.

direction caused sensory disturbances – emphasised the relationship between the senses and physiological regularity.[127] Sounds, sights, and smells thus resonate as medico-religious agents in the *Book* and situate Kempe not only as mystical bride but also as privileged receiver of divine prophylactics, healing her body and soul.

A transcendent physicality occurs through the literal site of the marriage bed when Kempe is married to the Manhood and they must, therefore, 'ly to-gedir & rest to-gedir in joy & pes' (90). Reiterating her renewed purity, that Christ has '*clene forȝoue þe alle thy sinnes*', he insists he must be 'homly wyth þe & lyn in þi bed wyth þe'.[128] The interaction must also be intimate and tender: 'þy mayst boldly take me in þe armys of þi sowle & kyssen my mowth, myn hed, & my fete as swetly as thow wylt' (90). The latent eroticism of this encounter reveals Kempe's progression towards the ultimate amalgamation of her flesh with Christ's, but also the way in which her spirituality remains firmly within the terms of a domestic lexicon. Though her mystical marriage symbolises the rejection of the sordid matter ('mukke') of the world, the *Book*'s insistence on synchronically embodied and transcendent union reveals a holy destination not yet attained. The particular significance placed on the Christic body by medieval religious women has been shown comprehensively, a tradition that Kempe conforms to fully in her rapturous partaking of the Eucharist.[129] *The Pore Caitif* author describes St Katherine during the Eucharistic ceremony as being 'moued of feruent will & brennyng loue as hir maister crist was moued'.[130] Nicholas Love's *Mirror* describes the sacrament as acting to 'kyndele mannus soule & enflawme it al holy'.[131] Comparably, the all-encompassing love that Kempe experiences through the Eucharist is a simultaneously unbearable incorporation of Christ in her soul: 'sche myth not *beryn* þe habundawns of lofe þat sche felt in þe precyows Sacrament, which sche stedfastly beleuyd was very God & Man in þe forme of breed' (138). This ecstatic and awful consumption of the sacrament is imbued with the heavy weight of love and loss, laden also with Christ's *bearing*, or birthing, of humanity.[132] While the sensory medication of spiritual marriage is efficacious, Kempe's reluctance to self-conceptualise beyond the physical consummation of Christ's body, and her doubt, as an 'vn-worthy wrech' (90), limits the

---

[127] Jacquart and Thomasset, p. 174.

[128] My emphasis.

[129] See Miri Rubin, *Corpus Christi: The Eucharist in Late Medieval Culture* (Cambridge: Cambridge University Press, 1991). Bynum states: 'reception of Christ's body and blood was a substitute for ecstasy – a union that anyone, properly prepared by confession or contrition, could achieve. To receive was to become Christ – by eating, by devouring and being devoured'. See Bynum, *Fragmentation and Redemption: Essays on Gender and the Human Body in Medieval Religion* (New York: Zone Books, 1989), p. 126.

[130] *The Pore Caitif*, p. 195.

[131] Nicholas Love, *The Mirror of the Blessed Life of Jesus Christ: A Reading Text*, ed. Michael G. Sargent (Exeter: University of Exeter Press, 2004), Capitulum xxxix, p. 149.

[132] MED s.v. beren: 1(a) To carry; to be a carrier or bearer; 3(a) To hold up; 9(a) To endure; 10(a) To give birth to.

analgesic power of her marriage to the Godhead and perpetuates the fear that she might yet encounter pain.

Kempe's struggle to conceptualise a totalised spiritual self is also evident when Christ assures her of a widow's status via the metaphorical 'death' of her husband after their vow of chastity and the publicly visible social shift. They are slandered by their neighbours after first remaining in cohabitation after the vow: 'þan þe pepil slawndryd hem & seyd þei vsyd her lust & her liking as þe dedyn be-forn her vow making' (179–80). As an enforcer of the solemn vow, the Church was obliged to monitor the committed couple, since Bernard of Clairvaux, for example, stated in a sermon that 'the Church forbids men and women who have taken a vow of chastity to live together'.[133] But Kempe receives divine assurance that she is a quasi-widow and should thus have faith that her suffering will be replaced by love:

> & 3et þu hast an-oþer gret cawse to louyn me, for þu hast þie wil of chastite as þu wer a widow, thyn husbond leuyng in good hele. Dowtyr, I haue drawe þe lofe of þin hert fro alle mennys hertys in-to myn hert. Sum-tyme, dowtyr, þu thowtyst it had ben in a maner vnpossybyl for to ben so, & þat tyme suffyrdyst þu ful gret peyne in þin hert wyth fleschly affeccyons. & þan cowdyst þu wel cryen to me, seying, 'Lord, for alle þi wowndys smert, drawe al þe lofe of myn hert in-to thyn hert'. Dowtyr, for alle þes cawsys & many oþer cawsys & benefetys which I haue schewyd for þe on þis half þe see & on 3on half þe see, þu hast gret cawse to louyn me (161).

This lack of faith in Christ's promise – 'þu thowtyst it had ben in a maner vnpossybyl for to ben so' – is anticipated earlier in the *Book* when a doubtful Kempe is told that she is a virgin in God's sight: 'þu art a mayden in þi sowle … & so xalt þu dawnsyn in Hevyn wyth oþer holy maydens & virgynes' (52). And even in her virgin–widow transformation, emancipated from the patri-archal construct of marriage and reborn from her postlapsarian body, medical treatises like the *Trotula* texts show how widowhood, too, carried risks to health, including uterine suffocation and the exacerbation of a cold constitu-tion through the lack of male heat in sexual union. *De secretis mulierum* also emphasises the inescapability of this type of pain, since the affliction happens most often to widows ('viduis').[134] In her post-sexual metamorphosis, then, Kempe is more susceptible to the painful conditions associated with chastity and is concurrently at a precarious point of spiritual transition.

Mystically instructed, just before the time of the vow, to wear white clothes when she ventures on her impending pilgrimage, Kempe evokes her spiritual immaturity as a holy women in transition.[135] Though it is '[God's] wyl þat

---

[133] Bernard of Clairvaux, Sermon 65, c. 4. From Elliott, *Spiritual Marriage*, p. 140.
[134] *De secretis mulierum*, trans. Lemay, p. 132. Albertus Magnus, *De secretis mulierum*, p. 113.
[135] Kempe's revelation about the wearing of white occurs during a mystical conversation in Chapter 15 about her future pilgrimages to Rome, Jerusalem and the shrine of St James at Santiago de Compostella. Since the first of her pilgrimages is in late 1413, to the Holy Land, and that the chapter mentions that this conversation occurs 'ij 3er er þan

[she] were clothys of whyte & non oþer colowr, for [she] xal ben arayd aftyr [his] wyl' (32), she ruminates on the othering that wearing such clothes would effect. Anxious that by dressing in an '*oþer* maner' to chaste women she will endure slander, Kempe not only intimates that most chaste women do *not* wear white, but also exposes her internal struggle with the social *otherness* of alienation and difference (32).[136] While Gunnel Cleve sees the white clothes as 'instrumental in bringing about some of the qualities that are considered essential in mystics' because wearing them makes her a subject of ridicule and teaches her obedience and submission to God's will, Kempe must already *be* a mystic, having received divine command to wear the clothes in the first place.[137] After approximately four years of oscillation between wearing and not wearing white, she prays during a visit to Norwich c. 1415 for a 'tokne of leuyn [lightning], thundyr, & reyn' from God to ascertain whether she should resume wearing such attire (103), and is told that she will receive such a sign within three days.[138] As the betokened storm appears within those three days, Kempe immediately finds the means of securing a white 'gowne ... an hood, a kyrtyl, & a cloke' (104) from a good local man, an ensemble that totally envelops her in white, her will strengthened by divine legitimation and the prophetic power that those clothes now signify.

Not only stark in their articulation of the peculiar, that the clothes are ordained through a quite literally thunderous revelation also suggests their potency as a fortification for chastity and untouchability. Like the mantle and ring of the vowess, they are, *because* of their bold declaration of otherness, identifiers of difference, of a holy woman in the making. Kempe's difference is regarded by Alastair Minnis as being 'set apart from other wives'.[139] Indeed, confused by her female identity, the Archbishop of York demands to know 'Why gost þu in white? Art þu a mayden?' That Kempe retorts, 'Nay, ser, I am no mayden; I am a wife' (124) reveals how she identifies still as a wife, recognising the incongruity of her garb (reassured through revelation that she is 'a mayden in [her] sowle' [52]) yet insisting on its legitimacy as a sign

---

sche went', this initial instruction must have occurred in c. 1411 when Kempe is in the transitional stage towards gaining her long-desired vow.

[136] While Mary Erler views the white clothes as a symbol of virginity, Sarah Salih disagrees, regarding white clothes as having been worn in differing contexts – often of transition – and thus as more complex in denotation. Salih notes, 'The use of white is not limited to virgins, but to people in carefully defined moments of transition, which are sometimes, in practice, moments of virginity, as in the case of the bride or the novice'. See Salih, *Versions of Virginity*, p. 220. See also Mary C. Erler, 'Margery Kempe's White Clothes', p. 79.

[137] Cleve, 'Semantic Dimensions in Margery Kempe's "Whyght Clothys"', p. 167.

[138] Mary Erler notes that the period of four years where the white clothes were variously worn and removed are an inherent part of her important life-transition. See Erler, 'Margery Kempe's White Clothes', p. 81. Barry Windeatt has calculated that the Friday of the storm was probably 24 May 1415. See Windeatt, *BMK*, p. 217, n. 3423.

[139] Alastair Minnis, *Translations of Authority in Medieval English Literature: Valuing the Vernacular* (Cambridge: Cambridge University Press, 2009), p. 128.

of holy individuation and elected status. As she kneels, in fear, in front of the archbishop, threatened with fetters and accused of being a 'fals heretyke', the clothes fulfil their own fortifying function as they hide her shaking hands beneath, enabling a modicum of authority and enclosure. Though she *is* slandered for the wearing of white ('sithen hath sche sufferyd meche despyte & meche schame' [104]), the clothes' othering produces a useful unease in her onlookers, uncertain as they are of *who she is*. They become, therefore, an efficacious shield, not unlike the private hair-shirt and invisible fortress that prevent John's carnal touch, and they stress her transformational liminality. Chastity and painful experience therefore continue to run concurrently, but the tribulation of public slander remains a worthwhile sacrifice with its own spiritual capital. Even so, the pain paradox of chaste living once again evokes MacKendrick's conception of the medieval body as unstable and thus more receptive to radicalised modifications of body and behaviour.[140] While Kempe's white clothes symbolise an identity fraught with ambiguity and a body-of-pain, then, they also provide her with a means of radicalisation, whence she can go in daring difference as Christ's bride and disciple. Having relinquished her reproductivity through her chaste marriage, Kempe's salvation will now be assured during the next phase of her life-course, when painful childbearing will be reactivated by her 'surrogacy' operations, the focus of the following chapter, and when she is finally 'redemyd fro euyr-lestyng peyne' (246). Since medieval culture insists upon the experiential imperative of female pain as a necessary route towards *imitatio Christi* and *imitatio Mariae*, it remains, therefore, a fruitful and inescapable prerequisite for Kempe's spiritual ascension.

---

[140] MacKendrick, 'The Multipliable Body', p. 109.

3

Lost Blood of the Middle Age:
Surrogacy and Fecundity

Unto this day *it dooth myn herte boote*
That I have had my world as in my tyme.
But age, allas, that al wole envenyme,
Hath me biraft my beautee and my pith.
Lat go. Farewel! The devel go therwith!
The flour is goon; ther is namoore to telle;
The *bren*, as I best kan, now moste I selle;
But yet to be right myrie wole I fonde.[1]

Alisoun of Bath's delight in having had agency over her 'world' and her 'tyme', her willingness to bid farewell to the refined and desirable 'flour' of youth in favour of the more essential, coarse, but enriched 'bren' of age, is a cogent metaphor. Unlike Margery Kempe's maturing, divine wisdom, Alisoun's specialism is marriage, about which she claims to be 'an expert in al myn age' (l. 174).[2] While many medieval literary representations of ageing women are pejorative portraits of malicious crones or 'spent' figures whose social efficacy terminates with their reproductivity, Alisoun's apparent ascent to the role of teacher and sage is not only an affront to St Paul's infamous ruling, but also an acknowledgement that, in her own words, '*Experience*, though noon auctoritee / Were in this world, is right ynough for me' (ll. 1–2).[3] The metaphor of grains as fecund is found in Paul's letters to the apostles, where the convergence of wheat and human generation is made explicit: 'And that which thou sowest, thou sowest not the body that shall be; but bare grain, as of wheat, or of some of the rest. But God giveth it a body as he will: and to

---

[1] My emphases. 'The Wife of Bath's Prologue', in Chaucer's *The Canterbury Tales*, ll. 472–9. From *The Riverside Chaucer*, p. 111.

[2] For studies that offer a comparison of Margery Kempe and The Wife of Bath, see M.C. Bodden, 'Take All My Wealth and Let My Body Go', in *Women and Wealth in Late Medieval Europe*, ed. Theresa Earenfight (New York: Palgrave Macmillan, 2010), pp. 33–49; Sheila Delany, 'Sexual Economics, Chaucer's Wife of Bath and *The Book of Margery Kempe*', in *Feminist Readings*, ed. Evans and Johnson, pp. 72–87; William Provost, 'Margery Kempe and Her Calling', and Janet Wilson, 'Margery and Alison: Women on Top', both in *Margery Kempe: A Book of Essays*, ed. McEntire, pp. 3–15 and pp. 223–7 respectively.

[3] My emphasis. 'The Wife of Bath's Prologue'. In the Epistle to Timothy, Paul declares that 'I suffer not a woman to teach, nor to use authority over the man: but to be in silence' (I Timothy 2:12).

every seed its proper body.'[4] This connection is medicalised in Hildegard of Bingen's *Causae et curae*, where maternal milk is understood to be processed by the digestion of grain: 'Milk also receives its whiteness from grain and other cooked foods. Grain has white flour, and food, in cooking, emits a white foam' (Nam et de cibo frumenti et de aliis coctis cibis lac albedinum capit, quia frumentum albam farinam habet et cibus, dum coquitur, albam spumam eicit).[5] Such ideas then become literalised into medical treatments for infertility. 'The Book on the Conditions of Women' advises that a treatment for barrenness should involve placing wheat bran ('cantabrum') into two pots of urine to determine the infertility of the male or female.[6] The Wife of Bath's fertile 'bran of *age*' is rich, therefore, with the essence of life and nourishment, associated not with the teleologies of human offspring or the refined product of bread-flour, but with its generative nucleus or seed: its procreative potentiality. That the recipe at the end of Margery Kempe's *Book* also contains seeds of spices such as fennel and anise further imbues such life-giving meanings of sustenance into Kempe's own text.

The preceding chapter of this study concluded at a significant turning point in Margery Kempe's life-course: her transition, at the age of forty, to a life of chastity and spiritual focus and an increasing detachment from domestic constraint. Here I want to explore a further, pivotal moment in her life cycle – that is, her middle age and post-reproductivity, in the sense of both the self-imposed post-reproductive state brought about by her vow of chastity, and, later, the biological state of menopause (considered in medieval medical texts to be around the age of fifty). The process of physiological menopause is *itself* one of transition and temporal development – from peri-menopause, through menopause, to post-menopause – and that metamorphosis of body and experience, the need to redefine the meaning of female blood and its concomitant absence, forms the basis of this chapter, as Kempe transforms into an 'older' agent of ministry and, particularly, surrogacy.

The linguistic foundation of this approach emphasises the cruciality of a 'surrogacy' reading, by which I mean the substitutional operations, redolent with Margery Kempe's own maternal history, through which she identifies during her post-reproductive life stage. The term 'menopause', deriving from the Greek *men* ('month') and *pausis* ('a cessation; a pause'), is conceived in Latin as *climactericus*, or 'climacteric', signifying the lengthier physiological event through pre- to post- menopause and meaning 'a critical period' and 'rung of a ladder'.[7] It thus denotes a *crucial* stage of female transition, resonant with the

---

[4] 1 Corinthians 15:35–8.

[5] *Hildegardis: Causae et curae*, ed. Kaiser (Liepzig: In aedibus B.G. Teubneri, 1903), Liber II, p. 111. Trans. from *Causes and Cures*, Throop, p. 91.

[6] 'The Book on the Conditions of Women', in *The Trotula*, pp. 94–5.

[7] OED s.v. menopause. OED s.v. climacteric: relating to a critical point or period. 2: *Physiol.* and *Med.* Designating a period of physical (and, often, psychological) change occurring in middle age and believed to indicate the onset of senescence; *spec.* menopausal.

textual motif of the ladder as a symbol of contemplative progression in medieval mystical texts and thus imbricated in the symbiosis of medieval corporeal life stages and spiritual development.[8] Rather than an indistinct phase, then, the temporality of middle age and menopause is unique as a locus of transition between youth and old age, and between the biological states of fecundity and post-reproductivity. The absence of a precise *medieval* term for menopause perhaps explains the limited scholarly attention that has been accorded to medieval women of this life juncture (medieval texts themselves address only the *symptoms* of menopause – the absence of the menses – without any conceptual formulation of the phase as meaningful for female health or status).[9] Here, I redress this void via a foregrounding of the socio-biological changes that, rather than signalling the somatic failure that is often homologised with menopause – the 'functionlessness' that Emily Martin has highlighted as a central anxiety – instead signal an emergent re-capacity.[10] Indeed, the way in which Kempe's 'maternal skills' are 'redirected' in her mid to later years towards a spiritual goal, as proposed by Liz Herbert McAvoy, and the potentiality of her *remade* virginity, as Sarah Salih argues, facilitate a 'maternal ministry' which is as performative as it is experiential.[11] The cooling and drying of the female body in the mid to later years – the effective *making male* of the menopausal woman – prior to the onset of physical and mental failure in older age, enables a powerful process of re-identification through which Kempe is able to achieve authority in voice, text, and painful understanding.

---

[8] See, for example, Bridget of Sweden's vision of a monk on a high rung of a ladder in *The Liber celestis of St Bridget of Sweden: The Middle English Version in British Library MS Claudius B i, together with a life of the saint from the same manuscript*, ed. Roger Ellis, vol. 1, EETS o.s. 291 (Oxford: Oxford University Press, 1987), p. 366. I am grateful to Laura Varnam for this observation.

[9] Exceptions are *The Prime of Their Lives: Wise Old Women in Pre-Industrial Europe*, ed. Anneke B. Mulder-Bakker (Leuven, Paris and Dudley: Peeters, 2004); *Middle Aged Women in the Middle Ages*, ed. Sue Niebrzydowski (Cambridge: D.S. Brewer, 2011); and Sue Niebrzydowski, *Bonoure and Buxom: A Study of Wives in Late Medieval English Literature* (Bern: Peter Lang, 2006). Colleen Donnelly's article, 'Menopausal Life as Imitation of Art: Margery Kempe and the Lack of Sorority', *Women's Writing*, 12 (2005), 419–32, in fact has little to say on the topic of menopause per se. See also Deborah Youngs, *The Life Cycle in Western Europe*, pp. 126–62; and Cordelia Beattie, 'The Life Cycle: The Ages of Medieval Women', in *A Cultural History of Women in the Middle Ages*, ed. Kim Phillips (London and New York: Bloomsbury Academic, 2013), pp. 15–38.

[10] Even modern medical discourse often employs unfavourable language such as 'fail' and 'decline'. See Emily Martin, 'Medical Metaphors of Women's Bodies: Menstruation and Menopause', in *Writing on the Body: Female Embodiment and Feminist Theory*, ed. Katie Conboy, Nadia Medina, and Sarah Stanbury (New York: Columbia University Press, 1997), pp. 15–41. On modern biological theories of menopause see Thomas B.L. Kirkwood and Daryl P. Shanley, 'The connections between general and reproductive senescence and the evolutionary basis of menopause', *Annals of the New York Academy of Sciences*, 1204 (2010), 21–9.

[11] Liz Herbert McAvoy, *Authority and the Female Body*, p. 51. Sarah Salih, *Versions of Virginity*, pp. 180–5.

In late Antiquity 'wise' women of forty and beyond often operated in a pseudo-priestly manner, as intermediaries between women and the male clergy. Such socio-religious permutations continued into the Middle Ages, particularly connecting spiritual development with post-reproductivity.[12] Like the fortified body of enclosure that Margery Kempe engenders as a strategic defence during her childbearing years, her middle-aged transformation to post-reproductive surrogate is an innovative route towards a holy life as an earthly wife and mother, and it is a trajectory characterised not in *spite* of her female biology, but, through the removal of reproductive functionality, because of it.[13] By replacing her lost 'fecundity' with a new fruitfulness and flourishing, a spiritual didacticism and willingness to become a surrogate for others becomes, I suggest, a central hermeneutic of the *Book*. This chapter will first explore the ontological 'regendering' of middle-aged women in light of the symbolic 'lost' blood of menstruation (post-vow) and the later 'lost' blood of menopause, before then exploring Margery Kempe's own mid-life fecundity. I thus look to the opportunities to be derived from the post-reproductive state as a phase of corporeal temperateness as opposed to it signifying the degeneration of the female experience, with recourse to the surrogacy hermeneutic that operates persistently in the *Book*. What, then, does female blood *mean* in the medieval imaginary? What are the implications for the 'menopausal' woman who, in a culture in which blood has multivalent meanings, loses the blood that has given her those meanings? And how do various forms of social and mystical surrogacy – wetnursing, godparenting, fostering, and image-substitution – empower Kempe to reproduce her lost maternity?

Middle Age and Menopause 'Made Male'

When Katharina Tucher, a wealthy and educated Bavarian woman of the fourteenth century, was negotiating her new life as an independent widow at the age of forty, she was told to 'behave like a man'.[14] Christine de Pizan, writing in her fortieth year, describes a dream in which Fortune 'touched me all over my body … I felt myself completely transformed … I found my heart strong and bold, which surprised me, but I felt I had become a true man'.[15]

---

[12] See Anneke B. Mulder-Bakker, 'The Age of Discretion: Women at Forty and Beyond', in *Middle Aged Women in the Middle Ages*, ed. Niebryzdowski, pp. 15–24 (p. 23).

[13] Other holy women who progressed to a spiritual life post-childbearing include Bridget of Sweden and Angela of Foligno. See Thomas Gascoigne, 'Lyfe of Seynt Birgette', in *The Myroure of Our Ladye*, pp. xlvii–lix; and Catherine Mooney, 'Angela of Foligno', in *Women and Gender in Medieval Europe: An Encyclopedia*, ed. Margaret Schaus (New York: Routledge, 2006), p. 21.

[14] Mulder-Bakker, 'The Age of Discretion', in *Middle Aged Women*, ed. Niebrzydowski, pp. 15–18.

[15] Christine de Pizan, *The Book of Fortune's Transformation*, from *The Prime of Their Lives*, ed. Mulder-Bakker, pp. xviii–xix.

After menopause, medieval women were considered freer, to have a more legitimised voice, to be in some ways defeminised or more male. Lynn Staley, writing on female authorship, regards a woman's change at menopause as a trigger for writing, as the end of the childbearing years carries with it a shift in authority and didactic validity which is manifested, as Kempe demonstrates, in an alternative form of production: the text.[16] But the medical rationale for the physiological masculinisation and fluidity of gender in the maturing woman reveals much about the multivalence of such a paradigm. Women were considered colder and moister than men during their reproductive years before succumbing to the cooling and drying that characterises the ageing process. Aristotle (b. 384 BC) saw the female as not only cooler than the male, but also, resultantly, less able to refine nutriments, producing therefore not the superior fluid of semen, but that of menstrual blood, which merely *nourishes* the foetus as opposed to *shaping* its form.[17] Galen (b. c. 129 AD) stated that women are less warm than males, and are thus imperfect and inferior: 'Now just as mankind is the most perfect of all animals, so within mankind the man is more perfect than the woman, and the reason for his perfection is his excess of heat, for heat is Nature's primary instrument.'[18] In the early eleventh century Avicenna observed that 'women are colder in temperature than men. This is why they are normally of a smaller build. They are, also, more moist because their greater cold leads to the excessive formation of excrements.'[19] The female constitution and her reproductive function are thus utilised to justify her inferiority. It follows, therefore, that the physiological changes that occur around the menopausal years provoke a physical and cultural shift in the perception of women aged forty and beyond. Though senescent cooling occurs in both the male *and* the female, the accompanying drying is assumedly more marked in the female since she is characterised as moist throughout her many reproductive years, as Hildegard of Bingen notes: 'From her fiftieth, or sometimes sixtieth, year, a woman dries up and is enfolded around her openings' ('A quinquagesimo vero anno aut interdum a sexagesimo femina circa fenestralia loca sua implicatur et crescit').[20] As such, the middle-aged, or older, woman, through a process of cooling and drying, not only relinquishes the physiological reproductive function to which she has hitherto been bound, but also becomes drier and therefore more 'male' in the process.[21]

---

[16] Lynn Staley, *Margery Kempe's Dissenting Fictions*, p. 36. See also Kate Cooper, 'The Bride of Christ, the "Male Woman", and the Female Reader in Late Antiquity', in *The Oxford Handbook of Women and Gender in Medieval Europe*, ed. Judith M. Bennett and Ruth Mazo Karras (Oxford: Oxford University Press, 2013), pp. 529–44.

[17] Aristotle, *Generation of Animals*, I, 2 and 17–23; II, 1–3. From Cadden, *Meanings of Sex Difference*, p. 23.

[18] *Galen On the Usefulness of the Parts of the Body*, ed. May, vol. 2, p. 630.

[19] Avicenna, *The Canon of Medicine*, adapt. Bakhtiar, vol. 1, p. 30.

[20] *Hildegardis: Causae et curae*, ed. Kaiser, Liber II, p. 106. Translation from *Causes and Cures*, trans. Throop, p. 87.

[21] Note the correlation with the state of virginity, considered to be an elevated modification of human sexuality. An espousal of virginity was valued in the Middle Ages with

Though the political ramifications of increased female agency brought about by a growing identification with the male are manifold, it is my aim here to illustrate how Margery Kempe exploits and takes ownership of such cultural understandings, reclaiming and refashioning her body. Within the patriarchal Middle Ages there were certain fissures of opportunity into which some holy women, their physiology modified in middle age, could slip. Furthermore, the concurrent cooling of the male body in senescence produced a parity whereby ageing men, in losing the heat of male 'vigour', were at the same time feminised, resulting in similar 'regendering' at this point in the life cycle.

Although this chapter is concerned with post-reproductivity in its literal and performative operations, the accepted age of biological 'menopause' in medieval medical texts is most frequently cited as fifty years, with variations from thirty-five to seventy-five, highlighting the temporal elasticity of this life-stage. The Salernitan physician Copho, living in the second half of the eleventh century, states in *Egritudines tocius corporis* that the menses 'are not present naturally before the twelfth year or after the fiftieth'.[22] *The Knowing of Woman's Kind in Childing* states menstruation to occur 'fro xv yere till sche be fifty wyntyr olde', the reason for the onset of menopause being securely linked to symptoms of cooling and drying: 'Ne þe women of [fifty] yere [of] age be-cause they be so dryed þat þe hote of þe blode is distroyde þat no superhabundant humvre may ryse in hem ne passe'.[23] Similarly, the *Sickness of Women* also considers the duration of the menstruating years to be 'into þe age of l wynter'.[24] It makes clear the overarching contingency of temperature and moisture for the retention of the menses, which occurs because 'as of hete other of colde of the matrice, other of hete or of cold of the humours that bien enclosed withinfurth in the matrice, other of grete drynes of hir complexioun'.[25] Variations are, however, in-built to medical writings.[26] My application of the female mid-life stage as connected to the drawn-out temporality of pre- to post- menopause chimes, then, with the implicit flexibility that these medical texts imply. Medieval writings often overlook the onset of middle

---

the 'highest patristic compliment: they were praised for becoming "male" or "virile"'. See Jane Tibbetts Schulenburg, 'The Heroics of Virginity: Brides of Christ and Sacrificial Mutilation', in *Women in the Middle Ages and the Renaissance*, ed. Rose, pp. 29–72 (p. 32). See also *Religion and Sexism: Images of Women in the Jewish and Christian Traditions*, ed. R.R. Ruether (New York: Simon and Schuster, 1974), pp. 150–83; and Jo Ann McNamara, 'Sexual Equality and the Cult of Virginity in Early Christian Thought', *Feminist Studies*, 3 (1976), 152–4.

[22] Darrel W. Amundsen and Carol Jean Diers, 'The Age of Menopause in Medieval Europe', *Human Biology*, 45 (1973), 605–12.

[23] *The Knowing of Woman's Kind in Childing*, p. 48.

[24] *Sickness of Women*, p. 485.

[25] Ibid., pp. 486–7.

[26] See the 'Book on the Conditions of Women', in *The Trotula*, pp. 72–3. Lifestyles according to the six non-naturals could also affect the individual life span. See Peregrine Horden, 'A Non-natural Environment', in *The Medieval Hospital and Medical Practice*, ed. Bowers, pp. 133–45. Monica Green emphasises the complexity of ascertaining a reliable 'age' for menopause. See *The Trotula*, p. 215, n. 85.

age.[27] Indeed, the most common taxonomy of human age was the dichotomy of *juventus* and *senectus*: *juventus* representing folly, passions, and pleasures, heat, moisture, and sanguinity, while *senectus* represented reason, gravity, moral responsibility, coldness, dryness, melancholia, and phlegm.[28] Such disinterest in the *process* of ageing – that stage which we might consider as middle age – suggests its culturally perceived insignificance: those of 'middle' age might be reasonably expected to be established, perhaps unremarkably, in their community, work, and domestic environments, and thus offer little interest for the more pressing socio-religious teleology of senescence and, ultimately, the afterlife. However, the 'prime' of life is regarded in the Middle English translation of the pseudo-Baconian *De retardation accidentum senectutis* ('On Tarrying the Accidents of Age'), as between forty and fifty: 'after that natural heete bigynnyth to mynush of necessite, and that tyme bigynneth after xlv or l yeere generaly'.[29] Citing Philip of Novara (b. 1195), Elizabeth Sears notes how the *moien age* was considered the time to 'be an example to others in wisdom, goodness, and strength of character'. Importantly, she emphasises 'the unusual use of the now standard designation of "middle age" to describe these years'.[30] Several medieval writers, including Bernard of Gordon (fl. 1283–1309) and Aldobrandino of Siena (d. c. 1296), regarded the onset of the body's cooling and drying process, and therefore its ageing, as occurring from around the age of forty.[31] For Vincent of Beauvais (c. 1194–1264) it is in fact the female menopause which marks the end of the fourth stage of life, *juventus*, referring to the 'inability of women to give birth after fifty as the indicator of the end of this stage'.[32] The cooling and drying of a maturing individual, and the existence of an often long period of *senium* thereafter, suggests, then, that medieval 'old' age is what modern categorisation might label 'middle' age. Medieval 'age taxonomies' of human experience, therefore, can provide a useful starting point for attempts to describe the female life stages, but it is within the site of experience itself – as attested by Chaucer's Alisoun – that authentic meaning, subjectively *un*classifiable, is situated.

Indeed, the wholly distinctive interval of women's middle age is embraced by Hildegard, who employs a poetics of fecundity when describing mature adulthood, underlining the reproductivity that I suggest to be characteristic of this powerful life stage:

[27] See *Middle Aged Women*, ed. Niebrzydowski, p. 1.
[28] See Robert Magnan, 'Sex and Senescence in Medieval Literature', in *Aging in Literature*, ed. Laurel Porter and Laurence M. Porter (Troy: International Book Publishers, 1984), pp. 13–51 (pp. 16–19).
[29] 'On Tarrying the Accidents of Age' (*De retardatione accidentium senectutis*), ed. Carol A. Everest and M. Teresa Tavormina, in *Sex, Aging, and Death in a Medieval Medical Compendium*, vol. 1, ed. Tavormina, pp. 133–247 (p. 157).
[30] Elizabeth Sears, *The Ages of Man*, pp. 101–2.
[31] See Shulamith Shahar, 'Who were Old in the Middle Ages?', *Social History of Medicine*, 6 (1993), 313–34. See also J.A. Burrow, *The Ages of Man: A Study in Medieval Writing and Thought* (Oxford: Clarendon Press, 1988).
[32] Shahar, 'Who were Old in the Middle Ages?', p. 320.

and in adulthood, when all the person's veins are full, it shows its strongest powers in wisdom; as the tree in its first shoots is tender and then shows that it can bear fruit, and finally, in its full utility, bears it.[33]

[at in plena ætate cum omnes venæ hominis plenæ sunt, fortissimas vires suas in sapientia declarat, sicut etiam arbor in primo germine tenera existens ac deinde fructum in se ostendens, tandem cum plentitudim militatis educit.]

During what Hildegard sees as the maturing years, the soul works in harmony with the body to nurture and extrapolate its wise potential, to produce the fruit of knowledge (as opposed to that of the womb), but in insistently feminine terms. Fertility, as St Ambrose (c. 339–397) attests, can persevere into one's maturing years, which are 'a time of moral behaviour, like the palm tree which only bears fruit as it ages, not in its youth'.[34] Drawing on traditional biblical images of abundance and fertility, images of shoots, vines, and greenness are metonymies for Christ and the land of Israel.[35] Such topoi of fruitfulness and nurture in Christian theology are what Grace Jantzen argues should be reclaimed as an alternative doctrine of salvation centred on maternal and natal flourishing, as opposed to its theological emphasis on death as salvific – as Jantzen puts it, a 'necrophilic imaginary'.[36] Yet Jantzen's call is anticipated some 600 years earlier by the author of *The Pore Caitif*, who sees the five martyrs Agnes, Lucy, Agatha, Cecilia, and Katherine as quasi-generative flowers: 'fyue rede rosis for martyrdom: & white lilies for clene chastite'. By these flowers, along with the roses of Christ and his four apostles, the reader can also be edified: 'make þou', the text exhorts, 'a gay garland & were it vpon þi heed of þi soule, þat is on þe principal resoun: þese flouris mai neuere faile ne fade … for … crist [is] þe briȝtest roos & spouse of oure soules'.[37] The hermeneutic of spiritual as opposed to biologically reproductive flowering, the ontological significance of 'lost blood' and its symbolic absence, afford maturing women like Margery Kempe an alternative trajectory towards a new fecundity.

---

[33] Hildegard von Bingen, *Scivias*, I, 4.17, PL, col. 425. Translation from *Hildegard of Bingen, Scivias*, trans. Mother Columba Hart and Jane Bishop (New York: Paulist Press, 1990), p. 120.

[34] Ambrose, *Wisdom* 4.9. From Albrecht Classen, 'Old Age in the Middle Ages and the Renaissance: Also an Introduction', in *Old Age in the Middle Ages and the Renaissance: Interdisciplinary Approaches to a Neglected Topic*, ed. Albrecht Classen (Berlin and New York: de Gruyter, 2007), pp. 1–84 (p. 40).

[35] 'Israel shall spring as the lily, and his root shall shoot forth … they shall blossom as a vine' (Hosea 14:3–7). '[T]hey of the city shall flourish like the grass of the earth' (Psalm 71:16). 'I the Lord have brought down the high tree, and exalted the low tree: and have dried up the green tree, and have caused the dry tree to flourish' (Ezechiel 17:24).

[36] Grace Jantzen, *Becoming Divine*, pp. 156–70 (p. 165). On the theology of female flourishing, see also Liz Herbert McAvoy, '"Flourish like a Garden": Pain, Purgatory and Salvation in the Writing of Medieval Religious Women', *Medieval Feminist Forum: A Journal of Gender and Sexuality*, 50 (2014), 33–60.

[37] *The Pore Caitif*, p. 197.

Losing Blood

Sche myth neyþer wepyn lowde ne stille but whan God wolde sende it hir, for sche was sumtyme so *bareyn* fro teerys a day er sumtyme half a day & had so gret peyne for desyr þat sche had of hem þat sche wold a ȝouyn al þis worlde, ȝyf it had ben hir, for a fewe teerys, er a suffyrd ryth gret bodily peyne for to a gotyn hem wyth. And þan, whan sche was so *bareyn*, sche cowde fynde no joye ne no comforte in mete ne drynke ne dalyawns but euyr was heuy in chere & in cuntenawnce tyl God wolde send hem to hir a-geyn, & þan was sche mery a-now (199).

The language of sterility and *bareyn*-ness that Margery Kempe employs when she mourns the loss of her ghostly weeping exposes the way in which the spiritual gift signifies her self-identified fecundity and sense of completion.[38] When she receives the gift of tears at Mount Calvary in the spring of 1414, during her pilgrimage to the Holy Land, she is aged forty-one and at a turning point in her life of piety following her long-desired vow of chastity. The cries, she says, 'enduryd many ȝerys aftyr þis tyme' (68), a fact that she clarifies later in the *Book*: 'þis maner of crying enduryd þe terme of x ȝer' (140). The productive value of this effusive weeping, reiterated by the 'peyne' triggered by its absence, reveals her tears to be a vital facet of her efficacy as an emerging holy woman and a fruitful replacement for the socio-biological productivity of her former incarnation as a wife and mother. It is remarkable, then, that the terminus of those ten years of demonstrative crying, c. 1424, locates Kempe at the age of fifty-one, and, according to the medieval medical sources illustrated above, at the precise age of menopause.

That the cessations of menstrual blood and boisterous weeping converge at this juncture is striking.[39] We shall see that Kempe proceeds thereafter to modify her productivity from the biological prescription of menstruation and the didactic and divine gift of tears to a new phase of substitutional mother-ing, and this engenders the surrogacy hermeneutic central to much of this book. For not only is Kempe now freed of the dysmenorrhoea of her fertile years and the tangible stain of Eve's legacy (Kempe makes many references throughout the text to her sinful state, presented as a given), she is also now characterised physiologically by less excess and superfluity, making her more measured and balanced, free to heal and to minister via a synthesis of bodily

---

[38] MED s.v. barain(e): barren (woman); childless; unproductive; non-bearing; intellectu-ally or morally sterile; destitute, devoid, bare.

[39] Even before the end of this ten-year phase, we are informed that after Kempe's pilgrim-ages to Jerusalem and Rome, her meditations are drawn further towards the Godhead as well as the Manhood. This evolution in her devotional practices is enriching (she is more 'illumynyd' and more 'feruent'), and yet her tears become more subtle and less laborious: 'ȝet had sche not þat maner of werking in crying as sche had be-for, but it was mor sotyl & mor softe & mor esy to hir spirit to beryn' (209).

and social modification.[40] Christ's words to Kempe that 'þu art to me a very modir & to al þe world' (91) thus become literally embodied, repositioning her as an authorised agent of a divine maternity predicated on a paradoxically post-reproductive condition. In the medieval imaginary, menopause is not noted in and of itself but, rather, is formulated as the absence, or cessation, of the menses.[41] As such, I suggest that the vast symbolic value of an event that marks an escape from the indomitably gendered postlapsarian burden holds equal importance to the physical effects of menopause on the body. Menstruation, for example, was considered by theologians to be a 'sickness' or 'infirmity'. Much scholarship exists on the 'stain' of menstruation. However, less consideration has been paid to the ways in which menopause might be regarded in some ways as a *cure* for the female blemish in the Middle Ages – a window into a life interval where, emancipated from the 'brand' of menstruation and the constraint of childbearing, the mature woman may be conceptualised as freer and, perhaps, purer.

Blood infuses diverse aspects of medieval culture; in science, medicine, theology, iconography, and art it is situated as the very essence of existence, a life-source both spiritual and corporeal. Medieval medical texts frequently rely on blood as an indicator of sickness or health.[42] Blood is the carrier of life, yet, conversely, its superfluity within the body can cause pain and illness, creating imbalance, excess heat, and infirmity.[43] Caroline Walker Bynum has interrogated the 'blood frenzy' that engulfed devotional art and poetry, iconography and vision, and the significance of the visuality of blood outside the body. The cultural capital of blood piety is exemplified by the Man of Sorrows image, which depicted a progressively bold and living Christ spouting cascades of blood.[44] Female mystics were reported as experiencing ecstasies triggered by the envisioned Christic body and the Eucharistic sacrament. The hagiogra-

---

[40] Kempe frequently reiterates the burden of her sins in the *Book*, interpreting others' adversity as 'þe skowrges of owyr Lord þat wold chastyse hir for hir synne' (11). The historical sin that provides Kempe with so much anguish at the beginning of the *Book*, and to which she refers on occasion, highlights the ongoing burden that it represents: 'Sche was schreuyn sum-tyme twyes or thryes on þe day, & in specyal of þat synne which sche so long had conselyd & curyd' (12).

[41] From the Early Modern era, medical writers began to write more specifically about menopause, largely pathologically. See Michael Stolberg, 'A Woman's Hell? Medical Perceptions of Menopause in Preindustrial Europe', *Bulletin of the History of Medicine*, 73 (1999), 404–28.

[42] See Bettina Bildhauer, *Medieval Blood* (Cardiff: University of Wales Press, 2006).

[43] Ibid., p. 25.

[44] Caroline Walker Bynum, *Wonderful Blood: Theology and Practice in Late Medieval Northern Germany and Beyond* (Philadelphia: University of Pennsylvania Press, 2007), p. 3. On the Man of Sorrows, see Hans Belting, *The Image and Its Public in the Middle Ages: Form and Function of Early Paintings of the Passion*, trans. Mark Bartusis and Raymond Meyer (New York: Caratzas, 1990); and Bernhard Ridderbos, 'The Man of Sorrows: Pictorial Images and Metaphorical Statements', in *The Broken Body: Passion Devotion in Late Medieval Culture*, ed. A.A. MacDonald, H.N.B. Ridderbos, and R.M. Schlusemann (Groningen: Egbert Forsten, 1998), pp. 145–81.

pher of Beatrice of Nazareth (d. 1268) described her as suffused with Christ's blood during the sacrament.[45] Such Eucharistic visions served to heighten the lay frenzy for blood relics, as Bynum asserts: 'Pilgrimages proliferated to places (such as Wilsnack, Daroca, Walldürn) where hosts supposedly bled or chalices turned to blood; older cult sites that claimed relics of Christ's blood from the Holy Land ... bloomed anew'.[46]

Influenced by this cultural milieu, Margery Kempe's own faith in the transubstantiation of the Eucharist is exhibited in her internalisation of Christ's edict that she should forsake the eating of flesh in order to receive his body more receptively: 'And in-stede of þat flesch þow schalt etyn my flesch & my blod, þat is þe very body of Crist in þe Sacrament of þe Awter' (17). Kempe exculpates herself from accusations of Lollardy by stating her rejection of sacramental materiality, insistent that she ingests Christ himself: 'I be-leue þat it is hys very flesch & hys blood & no material bred' (115). This metaphysical semiosis of blood inspires her many pilgrimages and devotional activity. She visits the Holy Blood of Hailes when she is about forty-four years old, a trip which prompts a characteristically emotive response: '[she] went forth to þe Blod of Hayles, & þer was schrevyn & had lowde cryes & boystows wepyngys' (110).[47] And, despite great sickness and infirmity in her older age at around the age of sixty, she is carried to Wilsnack in a wain to visit the Precious Blood, 'wyth gret penawns & gret disese', all the while affirming God's role in facilitating the journey and the miracle of the blood: 'thorw þe help of owr Lord sche was browt to Wilsnak & saw þat Precyows Blod which be miracle cam owt of þe blissful Sacrament of þe Awtere' (234–5). The blood of the relics thus becomes a central focus for Kempe's devotional rebirth and an antidote to the bodily suffering of her advancing years. After menopause, the multivalent meanings of blood thus become epistemologically refocused, adopting a layering of spiritually fertile signification.

As the medieval iconography of Christ's crucifixion illustrates, blood represents a tension between the living and the dead, the wounds depicted as fresh and mobile, dripping with red blood. Blood's loss, or outpouring, is life lost, but blood is also life's carrier, empowered to regenerate and restore. It thus simultaneously evokes suffering, liberation, and fertility. Indeed, folk practices suggest the cultural connotations of blood with fecundity, the Eucharistic host reported to have been stolen from village churches as a talismanic reappropriation to assist with conception or farming.[48] Medieval traditions also include blood as a cure for infirmities such as blindness. For Bartholomaeus Anglicus, blood is also maternal – it 'nourische[s]' the body's members and travels

---

[45] From *The Life of Beatrice of Nazareth*, in Bynum, *Wonderful Blood*, p. 4.

[46] Ibid., p. 5.

[47] It is possible to date this trip to Hailes to 1417, because there is mention in this chapter of the death of Bishop Peverell, whose demise in 1419 was prophesied two years prior. See *BMK*, p. 309.

[48] See Bynum, *Wonderful Blood*, p. 155.

through the veins, 'souken þerof as it were of here modir, fedinge of blood'.[49] The notion of blood as an independent presence with its own detached and mobile meanings – able to be divided, changed, to transcend boundaries, to create the loss or regeneration of life – imbues it with a complexity that precludes straightforward significations of human pain and suffering in the medieval imaginary. Medieval medicine teaches of blood's nourishing prop-erties since the growing foetus is fed by uterine blood and the transformed blood of breastmilk (medieval scientific theory adopted the Galenic notion of dealbation, where breastmilk was considered to be reformed blood).[50]

The implications of the gendered menstrual blood from which Christ also originated in his human form therefore posed a great theological dilemma, at the same time as Marian devotion was flourishing.[51] Thomas Aquinas, however, reconciled the potentially corrosive influence of female blood on the Christ Child: 'This, however, did not take place in Christ's conception: because this blood was brought together in the Virgin's womb and fash-ioned into a child by the operation of the Holy Ghost. Therefore is Christ's body said to be "formed of the most chaste and purest blood of the Virgin"' ('Sed hoc in conceptione Christi non fuit, quia operatione spiritus sancti talis sanguis in utero virginis adunatus est et formatus in prolem. Et ideo dicitur corpus Christi ex castissimis et purissimis sanguinibus virginis formatum').[52] The inimitable Virgin Mary's blood is purified by the Holy Ghost and is thus clean, though the blood of gestation remained as vital for Christ as for all humans, repurposed as it was in the salvific blood of the Passion. The ontological movement of blood between bodies and genders – and, indeed, its loss – illustrate the dynamic ways in which it is conceptually reimagined in the Middle Ages.[53] The praxis of regular phlebotomy, for example, as part of a seasonal health regimen in monastic houses was conducted from the ninth century.[54] The *Ancrene Wisse* also recommends quarterly blood-lettings for

---

[49] *On the Properties of Things*, p. 279.

[50] See Cadden, *Meanings of Sex Difference*, pp. 117–30.

[51] On the dilemma of the Virgin Mary's menstrual blood, see Bynum, *Wonderful Blood*, pp. 158–9 and Miri Rubin, *Mother of God: A History of the Virgin Mary* (London: Penguin Books, 2010), p. 26.

[52] Thomas Aquinas, *Summa Theologiae*, III, 31.5, reply to Objection 3. Translation from <http://www.ccel.org/ccel/aquinas/summa> [accessed 20 January 2019].

[53] This phenomenon can also be seen through the myth of male menstruation. See Gianna Pomata, 'Menstruating Men: Similarity and Difference of the Sexes in Early Modern Medicine', in *Generation and Degeneration: Tropes of Reproduction in Literature and History from Antiquity to Early Modern Europe*, ed. Valeria Finucci and Kevin Brownlee (Durham and London: Duke University Press, 2001), pp. 109–52; Irven M. Resnick, 'Medieval Roots of the Myth of Jewish Males Menses', *The Harvard Theological Review*, 93 (2000), 241–63; Willis Johnson, 'The Myth of Jewish Male Menses', *Journal of Medieval History*, 24 (1998), 273–95; and Steven F. Kruger, 'Becoming Christian, Becoming Male?', in *Becoming Male in the Middle Ages*, ed. Jeffrey Jerome Cohen and Bonnie Wheeler (New York and London: Garland Publishing, 2000), pp. 21–41.

[54] See the Introduction to 'A Latin Technical Phlebotomy and Its Middle English Translation', ed. Linda E. Voigts and Michael R. McVaughs, *Transactions of the American*

its anchoritic audience so as to maintain correct humoral balance and achieve salvific cleansing.[55] Such non-menstrual bleeding, enacted in a 'menstruating' and purgative way, is indicative of its purificatory potentiality.[56] Blood, then, is a symbol at once of fertility and affirmation, of pain, pollution, and loss. It is also transcended, 'Because the life of the flesh is in the blood: and I have given it to you, that you may make atonement with it upon the altar for your souls, and the blood may be for an expiation of the soul.'[57]

The dichotomy of pain and purgation that menstruation affords women therefore illuminates the productive absence of that menstruation in the middle-aged woman. *The Knowing of Women's Kind in Childing* states, paradoxically, that 'The flourys of women ys anguysch.'[58] Female bleeding is itself here an affliction, a synthesis of science and theology emphasised through the description of the blood as a 'mortall poyson', or 'corrupte'. Such evils, of course, require purgation, as the text outlines: 'And so þis purgation ys *ordende* to women & ys clepid menstrual be-cause hit commyth euery monyth onys.'[59] Women are thus not merely contaminated by 'euyll' blood, but are divinely ordained to be so. The *Sickness of Women* lists several explanations for the retention of the menses and the profound bodily afflictions and disordered behaviours that the 'condition' causes:

> And long witholdyng of this bloode maken wymmen otherwhile to falle into a dropesy, oþerwhiles makith hem to have the emerawdis [haemorrhoids], otherwhiles it grevith the herte and the lunges and makith hem to have the cardiacle [heart disease], and otherwhiles it affraieth the herte so moche that it makith hem to fallen doun in a swoun as though thei hadden þe fallyng evil and thei liggen in that sikenes a day or two as though thei wern dede. And otherwhiles thei han scotayne [dizziness] with grete stonyeng [confusion] in the brayne and whan that al thyng tournyth vp-so-doun.[60]

Inert female menstrual blood is thus regarded as potentially destructive to the woman herself. Like the religiosity of *The Knowing of Woman's Kind in Childing*, the *Sickness of Women* depicts the 'falling sickness' as 'þe falling *evil*' (my emphasis), ascribing it with a latent maleficence born from the reten-

---

Philosophical Society, 74 (1984), 1–69 (pp. 1–34). See also Pedro Gil-Sotres, 'Derivation and Revulsion: The Theory and Practice of Medieval Phlebotomy', in *Practical Medicine from Salerno to the Black Death*, ed. Luis Garcia-Ballester, Roger French, Jon Arrizabalaga, and Andrew Cunningham (Cambridge: Cambridge University Press, 1994), pp. 110–47.

[55] See Part 8 of the *Ancrene Wisse: A Corrected Edition of the Text in Cambridge, Corpus Christi College, MS 402, with Variants from other Manuscripts*, vol. 1, EETS o.s. 325, ed. Bella Millett, with glossary and notes by Richard Dance (Oxford: Oxford University Press, 2005).

[56] On this practice, see McAvoy, 'Bathing in Blood', in *Medicine, Religion and Gender in Medieval Culture*, ed. Yoshikawa, pp. 85–102 (pp. 95–6).

[57] Leviticus 17:11.

[58] *The Knowing of Woman's Kind in Childing*, p. 46.

[59] My emphasis. *The Knowing of Woman's Kind in Childing*, p. 54.

[60] *Sickness of Women*, p. 487.

tion of such noxious blood. Furthermore, the disorder caused is reiterated through the affliction of dizziness ('scotayne') and confusion ('stonyeng'), whereby physical malady is compacted by the inversion of reality, and so 'al thyng tournyth vp-so-doun'. Such disorientation is not only testament to the potency attributed to menstrual blood and its unnatural entrapment in the body in medieval culture, but also resonates strikingly with the Proem's first assertion that Margery Kempe's own lifelong condition followed a similar path of 'alle þis thyngys turnyng vp-so-down' (1).

Given the ambivalence in medieval culture towards the 'poisoning fertility' of menstrual blood, several holy women ceased to menstruate as part of an increasing desire to enclose and to control their bodies. Thomas of Cantimpré (1201–72) recorded Lutgard's menstrual cessation and Colette of Corbie's biographer states that she never menstruated: 'a special grace not heard of in others'.[61] A short medical treatise known as 'The Nature of Women' states that 'Wommen of relegion purge noght because of rysyng o nyght and synggyng and ocupacyon in her seruyse her blod wastyth'.[62] Amenorrhoea (the absence of the menses), then, was a desirable trajectory towards sanctification, marking a twofold process of pain removal where the 'anguysch' of menstruation and the spiritual 'pain' of Original Sin were simultaneously eroded and replaced with a state of purified closure. The value of female blood inside or outside the body was imbued with multiple dichotomies: its generative necessity yet capability to destroy; its latent pollution and potential to heal; its existence as a mark of sin and vital means of purgation. The medieval body, then, is permeated by multiple significations, not least the ways in which blood can be divided, reused, redefined, and, by default, made meaningful through its absence. Margery Kempe thus reaches beyond an *imitatio Christi* in her post-reproductive metamorphosis, engendering a transformed fecundity entrenched in her maturing female body. Her surrogate and 'nursing' devotions are further cemented through the inherent connection between female blood and breastmilk in medieval culture as metonymies for divine motherhood. Through menopause – through *losing* blood – she will achieve the same state of somatic closure for which the holy women of her age strove, as more enclosed, more measured, more devout, and more authorised to act on earth as God's surrogate.

---

[61] From Bynum, *Holy Feast and Holy Fast*, pp. 122 and 138.
[62] 'The Nature of Women', in London, British Library, MS Egerton 827, s. 14, fols 28v–30v. This Middle English excerpt is an abbreviated translation of a longer Latin adaptation of Musico's *Gynaecia*, extant only in one copy: Paris, Bibliothèque Nationale, MS lat. 15081 (s. 13–14), fols 86vb–89va, entitled (misleadingly) *Trotula de naturis mulierum*. The Middle English extract, 'The Nature of Women', is edited by Monica Green in 'Obstetrical and Gynecological Texts in Middle English', in *Women's Healthcare in the Medieval West*, IV, pp. 53–88 (pp. 83–8). Compare this with the similar example from *The Knowing of Woman's Kind in Childing* in Chapter 2 of this study, p. 78.

Lost Blood of the Middle Age

Surrogacy as a New Fecundity

The surrogacy hermeneutic that I see as a central operation in the *Book* is anticipated during Margery Kempe's vision of the Nativity, when she becomes a handmaiden to the Virgin Mary. Such emphasis on Christ's infancy was inspired by the 'connection medieval culture drew between Christ's Passion and his infancy', for example in the diptychs that juxtaposed the Virgin Mary with the timeless suffering of the Man of Sorrows.[63] In fact, several of the activities in which Kempe engages mystically are rooted in the everyday rituals of childbirth and lying-in.[64] Such activities are close in nature to those that Poor Clare, the nun to whom the thirteenth-century *Meditationes vitae Christi* were addressed, was urged to undertake. They are 'spiritual exercises' which illustrate not only Kempe's knowledge of such texts but, moreover, the eschatological currency of mothering.[65] In Nicholas Love's *The Mirror of the Blessed Life of Jesus Christ*, Christ's birth is described with brevity and painlessness: 'when tyme of þat blessed birþe was come ... [Jesus went] oute of þat wombe without trauile or sorowe'.[66] The midwife in Love's account is, in fact, the Holy Ghost, as Mary is described as 'swetly clippyng & kissing [Jesus], [and she] leide him in hir barme, & with a full pap, *as she was taght of þe holi gost*, weshe him alle aboute with hir swete milke, & so wrapped him in þe kerchif of her hede, & leide him in þe crach'.[67] With similar brevity, the apocryphal Infancy Gospel of St James, which circulated widely in the Middle Ages, describes the very sudden birth of Christ: 'an intense light appeared inside the cave, so that their eyes could not bear to look. And a little later that light receded until an infant became visible; he took the breast of his mother Mary.'[68] In Margery Kempe's visionary account, the painlessness of Mary's labour is emphatic; indeed, the *Book* passes over the event of childbirth in utter silence, rendering Mary's experience of childbirth antithetic to Kempe's own labouring trauma, a trauma so foundational for her identity that it is recalled in the earliest pages

---

[63] See Kathy Lavezzo, 'Sobs and Sighs Between Women: The Homoerotics of Compassion in *The Book of Margery Kempe*', in *Premodern Sexualities*, ed. Louise Fradenburg and Carla Freccero (New York and London: Routledge, 1996), pp. 175–98 (p. 182). See also Richard Kieckhefer, *Unquiet Souls: Fourteenth-Century Saints and Their Religious Milieu* (Chicago: University of Chicago Press, 1984), pp. 106–7.
[64] See Hellwarth, *The Reproductive Unconscious*, p. 50.
[65] See Gail McMurray Gibson, *The Theatre of Devotion*, pp. 49–51.
[66] Nicholas Love, *The Mirror of the Blessed Life of Jesus Christ*, p. 38.
[67] Ibid. My emphasis.
[68] 'Infancy James 19:15–16', in *The Infancy Gospels of James and Thomas*, ed. Ronald F. Hock (Santa Ross: Polebridge Press, 1995), p. 67. On the influence of the apocryphal gospels see R. Trombley and A. Carr, 'Birth of the Virgin', and 'Presentation of the Virgin', in *The Oxford Dictionary of Byzantium*, ed. Alexander p. Kahzdan (Oxford: Oxford University Press, 1991), vol. 1, p. 291, and vol. 3, p. 1715 respectively.

of the *Book*.[69] In her vision of Mary's childbirth, however, Kempe is in full control, implying some midwifery expertise:

> And þan went þe creatur forth wyth owyr Lady to Bedlam & purchasyd hir herborwe euery nyght wyth gret reuerens, & owyr Lady was receyued wyth glad cher. Also sche beggyd owyr Lady fayr whyte clothys & kerchys for to swathyn in hir Sone whan he wer born, and, whan Ihesu was born, sche ordeyned beddyng for owyr Lady to lyg in wyth hir blyssed Sone. And sythen sche beggyd mete for owyr Lady & hir blyssyd chyld. Aftyrward sche swathyd hym wyth byttr teerys of compassion, hauyng mend of þe scharp deth þat he schuld suffyr for þe lofe of synful men, seying to hym, 'Lord, I schal fare fayr wyth ȝow; I schal not byndyn ȝow soor. I pray ȝow beth not dysplesyd wyth me' (19).

As a replacement wet nurse, and nurturing provider, Kempe begs food for the Virgin and the Christ Child. She undertakes the medieval custom of swaddling the newborn with characteristic emotion, swathing him not in sheets of fabric, but in her 'byttr' tears of compassion, a pseudo-maternal performance that mirrors Mary's anguish at the foot of the cross. And the 'byndyn' that she acknowledges will follow, will be gentle, not 'soor'.[70] In adopting the role of merciful nurse, Kempe is strategically distanced from the future torture and pain that are symbiotic with Christ's birth – the 'scharp deth' about which she is mindful throughout the episode – imagining herself instead as a balsam with which to soften the impending persecution.

The mystical drive to nurse and to feed the Virgin and the infant Christ is likely borne from the common medieval practice of wet nursing, described in most medical texts as a 'given'. *The Knowing of Woman's Kind in Childing* states that after childbirth one should 'tak a norse for hym to kepe þe chylde'.[71] The treatise also advises against allowing the mother to feed her own baby in the early days owing to the purgative effects of the labour. Instead, 'svmme say þat hyt were good for a chyld to drynk þe mylk of ix women be-foore he drank eny of hys modere'.[72] The 'Book on the Conditions of Women' also assumes the presence of a nurse: 'let the child's nurse anoint its

---

[69] The painlessness of Christ's birth is frequently emphasised in medieval writings. In St Bridget of Sweden's vision, Mary is 'rapt into hye contemplacyon ... Then she being thus in prayer ... sothenly in a moment and in the twynklynge off an ey she had borne her chylde ... And that maner off the byrth was so sothenly and so wisely done that I myght not discerne nor perceive how er what membyr off her body she had borne her chylde wythall'. From *Women's Writing in Middle English*, 2nd edn, ed. Alexandra Barratt (Harlow: Longman, 2010), p. 92.

[70] On medieval swaddling praxes see William F. MacLehose, *A Tender Age: Cultural Anxieties over the Child in the Twelfth and Thirteenth Centuries* (New York: Columbia University Press, 2008), pp. 19–20.

[71] *The Knowing of Woman's Kind in Childing*, p. 72.

[72] Ibid. The treatise also states that 'þan [ie. after nine other women's milk] hys modere mylk ys best for hym' (p. 72). Whilst the mother's own milk is recommended from this point, the number of other women who are suggested to feed the baby after birth suggests that wet nursing was considered actively beneficial for the health of the child.

tongue frequently with honey and butter' ('nutrix eius linguam frequenter cum melle et butyro ungat').[73] The writer of 'On Treatments for Women' emphasises the importance of preventing the resumation of menses in the wet nurse for her efficacious milk production: 'let her ... beware provoking her own menses [through sexual activity]' ('et menstruorum prouocationem sibi cauet').[74] Such assumptions about the presence of wet nurses firstly indicate the practice of wet nursing as a cultural essential, particularly for the urban upper classes. This is something that Valerie Fildes has termed 'an ancient, deeply-ingrained and widely accepted social custom', which increased from the eleventh century in western Europe and was common by the late Middle Ages.[75] Such cultural normalcy is also evident in Bernard of Gordon's *Regimen sanitatis*, which judgementally states that wet nursing is often required because 'women nowadays are too delicate or too haughty or they do not like the inconvenience'.[76] The status of wet nurses as necessarily non-reproductive – women who have given birth but whose subsequent wet-nursing role is contingent on their surrogacy as opposed to their maternity – hinges upon the concomitant dormancy of the menstrual cycle (or, more importantly, the rejection of reproductive potential). This model, then, is strikingly accessible to Kempe in middle age, opening an adoptive pathway that enables her gradual transformation towards maternal substitution.[77]

The surrogacy hermeneutic develops more prominently on Kempe's pilgrimage to Rome in 1414–15, when she is in her early forties. As she journeys with Richard, a broken-backed man whom she persuades to accompany her, she encounters two Grey Friars and a woman, who had with them

---

73 'Book on the Conditions of Women', in *The Trotula*, pp. 108–9.

74 'Book on the Conditions of Women', in *The Trotula*, pp. 110–11.

75 Valerie Fildes, *Breasts, Bottles and Babies: A History of Infant Feeding* (Edinburgh: Edinburgh University Press, 1986), p. 100. See also *Medieval and Renaissance Lactations: Images, Rhetorics, Practices*, ed. Jutta Gisela Sperling (London and New York: Routledge, 2013); Sarah Blaffer-Hrdy, 'Fitness Tradeoffs in the History and Evolution of Delegated Mothering with Special Reference to Wet-Nursing', *Ethology and Sociobiology*, 13 (1992), 409–42; Luke Demaitre, 'The Idea of Childhood and Child Care in Medical Writings of the Middle Ages', *Journal of Psychohistory*, 4 (1977), 461–90; Leah Otis, 'Municipal Wet Nurses in Fifteenth-Century Montpellier', in *Women and Work in Pre-Industrial Europe*, ed. Barbara Hanawalt (Bloomington: Indiana University Press, 1986), pp. 83–93; and Christine Klapisch-Zuber, *Women, Family and Ritual in Renaissance Italy*, trans. Lydia Cochrane (Chicago and London: University of Chicago Press, 1985), pp. 132–64.

76 Fildes, *Breasts, Bottles and Babies*, p. 47.

77 The practice of wet nursing in medieval Europe was commonplace not only amongst the nobility but also the upper echelons of the urban population who regarded it as a symbol of status. See Shulamith Shahar, *Childhood in the Middle Ages* (London and New York: Routledge, 1990), p. 61, and pp. 55–76. Since Margery Kempe was of the wealthy merchant class, it is probable that she would have employed wet nurses for her own children. Kempe's father was John Brunham, several times mayor of Lynn and Member of Parliament, and Kempe boasts to her husband in the early stages of her text that 'sche was comyn of worthy kenred' (9). On Kempe's 'worthy kin' see Susan Maddock, 'Margery Kempe's Home Town and Worthy Kin', in *Encountering the Book of Margery Kempe*, ed. Kalas and Varnam (forthcoming).

'an asse þe which bar a chyst & an ymage þerin mad aftyr our Lord' (77). This Christ-image – embodying the popular medieval devotion to the infant Christ – becomes a focus of female reverence on the journey, a multilayered worship-performance whereby the mothering, as well as the doll, provoke Kempe's boisterous sobs:[78]

> And þe woman the which had þe image in þe chist, whan þei comyn in good citeys, sche toke owt þe image owt of hir chist & sett it in worshepful wyfys lappys. & þei wold puttyn schirtys þerup-on & kyssyn it as þei it had ben God hym-selfe. &, whan þe creatur sey þe worship & þe reuerens þat þey dedyn to þe image, sche was takyn wyth swet deuocyon & swet meditacyons þat sche wept wyth gret sobbyng & lowde crying. & sche was meuyd in so mych þe mor as, whil sche was in Inglond, sche had hy meditacyons in þe byrth & þe childhode of Crist, & sche thankyd God for-as-meche as sche saw þes creaturys han so gret feyth in þat sche sey wyth hir bodily eyelych as sche had be-forn wyth hir gostly eye. Whan þes good women seyn þis creatur wepyn, sobbyn, & cryen so wondirfully & mythtyly þat sche was nerhand ouyrcomyn þerwyth, þan þei ordeyned a good soft bed & leyd hir þerup-on & comfortyd hir as mech as þei myth for owyr Lordys lofe, blyssed mot he ben (77–8).

Kempe's emphatic crying at the sight of the wives' nurturing devotions to the Christ-doll has been interpreted by Kathy Lavezzo as a homosocial event: the doll is not only 'a conduit for the ladies' original maternal desires but it enables the condensation of a number of female same-sex fantasies', including a desire for the holy mother, Mary.[79] Lavezzo's Freudian reading of this episode appropriates the doll image with a tradable value, regarding it as a 'commodity' which facilitates a 'traffic in Christ', allowing the women to access their feminine needs and desires. While the doll does allow for a symbolic performance between women, shared through their socio-maternal identification with childrearing, it also facilitates a displacement strategy where Kempe's reciprocal, surrogate activities illustrate her conflicting metamorphosis as a middle-aged holy woman. Indeed, it is salient that the Christ-doll is offered to the local *wyfys* specifically, and, given that she has recently abrogated her own life as a wife and mother in favour of chastity and pilgrimage, Kempe's tears may also reveal a latent grief for her own surrendered reproductivity, especially since, as McAvoy has persuasively argued, she has probably left a baby back in England.[80]

---

[78] Hope Emily Allen suggests that a chapel in St Margaret's in Lynn may have stimulated her devotion to the Infancy of Christ. See *BMK*, ed. Meech and Allen, p. 297, n. 77/17.

[79] Kathy Lavezzo, 'Sobs and Sighs between Women', in *Premodern Sexualities*, ed. Fradenburg and Freccero, p. 186. For an explanation of maternal and nuptial liturgy and female performances, see Bynum, *Fragmentation and Redemption*, p. 198. See also Ursula Schlegel, 'The Christchild as Devotional Image in Medieval Italian Sculpture: A Contribution to Ambrogio Lorenzetti Studies', *The Art Bulletin* 52 (March 1970), 1–10; and Elizabeth Petroff, *Medieval Women's Visionary Literature* (Oxford: Oxford University Press, 1986), p. 54, n. 22.

[80] See McAvoy, *Authority and the Female Body*, p. 56. See also McAvoy's response to Laura L. Howes' article, 'On the Birth of Margery Kempe's Last Child', *Modern Philology*, 90

Kempe's reaction to God's disclosure of her most recent pregnancy was one of dismay, as it would encumber her literal and spiritual journey: 'how xal I þan do for kepyng of my chylde?' (48). God promises that he 'xal ordeyn for an kepar' (48) for the child so that Kempe may be free to continue with her planned pilgrimage to the Holy Land. It is probable that the 'kepar' would have been a wet nurse, caring for the child in her own home in Kempe's physical absence. But once Kempe is 'newly delyueryd of [the] chyld', she is divinely informed that 'sche xuld no mor chyldren beryn' (38). Christ's declaration is qualified immediately with '& þerfor he bad hyr gon Norwych' to disclose his approval of the vicar of St Stephen's, juxtaposing Kempe's liberation from reproductivity with her spiritual elevation as God's own legate. The *Book* is silent about this last, forsaken baby, a narrative side-lining that implies that abandoning the child was a necessary religious sacrifice.[81] However, I do not think that a sacrificial narrative is what Kempe strives for here, although this does play a part in her wider imitation of the Virgin. Many scholars have considered the reasons for the narrative absence of her children in the *Book*, especially as she gave birth to so many. Given her merchant social class and that class's custom of employing wet nurses, the absence of children in the *Book* (save her adult son) is most likely due to her habitual use of wet nurses throughout her reproductive lifespan. As children were generally weaned at the age of two, infants required a wet nurse for some time. Kempe, therefore, might have had only limited relationships with her children, especially in their early years.[82] Moreover, once her economic focus transitioned to the spiritual, the employment of wet nurses would be a pragmatic necessity for the enaction of pilgrimage and contemplation. The almost total subordination of child-narratives within the *Book* is thus a product of two powerful forces: the social trend of entrusting one's children to surrogates, and Kempe's own motivation to construct a spiritually rooted life/text narrative.

Medical texts held that a wet nurse must be reasonably close to childbirth in order to be efficacious. Avicenna had stipulated that 'the nurse's own baby should neither be quite grown up, nor less than one or two months old', and that she must have given birth to a boy, carried to 'full term'.[83] This understanding persists into later medieval medical writings: the 'Book on the

---

(1992), 220–5. McAvoy contests Howes' claim that Kempe gave birth to her last child en route to the Holy Land. See McAvoy, 'Margery's Last Child', *Notes and Queries*, 46 (1999), 181–3.

[81] On child sacrifice, see Barbara Newman, *From Virile Woman to Woman Christ: Studies in Medieval Religion and Literature* (Philadelphia: University of Pennsylvania Press, 1995), pp. 76–107.

[82] The propensity for wet nurse usage amongst the upper and prosperous urban classes meant that these women would often give birth 'to their fullest biological capacity', largely because the employment of wet nurses resulted in them losing the natural (albeit unreliable) contraceptive effect offered by lactation. Kempe's fourteen children are thus further suggestive of her systematic use of wet nurses. See Shahar, *Childhood in the Middle Ages*, p. 64 and p. 70.

[83] Avicenna *Canon*, adapt. Bakhtiar, vol 1., pp. 364–5.

Conditions of Women' states that the wet nurse must be 'not too close to her last birth nor too far removed from it either' ('que non sit patui uicina neque multum remota').[84] *The Knowing of Woman's Kind in Childing* requires her to have 'twyes trauelyd of chyld'.[85] Given that Kempe herself is apparently recently delivered of a child when in Rome, and the fact that the terminus of her reproductive life is officially sanctioned by Christ, she paradoxically meets certain medical wet-nursing requirements. The surrogacy strategies that are developed in the Holy Land are thus teleological responses to both the socio-medical perception of the postpartum female body as being 'ripe' for nursing, and the cultural preference for the employment of wet nurses. Furthermore, the ubiquitous iconography of the Virgin and child, the infant Christ often portrayed as nursing at the breast, would resonate more power-fully after Kempe's conversion and desire for Marian identification.[86]

The surrogate praxes in the *Book* are performed, then, in a paradoxically post-reproductive, medicalised, and holy framework. As medical texts attest, the health of the nurse was paramount – she must have the correct diet, physical condition, and behaviour (including sexual abstinence) – because breastmilk was thought to have pathological potential at the same time as being vital and nourishing. *The Knowing of Woman's Kind in Childing* advises that the nurse should be:

> yong & in good stat, þat hath twyes trauelyd of chyld, þat be of good [colour] & hath large brestys & not to schort pappys & þat þe openynge of them be not to wyde, & wel a-vysd & not wrathfoll, & þat sche lovyth þe chylde with all here hert ne þat sche be not dronklew of ouer-moche drynk, but euer let here ete wele & lette here sume tyme travayle þat sche fall not costyff [constipated]. And þat sche entermet not of dedeuyt [sexual pleasure] of dewery [love-making], for of þat my3ght fall here purgacyon & tak a-way here mylk & mak hym dry.[87]

This example cites youth as a precondition of wet nursing, precluding Kempe in the literal sense. However, as well as having recently given birth, she also fulfils several other criteria – increased wisdom, the absence of anger, love in her heart, and sexual abstinence – demonstrating her multivalent suitability as a surrogate. Furthermore, the imbrication of physical and moral health indicates what William MacLehose terms 'a symbiosis between nurse and infant'.[88] Such symbiotic potentiality illuminates Margery Kempe's imitation of the surrogate model in Rome as a deliberate harnessing of the intimate and

---

[84] 'Book on the Conditions of Women', in *The Trotula*, pp. 110–11.
[85] *The Knowing of Woman's Kind in Childing*, p. 72.
[86] This iconography included representations of the *Virgo lactans*, and Eve nursing her child, portrayed for example, on the bronze doors at Hildesheim and Verona. See Mary McLaughlin, 'Survivors and Surrogates: Children and Parents from the Ninth to the Thirteenth Centuries', in *Medieval Families*, ed. Neel, pp. 20–124 (p. 115). On Bridget of Sweden's own nursing of her children, see Morris, *St Birgitta of Sweden*, p. 52.
[87] *The Knowing of Woman's Kind in Childing*, p. 72.
[88] MacLehose, *A Tender Age*, p. 24. See also MacLehose, 'Nurturing Danger: High

social role of the nurse for fostering a closer connection to the infant Christ.[89] In exploiting the wet-nursing subtext, a deeper bond with the Christ Child, to whom she must therefore be inextricably tied, is established.[90]

Given these surrogate qualifications and resonances, Kempe's geographical and personal odyssey imposes manifold significances on the effigy of Jesus, stirring in her a pain that evokes not only the infant Christ, but perhaps also the maternal sacrifice that complete devotion expiates. The women's mothering of the doll, which mirrors the Virgin Mary's mothering of the Christ Child, is doubly re-enacted by the wives' re-mothering of Kempe, who 'wepyn, sobbyn, & cryen so wonderfully & mythtyly' (78) that she prompts the women to attend to her, laying her on a bed and comforting her. The pain of the Passion and the Virgin's lamentation, signified materially by the Christ-doll, is displaced to Kempe, whose own suffering becomes the primary image of the episode, locating her fully as a privileged surrogate of Christic and Marian pain, herself requiring nursing by God's wifely disciples.

Kempe's piety towards the Christ Child develops during a visit to the Dominican house in Lynn during a life-phase that Santha Bhattacharji terms her 'quieter' years, between 1418 and 1433.[91] In the Chapel of Our Lady (which contained a magnificent image of the Virgin Mary), she experiences a dream-like vision. In a mimesis of the mystical swaddling of the Christ Child and the literal swaddling of the Christ-doll, she takes 'gostly joye' in witnessing the Virgin swathing her son with the lightest touch:

> & sodenly sche sey, hir thowt, owr Lady in þe fairest syght þat euyr sche say, holdyng a fayr white kerche in hir hand & seying to hir, 'Dowtyr, wilt þu se my Sone?' & a-non forth-wyth sche say owr Lady han hyr blissyd Sone in hir hand & swathyd hym ful lytely in þe white kerche þat sche myth wel be-holdyn how sche dede. Þe creatur had þan a newe gostly joye & a newe gostly comfort, wheche was so meruelyows þat *sche cowde neuyr tellyn it as sche felt it* (209).

The ineffability of the vision – she could 'neuyr tellyn it as sche *felt* it' – illustrates the visceral profundity with which Mary's motherhood is appropriated in *imitatio Mariae*. Indeed, that the Virgin herself requests that Kempe

Medieval Medicine and the Problem(s) of the Child', in *Medieval Mothering*, ed. Parsons and Wheeler, pp. 3–25.

[89] The importance of this symbiosis can be seen through the power with which wet nurses were accorded. Aldobrandino of Siena states that she 'should be healthy, as far as one can tell, for sickly nurses kill children straight away'. See *Medieval Medicine: A Reader*, ed. Wallis, pp. 497–8.

[90] By the early thirteenth century wet nurses also mothered, or 'nannied', their charges. See McLaughlin, 'Survivors and Surrogates', in *Medieval Families*, ed. Neel, p. 117.

[91] On the image of the Virgin, see Meech and Allen, *BMK*, p. 338, n 209/15–16. Prior to this account, Kempe has just mentioned her pilgrimages to Jerusalem and Rome and her vow of chastity (209). The immediacy of this recollection, and the likelihood of some chronology in the narrative recollection, as well as the fact that this visit occurs back in Lynn, suggests that the event occurs between 1418 and 1433 (and thus when she was aged between 45 and 60). See Bhattacharji, *God is an Earthquake*, pp. 18–21.

witness the tending of her son immerses her more indispensably within the event and reinforces the mothering imperative that underlies her surrogate strategies. Divine confirmation is received on her way home from a visit to see the Abbess of Denney, where she feels 'heuy' that the boats have all departed and she may fail to do God's bidding.[92] In comfort, 'owr Lord mad a maner of thankyng to hir, for-as-meche as sche in contemplacyon & in meditacyon had ben hys Modyrs maydyn & *holpyn to kepyn hym in hys childhood* & so forth in-to þe tyme of hys deth' (203). Such mystical recognition of Kempe's duties as his handmaid and nurse ('keeping' Jesus in the same way that a 'keeper' was secured for her own child) depicts them as valuable services, practically and spiritually. Furthermore, during the extended private sermon that follows between God and Kempe, the words 'seruyse', 'seruyn', or 'serue' frequently repeat, connecting her surrogate duties with service to God, and therefore presenting them as valid offerings for spiritual promotion.[93] Indeed, the Church's support of exogamy extirpated 'the custom of adoption practised in Rome … introducing in its stead, spiritual parentage as represented by the godparents, and with it a new system of spiritual affinity': a promotion of the very spiritual surrogacy through which Kempe accesses her holy ambitions.[94]

Nowhere is Kempe's desired surrogacy more evident than in a brief passage within the same few pages of narrative as the infancy visions. Suggesting a

---

[92] In attempting to situate this episode within Kempe's life span, there are two significant factors to consider. First, as Hope Emily Allen has indicated, the request from the abbess for Kempe's visits, would have been considered weighty. As this house of Franciscan nuns was a strict enclosure, such visits would require formal, 'sometimes papal', permission. This suggests that Kempe was at an advanced enough stage in her life and spiritual maturity to be invited on these terms. Second, Kempe mentions that the visit takes place during 'pestylens-tyme' (202). While the precise epidemic or date is uncertain, several epidemics occurred during the first third of the fifteenth century, including a pestilence mentioned in the *Annales Monasterii de Bermundeseia*, in Norfolk specifically, in 1420. Other possible matches are 1427 and 1431. Even at the earliest date of 1420, this would position Kempe at the age of 47, and therefore at a likely peri-menopausal or menopausal life stage. See Allen, *BMK*, p. 337, n. 202/6 and n. 202/16.

[93] The value placed on Kempe's surrogate duties reflects a society where high mortality levels necessitated surrogates of various kinds. Siblings, aunts, uncles, institutions like foundling hospitals and private adoptions were sources of guardianship. Factors such as epidemics and plagues, famine, poverty and malnutrition meant that children who themselves survived these earthly challenges would be likely to be orphaned or semi-orphaned at a young age. See McLaughlin, 'Survivors and Surrogates', in *Medieval Families*, ed. Neel, p. 65. On the medieval population, see Josiah Cox Russell, 'Medieval Population', *Social Forces*, 15 (1937), 503–11. See also Pamela Nightingale, 'Some new evidence of Crises and Trends of Mortality in Late Medieval England', *Past & Present*, 187 (2005), 33–68; and Mary E. Lewis and Rebecca Gowland, 'Brief and Precarious Lives: Infant Mortality in Contrasting Sites from Medieval and Post-Medieval England (AD 850–1859)', *American Journal of Physical Anthropology*, 134 (2007), 117–29. The emergence of foundling homes spread rapidly. Pope Innocent III established foundling hospitals in Saxia, the legacy of which Kempe may have been aware. See McLaughlin, 'Survivors and Surrogates', in *Medieval Families*, ed. Neel, p. 122.

[94] Shulamith Shahar, *Childhood in the Middle Ages*, p. 73.

similar chronology because of its concurrent recollection, the passage depicts the Christ Child suckling at the Virgin's breasts *within* Kempe's soul, positioning her as a vessel of divine sustenance, sanctioned to internalise, to almost ingest, the ultimate mother–child relationship: 'And also, dowtyr, þu clepist my Modyr for to comyn in-to þi sowle & takyn me in hir armys & leyn me to hir brestys & ȝeuyn me sokyn' (210). The enclosure that Kempe provides for the nursing Jesus within her own soul-womb is a surrogacy that transmogrifies the bodily borders of motherhood in a totalised possession of the infant Christ.[95]

Such contemplative experiences were no doubt inspired by the popular medieval iconography of Christ's own maternity. The Israelites are frequently shown in the Old Testament to be conceived in God's womb, being fed with God's milk.[96] Maternal imagery increased from the eleventh century, in writings such as those of Anselm of Canterbury (1033–1109) and Julian of Norwich, whose affective piety focused on the accessibility of God through his humanity and maternity.[97] Julian writes:

> The moder may geve her childe sucke her milke. But oure precious moder Jhesu, he may fede us with himselfe, and doth full curtesly and full tenderly with the blessed sacrament that is precious fode of very life … The moder may ley her childe tenderly to her brest. But oure tender mother Jhesu, he may homely lede us into his blessed brest by his swet, open side, and shewe us therein perty of the godhed and the joyes of heven, with gostly sekernesse of endless blisse.[98]

For Julian, Christ suckles his *even cristen* with the sustenance of his sweet, wounded body, made literal through the sacrament which engenders a particularly affective response from Margery Kempe in the *Book*. Guerric, Abbot of Igny (d. 1157), describes Christ as having 'breasts … He is a father in virtue of natural creation … He is a mother, too, in the mildness of his affection, and a *nurse*' (my emphasis).[99] A Middle English translation of Aelred's *De institutione inclusarum*, originally written for a female recluse, indicates familiarity with a surrogacy hermeneutic, as it advises the reader to meditate on

---

[95] Other holy models of maternal nursing may have provided Kempe with the desire to replicate the maternal feeding that she may have previously bypassed. Catherine of Siena's mother had twenty-four children, but she reportedly only breastfed Catherine. Bernard of Clairvaux was breastfed by his mother. See Fildes, *Breasts, Bottles and Babies*, p. 48.

[96] 'That you may suck, and be filled with the breasts of her consolations: that you may milk out, and flow with delights, from the abundance of her glory. For thus saith the Lord: Behold I will bring upon her as it were a river of peace, and as an overflowing torrent the glory of the Gentiles, which you shall suck; you shall be carried at the breasts, and upon the knees they shall caress you'. Isaiah 66:11–12.

[97] See Caroline Walker Bynum, *Jesus as Mother*, p. 130.

[98] 'A Revelation of Love', Ch. 60, in *The Writings of Julian of Norwich*, ed. Watson and Jenkins, p. 313.

[99] From the second sermon for SS. Peter and Paul, chap. 2, *Sermons* 2: 384–6. In Bynum, *Jesus as Mother*, p. 122.

the Christ Child playing, on 'hou seruisable he was to his moder, and anoþer tyme how swet and gracious he was to his nursche'.[100] 'Nursche' in this context denotes Joseph, and thus 'foster-father': another type of surrogate and illustrative of the elasticity of the concept in the medieval imaginary.[101] The transference between bodily fluids in medical theory – breast milk is transformed menstrual blood, as we have seen – extends therefore to theological understanding: Christ's blood, in the form of wine, means that water and milk flow between and within each other, constructing an overarching nursing motif.[102] This connection is revealed to Kempe at an early stage of her spiritual journey when God ravishes her spirit and ordains her to forego the eating of meat. Instead, she 'schalt etyn my flesch & my blod, þat is þe very body of Crist in þe Sacrament of þe Awter' (17). On describing these revelations to the anchorite at the Friar Preachers, he articulates the very transformation that medico-culture prescribes, by stating, 'Dowtyr, 3e sowkyn euyn on Crystys brest, and 3e han an ernest-peny of Heuyn' (18). As receiver of Christ's milk, blood, and body, and thus now in a state of evolving grace, Kempe is both recipient of divine sustenance and authorised provider, given her promised place in heaven.[103]

As well as her visionary acts of surrogacy, Kempe's affective piety translates to earthly infants. In Rome a poor woman calls her into her house, offering her rest and a drink. Beyond this act of kindness, Kempe is moved by the nursing infant there:

> & sche had a lytel manchylde sowkyng on hir brest, þe which sowkyd o while on þe moderys brest; an-oþer while it ran to þis creatur, þe moder syttyng ful of sorwe & sadness. Þan þis creatur brast al in-to wepyng, as þei sche had seyn owr Lady & hir sone in tyme of hys Passyon, & had so many of holy thowts þat sche myth neuyr tellyn þe haluendel, but euyr sat & wept plentyvowsly a long tyme þat þe powr woman, hauyng compassion of hir wepyng, preyd hir to sesyn, not knowyng why sche wept. Þan owr Lord Ihesu Crist seyd to þe creatur, 'Thys place is holy' (94).

[100] *Aelred of Rievaulx's De institutione inclusarum: Two Middle English Translations*, ed. John Ayto and Alexandra Barratt, EETS o.s. 287 (London, New York and Toronto: Oxford University Press, 1984), ll. 639–41, p. 41.
[101] MED s.v. noriีce, 1(a) A wet nurse; nursemaid, governess; foster mother; foster parents; (b) a man who takes care of a child, foster father; a tutor; as a foster father. On the use of terms 'foster-brother' and 'foster-father' to express transcendent relationships, see John Eastburn Boswell, 'The Abandonment of Children and the Ancient and Medieval Family', in *Medieval Families*, ed. Neel, pp. 234–72. The term *fostermoder* can refer more to a surrogate mother than to a wet nurse. See Danièle Alexandre-Bidon and Didier Lett, *Children in the Middle Ages: Fifth to Fifteenth Centuries*, trans. Jody Gladding (Notre Dame, Indiana: University of Notre Dame Press, 1999), pp. 18–20.
[102] See Bynum, *Jesus as Mother*, p. 122 and pp. 132–3; and Cadden, *Meanings of Sex Difference*, pp. 119–30.
[103] Miraculous tales about women beyond childbearing age suddenly being able to lactate might also have entered Kempe's frame of reference, given the religious works to which she had access via her confessors. See Fildes, *Breasts, Bottles and Babies*, p. 53.

The image of the breastfeeding infant provokes a displaced devotion to the Christ Child, transcending the very human activity of the nursing mother to one of spiritual signification. As in the Christ-doll episode, Kempe's weeping becomes the primary focus, causing the mother, already full of 'sorwe & sadnes', presumably because of her poverty, to show her compassion to Kempe, praying her to cease her distressing lamentation.[104] The scene is an edifying one, however, as Kempe leaves to continue her sojourn around Rome, bearing witness to further destitution and 'thank[ing] God hyly of þe pouerte þat sche was in, trostyng þerthorw to be partynyr wyth hem in meryte' (94). Here Kempe literally follows in the footsteps of Bridget of Sweden, who, after the death of her husband, Ulf, and concomitant post-reproductivity, 'went in pylgremage to Rome' at the age of forty-two, 'ther to abyde in the lyfe of penaunce', and 'she lyuyd the resydue of hir lyfe in the cyty of Rome'.[105] The impoverished, nursing mother thus becomes a reverential model through her projection of the Mary-and-child image, sharing her milk with Kempe and facilitating her access to God's salvific maternity.

Replacement or surrogate strategies occur elsewhere in Rome, when, after her mystical marriage to the Godhead, Kempe reacts emotively to any sighting of a boy child, kissing him '*in þe stede of Criste*':

> Sche was so meche affectyd to þe manhode of Crist þat whan sche sey women in Rome beryn children in her armys, ȝyf sche myth wetyn þat þei wer ony men children, sche schuld þan cryin, roryn, & wepyn as þei sche had seyn Crist in hys childhode. And, yf sche myth an had hir wille, oftyn-tymes sche wolde a takyn þe childeryn owt of þe moderys armys & kissed hem in þe stede of Criste (86).

Margery Kempe retains her desire to achieve substitutional access to the Christ Child when back in Lynn during the years spent at home after her pilgrimage to Rome between 1415 and 1424, and when the boisterousness of her tears decreases. On meeting a group of women with children in their arms, Kempe enquires:

> ȝyf þer wer any man-childe a-mongys hem, & þe women seyd, 'Nay'. Þan was þe mende so raueschyd in-to þe childhood of Crist for desir þat sche had for to see hym þat sche mith not beryn it but fel downe & wept & cryid so sor þat it was merueyl to her it (200).

Such grief and melancholic lamentation are provoked by Kempe's unfulfilled longing to *see* the Christ Child – to experience, kiss, and embrace the manhood of God corporeally, to retain his tangible presence.

---

[104] We are reminded by this weeping that Kempe is still in her early forties and not yet subject to the 'drier' time of the age of full menopause, at around fifty, nor the cessation of her tears at the age of fifty-one.

[105] Thomas Gascoigne, 'Lyfe of seynt Birgette', in *The Myroure of Our Ladye*, pp. xlvii–lix (p. li and p. lvi).

Margery Kempe's self-appointed role as surrogate is externally enforced and validated in Rome. Relying on people's charity for her meals, she meets a man named Marcelle, who 'bad hir to mete' for two days of the week, and whose wife was 'gret wyth childe' (93–4). Her spiritual demeanour clearly stirred feeling in others, as the couple were 'hyly desiring to haue had þis creatur to godmodyr to hir childe whan it had ben born', despite the fact that 'sche abood not so long in Rome' (94). In the sharing of food, brought about by an act of Christian charity, Kempe affirms the couple's faith through her symbolic situation as an impoverished pilgrim and speaker of God's word. The impact of her company and ministry is not only a foreshadowing of things to come, but also displays the couple's desire to consolidate this new relationship in God through the appointment of Kempe as their child's ordained godmother. Kempe thus becomes not only a surrogate parent, but also a surrogate for God on earth through the godparent's didactic position of wisdom and spiritual understanding.[106] This broader medieval paradigm of godparenting as a form of surrogacy was considered so solemn that failure to fulfil one's godparent duties was considered a sin. It was a precondition of the role that the chosen godparent had great knowledge of the tenets of the faith, as they became, in Shahar's words, a 'spiritual relative'.[107] The tradition of spiritual kinship developed from the early Middle Ages and was important because 'the medieval family sustained itself and its members by fostering an alternative network based on the voluntary tie of godparenhood to save some people from the problems [of family failure]'.[108]

Indeed, the corpus of medical texts emphasises the importance of morality in the wet-nurse surrogate. Avicenna believed that the nurse should be of 'good moral character'.[109] This is echoed in *The Knowing of Woman's Kind in Childing*, which requires the nurse to be 'wel-a-vysed & not wrathfoll & þat sche lovyth þe chylde with all here hert', and that 'sche entermet not of dedeuyt of dewery [sexual pleasure from love-making]' (72).[110] Similarly, Bartholomaeus Anglicus insists that 'þe *vertu* of þe norische [nurse]' is paramount, 'For of good *disposicioun* of milke foode comeþ good disposicioun of þe childe', an ideology that conflates the nurse's temperament and moral fortitude with the child's healthy physiology and constitution.[111] Even

---

[106] On godparents and spiritual kinship, see Joseph H. Lynch, *Godparents and Kinship in Early Medieval Europe* (Princeton: Princeton University Press, 1986). See also Rob Lutton, 'Godparenthood, Kinship, and Piety in Tenterden, England 1449–1537', in *Love, Marriage and Family Ties in the Later Middle Ages*, ed. Isabel Davis, Miriam Müller, and Sarah Rees Jones (Turnhout: Brepols, 2003), pp. 217–34.

[107] See Shulamith Shahar, *Childhood in the Middle Ages*, pp. 117–18.

[108] Steven A. Epstein, 'The Medieval Family: A Place of Refuge and Sorrow', in *Medieval Families*, ed. Neel, pp. 405–28 (p. 417).

[109] Avicenna, *Canon*, 15.2.2., vol. 1, adapt. Bakhtiar, p. 362.

[110] *The Knowing of Woman's Kind in Childing*, p. 72.

[111] My emphasis. *On the Properties of Things*, vol. 1, p. 299.

emotional health and happiness when feeding are influential: 'fede hym whan he ys mery [happy] & þan schall none corrupcyon hym greve ne entire with-in hym'.[112] The symbiotic moral, nutritional, and dispositional characteristics of the nurse and the infant thus illustrate the vast spiritual and salvific potentiality of the surrogate, a paradigm in which Kempe becomes immersed.

It is striking, therefore, that Margery Kempe, in her middle years of maturation, embodies the totality (bar youth) of these wet-nursing virtues. Her vowed chastity, mystical perspicacity, and correlative wisdom position her as a prime candidate for the intermediary status of the nurse.[113] She thus constitutes a fusion of mature-nursing credentials based on the medieval value system of routine surrogate use, her new status as godparent a formalisation of this powerful nexus. Such a status is compounded by the fact that, at least in London, civic law held that on the death of a male citizen, his underage children became the responsibility of the mayor and aldermen.[114] Since Margery Kempe's father was elected mayor of Lynn five times and was alderman of the Holy Trinity Guild from 1394 to 1401, it is probable that she was familiar with questions of guardianship and surrogacy in civic as well as spiritual terms.[115] A 'surrogate ministry' thus evolves where her familial experience, moral character, and privileged insight into the word of God itself 'foster' spiritual privilege.[116] The godparent surrogacy occurs again in Rome when a gentlewoman asks Kempe to be 'godmodyr of hir childe', whom she names 'aftyr Seynt Brigyt, for they haddyn knowlach of hir in hir lyue-tyme' (94). The simple narrative qualification '& so sche dede' suggests the matter-of-factness with which Kempe dictated the decision to accept another godchild to her amanuensis, the short sentence indicating the instinctiveness with which she adopts the role. The Bridgettine connection adds power to her decision, of course, enabling Kempe not only to tread more forcefully in St Bridget's footsteps and to forge relationships with her acquaintances, but also to become a surrogate to Bridget's namesake. In direct application of the vision that situates Kempe as handmaid to the Virgin and Christ Child, here she imitates another holy mother – St Bridget – via the spiritual mothering accorded to the godmother.

---

[112] *The Knowing of Woman's Kind in Childing*, p. 74.

[113] On the correlative dangers of sub-standard nursing see *The Knowing of Woman's Kind in Childing*, p. 76; and the 'Book on the Conditions of Women', in *The Trotula*, pp. 110–11. See also MacLehose, *A Tender Age*, pp. 26–8.

[114] See Caroline M. Barron and Claire A. Martin, 'Mothers and Orphans in Fourteenth Century London', in *Motherhood, Religion, and Society in Medieval Europe, 400–1400*, ed. Conrad Leyser and Lesley Smith (Farnham: Ashgate, 2011), pp. 281–96 (p. 281).

[115] On Margery Kempe's father, John Kempe, see Goodman, *Margery Kempe and Her World*, p. 49. On Margery Kempe's own possible godmother, see Susan Maddock, 'Margery Kempe's Home Town and Worthy Kin', in *Encountering the Book of Margery Kempe*, ed. Kalas and Varnam.

[116] Liz Herbert McAvoy employs this term in *Authority and the Female Body*, p. 51.

Christ's own estimation of the surrogacy matrix is evident in the biblical account of the time leading up to his crucifixion: 'When Jesus therefore had seen his mother and the disciple standing whom he loved, he saith to his mother: Woman, behold thy son. After that, he saith to the disciple: Behold thy mother. And from that hour, the disciple took her to his own.'[117] Such adoption is transferred to Kempe, who has accrued 'gret fauowr a-mong the pepyl' (94) in Rome. An English priest, who had heard of her in England and 'longyd hyly to spekyn [with her] 3yf God wolde grawntyn hym grace' (96), directly requests her maternal ministrations: 'Þan be inqwyryng he cam in-to þe place wher þat sche was, & ful humbely & mekely *he clepyd hir modyr*, preying hir for charite to receyuen hym as hir sone. Sche seyd þat he was wolcom to God & to hir as to hys owyn modyr (96). The pseudo-family dynamic of the relationship is also reciprocal; the priest, who 'wolde … no lengar suffyr hir to beggyn hir mete', insists that she eat meals with his company (96–7). Kempe, meanwhile, recognises in him a willing recipient of her teaching and revelations: '& þan sche, discuryng þe preuyte of hert, reuelyd what grace God wrowt in hir sowle thorw hys holy inspiracyon & sumwhat of hir maner of leuyng' (96). Thereafter, they employ the proper nouns *Modyr* and *Sone* as their forms of address to each other as active participants in a surrogate mother–child template.[118] Indeed, when the priest becomes afraid of threats from enemies during their passage back to England, Kempe responds with a fusion of mothering and spiritual discernment: 'Nay, sone, 3e schal far ryth wel & gon saf be þe grace of God' (100–1). He is reassured by her ministry and Kempe is happy to have the company of an adopted son, 'trusty[ng] meche in hir felyngys and mad hir as good cher be þe wey *as 3yf he had ben hir owyn sone born of hir body*' (101). Like the infant boys in Rome whom Kempe 'kisse[s] in þe stede of Criste' (86), the priest becomes not only a substitute for her own children, left resolutely in England as symbols of a past reproductive life, but also a surrogate child *in þe stede of Criste*, a figure through whom she can project her love and tenderness towards the divine.

This episode serves to exemplify the multivalent ways in which Kempe develops her surrogacy, utilising its cultural and spiritual capital on her trajectory towards holiness. However, after the Easter of 1415 Kempe departs from Rome and arrives in Norwich, where the spiritual merit of her pilgrimage is placed under scrutiny by an anchorite, possibly of the name Thomas Brakleye.[119] Despite the anchorite having once been a faithful supporter, recent gossip and 'euyl langage' turn him against her, causing him to ask

---

[117] John 19:26.

[118] 'The term *fostermoder*, found very frequently in Anglo-Saxon literature from the High Middle Ages, undoubtedly refers more to a surrogate mother than to a wet nurse'. See Alexandre-Bidon and Didier Lett, *Children in the Middle Ages: Fifth to Fifteenth Centuries*, trans. Jody Gladding (Notre Dame, Indiana: University of Notre Dame Press, 1999), esp. pp. 18–20.

[119] Probably May 1415, when Kempe was forty-two. On the chronology and an explanation of the anchorite's identity see Windeatt, *BMK*, p. 214, n. 3352 and p. 216, n. 3389.

'wher sche had don hir chylde þe which was begotyn & born whil sche was owte, as he had herd seyde' (103).[120] Kempe answers somewhat ambivalently in response to this accusation of sexual incontinence and procreation, stating, 'Ser, þe same childe þat God hath sent me I haue browt hom, for God knowyth I dede neuyr sithyn I went owte wher-thorw I xulde haue a childe' (103). I contend that Kempe's somewhat clouded response, the 'childe' whom she has 'browt hom', is not intended to denote the literal fruit of her womb, but rather the progeny of godchildren and surrogate children that she has gained on her travels. Indeed, she *has* begotten offspring, and she *has* fulfilled God's command to 'increase and multiply' (Genesis 1:22), using an alternative form of holy surrogacy that is entirely in keeping with her spiritual maturation. At the age of forty-two and having now undertaken the most significant journey of her life, she reveals a fecundity that is not bound up with corporeal efficacy, but with the ability to reproduce her motherly devotion and to reveal God's will in the souls of others.

Just two years later, aged forty-four, Kempe is given the opportunity to divulge her understanding of Genesis 1:22 when, in York, she is challenged by a 'gret clerke' as to the meaning of the scripture 'Crescite & multiplicamini' (121):[121]

> Ser, þes wordys ben not vnderstondyn only of begetyng of chyldren bodily, but also be purchasyng of vertu, which is frute gostly, as be heryng of þe wordys of God, be good exampyl ӡeuyng, be mekenes & paciens, charite & chastite, & swech oþer, for pacyens is more worthy þan myraclys werkyng (121).

Though the undertones of the clerk's question may imply that he suspects her of sexual incontinence, her response is just as measured as was that she gave in Norwich.[122] Making the distinction between bodily and spiritual generation, and carefully listing examples of ghostly fruits, she reveals an oratory skill and spiritual wisdom that effectively rebuff the clerk as posing an arbitrary and spurious question. She recalls, perhaps, God's reassurance after his disclosure that she was pregnant with her last child, that he 'wyl þat þow bring me forth more frwte' (48), implying that her future will entail spiritual generation. Not only does she prove herself a maturing teacher, but her knowledge of divine fruit also suggests a refocusing of the reproductive mode by which she, along with all the other wives and mothers denied free access to a spiritual life, has been hitherto defined. Maternal reproductiv-

---

[120] See Howes, 'On the Birth of Margery Kempe's last Child', p. 224, and McAvoy, *Notes and Queries*, pp. 181–3, for a refutation. On the edification of slander, see Olga Burakov Mongan, 'Slanderers and Saints: The Function of Slander in *The Book of Margery Kempe*', *Philological Quarterly*, 84 (2005), 27–47.

[121] On this episode and the accusation of Lollardy, see Alistair Minnis, *Translations of Authority*, pp. 112–29.

[122] Windeatt discusses the implications of the clerk's question and the cultural anxiety in the late Middle Ages about the potential exploitation of Genesis 1:22 for 'free love' and immorality in *BMK*, p. 243.

ity is replaced, insistently, with holy productivity. Now she will embody these virtues and generate new fruits for preaching and healing, in effect transforming her anachronistic body into one of new fecundity, capable of absorbing others' pain instead of her own, and with which a powerful *re*productivity will be born.

4

Margery Medica:
The Healing Value of Pain Surrogacy

When Margery Kempe faces the most dangerous illness of her lifetime –
the postpartum trauma that threatens her with psychosomatic annihilation
– she is cured not by physicians or medicines, but by the appearance of a
'most bewtyuows' Christ, whose blessed 'chere' effects her instant stabilisation and return to the concerns of the household. In a broader healing
paradigm, Kempe would have later received the sacrament during the
purification rite, also known as women's Churching after childbirth, when
the medicating effect of Christ's body in communion encapsulates the
transformative potentialities of holy flesh.[1] Through this lesson in spiritual
medicina Kempe's curative understanding is established, as she places her
faith in the efficacy of divine treatment. This faith is dramatically tested
many years later when a stone and piece of wood from the vault in St
Margaret's Church fall onto her back, a blow so terrible that she 'ferd as
sche had be deed a lytyl whyle' (21). On crying, 'Ihesu mercy … hir peyne
was gon' (21–2).[2] That this injury is likely to have occurred on 9 June
1413, just two weeks before Margery and John Kempe's vow of chastity,
illustrates how crucial Kempe's surety in God's medicine is.[3] For this pain
removal and divine rescue coincide with the vow that, in its Godly ordination, symbolises another type of cure for Kempe's corporeal scourge, and
sets her more fixedly on her own path as a physician.

The discourse of *Christus medicus*, or Christ the Physician, was ubiquitous
in the Christian Middle Ages, originating from biblical depictions of God
as the healer of body and soul.[4] The etymology of the term 'doctor' is in

---

[1] See Naoë Kukita Yoshikawa, 'Mysticism and Medicine: Holy Communion in the
Vita of Marie d'Oignies and *The Book of Margery Kempe*', in *Convergence / Divergence*,
ed. Renevey and Yoshikawa, *Poetica*, 109–22. See also David Cressy, 'Purification,
Thanksgiving and the Churching of Women in Post-Reformation England', *Past
& Present*, 141 (1993), 106–46; Angela Florschuetz, 'Women's Secrets: Childbirth,
Pollution, and Purification in Northern Octavian'; Gail McMurray Gibson, 'Blessing
from Sun and Moon', in *Bodies and Disciplines*, ed. Hanawalt and Wallace, pp. 139–54;
and Gibson, 'Scene and Obscene'.
[2] Note the same, powerful invocation of the Name of Jesus that helped Kempe in her
avoidance of marital sexual union in Chapter 2 of this study, p. 85.
[3] Barry Windeatt has dated this incident in relation to two other events. See *BMK*, ed.
Windeatt, p. 82.
[4] On *Christus Medicus*, see the rulings of the Fourth Lateran Council of 1215. See also
Henry of Lancaster, *Le livre de seyntz medicines: The Book of Holy Medicines*, trans.

127

fact fused with religious teaching in the late Middle Ages, emphasising the conceptual crossover between spirituality and medicine that Kempe understands and manifests.[5] Ideas about the medicinal qualities of the Eucharist were also widely disseminated through preaching in the late Middle Ages.[6] The Book of Ecclesiasticus states:

> Honour the physician for the need thou hast of him: for the most High hath created him. For all healing is from God, and he shall receive gifts of the king. The skill of the physician shall lift up his head, and in the sight of great men he shall be praised ... My son, in thy sickness neglect not thyself, but pray to the Lord, and he shall heal thee (38:1–9).

The interrelation of sin and disease was an idea that was predicated upon the pre-Cartesian understanding of the body and soul as unified entities, meaning that sin could be interpreted as the root of sickness, and confessional cleansing as an efficacious remedy.[7] Theologians like St Augustine often used the motif of *Christus medicus*, suggesting that the Passion of Christ was the most apposite medicine for the treatment of sick bodies and souls, a concept that was later developed in terms of the power of the Eucharist as a healing device.[8] Illustrating what Naoë Kukita Yoshikawa regards as the 'symbiotic relationship between medicine and religion', Henry of Lancaster's *Le livre de seyntz medicines* depicts the healing of Henry's wounds by Christ the Physician and also the Virgin, his nurse.[9] Concomitantly, Diane Watt has argued for the widespread medieval belief in Mary the Physician, or *Maria medica*, which validated the role of the woman as healer and which, she suggests, was an important model for Margery Kempe's healing practices.[10] Indeed, as Monica Green has shown, while women were increasingly excluded from formalised, textual forms of medicine, their silent and uncategorised medical work

---

Catherine Batt (Tempe: Arizona Centre for Medieval and Renaissance Studies, 2014); Naoë Kukita Yoshikawa, 'Introduction', in *Medicine, Religion and Gender in Medieval Culture*, ed. Yoshikawa, pp. 1–24; Yoshikawa, 'Holy Medicine and Diseases of the Soul: Henry of Lancaster and *Le livre de seyntz medicines*', *Medical History*, 53 (2009), 397–414; *Religion and Medicine in the Middle Ages*, ed. Biller and Ziegler; Rawcliffe, *Medicine for the Soul: The Life, Death and Resurrection of an English Medieval Hospital*; and John Henderson, *The Renaissance Hospital: Healing the Body and Healing the Soul* (New Haven and London: Yale University Press, 2006).

[5] OED: s.v. doctor (n) 3(a) the Doctors of the Church, certain early 'fathers' distinguished by their eminent learning; 5(a) A person who is proficient in knowledge of theology: a learned divine. 6(a) A doctor of medicine. The Latin term 'to teach' is *docere*.

[6] See Yoshikawa, 'Mysticism and Medicine' in *Convergence / Divergence*, ed. Renevey and Yoshikawa, *Poetica*, 109–22.

[7] See Yoshikawa, 'Introduction', in *Medicine, Religion and Gender in Medieval Culture*, ed. Yoshikawa, p. 9.

[8] Ibid., p. 10. See also R. Arbesmann, 'The Concept of *Christus medicus* in St Augustine', *Traditio*, 10 (1954), 1–28.

[9] See *Le livre de seyntz medicines*, ed. Batt.

[10] Diane Watt, 'Mary the Physician: Women, Religion and Medicine in the Middle Ages', in *Medicine, Religion and Gender in Medieval Culture*, ed. Yoshikawa, pp. 41–69.

continued.[11] Bridget of Sweden, for example, was known to have founded a hospital near her home where she tended the sick.[12] It is a tradition encapsulated by a popular medieval lyric: 'On o ledy min hope is, / Moder and virgine; / We shulden into hevene bliss / Thurgh hire medicine.'[13] The model of the Virgin as mother and female healer is of particular appeal for the holy woman who, in mystical desire, seeks to share Mary's pain at the foot of the cross in the hope of attaining that 'hevene bliss' of eschatological rapture.

This chapter is concerned with the development of the surrogacy hermeneutic in *The Book of Margery Kempe* in relation to Kempe's strategies as a physician and healing agent of God. I argue that her acts of healing denote not only an emulation of *Christus medicus* but also the spiritual flourishing that situates that healing as a further example of re-productivity, and what I term *pain surrogacy*. Kempe's experience, or *knowledge*, of pain is translated to this pain surrogacy – that is, her willing receipt and support of pain that does not originate in the self. In this way pain surrogacy partially deviates from the aspiration to *imitatio Christi* since I conceptualise the hermeneutic as, by its very nature, being rooted in the maturing female body, taking as its subject both divine and earthly sufferers. Rather than the rarefied desire to experience Christ's anguish singularly, pain surrogacy is a necessarily maternal activity legitimised through the female mystic's physiology and capacity to (re)experience, or to *bear*, productive and physical pain. In considering the broader function of the medieval nurse and the multivalent ways in which Kempe utilises domestic, medical, and religious discourses of healing, I contend that her mid to later years signify a therapeutic development. Through the continued activities of healing and her painful transition from wife to widow, she embraces others' pain in order to achieve Christic union. Much of the pain described in the *Book* belongs to others – both mortal and divine – indicating, as I will show, Kempe's evolving understanding and sharing of painful experience.

The Multivalent Medicament of Milk

As well as being a nourisher and symbol of surrogacy, the medieval 'nurse' was accorded further power: that of healer and prophylactic agent. The idea of the

[11] Monica Green, *Making Women's Medicine Masculine*, p. 290. See also Green, 'Documenting Medieval Women's Medical Practice', in *Practical Medicine from Salerno to the Black Death*, ed. García-Ballester et al., pp. 322–52.

[12] Bridget Morris, *St Birgitta of Sweden*, p. 53. On the medical practice of the Swedish female enclosed, see Johanna Bergqvist, 'Gendered Attitudes Towards Physical Tending Amongst the Piously Religious of Late Medieval Sweden', in *Medicine, Healing and Performance*, ed. Gemi-Iordanou et al., pp. 188–225.

[13] IMEV 2359: 'Now skrinketh rose and lilie-flour'. No. 193, in *Middle English Lyrics: Authoritative Texts, Critical and Historical Backgrounds, Perspectives on Six Poems*, ed. Maxwell S. Luria and Richard L. Hoffman (New York and London: W.W. Norton, 1974), pp. 181–2.

'nurse' in the Middle Ages was understood as ambiguous, encompassing not only the wet nurse as a nourisher and curative intermediary, but also the nurse-maid, governess, or foster parent. Kempe's 'nursing' activities are regarded here as concomitantly multivalent and surrogate, influenced by a wider cultural milieu which imbued breastmilk, especially, with healing potential.[14] Bartholomaeus Anglicus recommends that the nurse 'vsiþ medicines to bringe þe childe to couenable state ʒif he is seeke'.[15] The accepted view of the child's weak body, based on Arabic authority, meant that the nurse was often used as a treatment intermediary, her body used as a conduit for medical remedies to be passed to the infant. Avicenna, for instance, recommended that the first step towards the child's health was to maintain a healthy regimen for the wet nurse.[16] The Arabic authors also prescribed curative foods to be administered to the child via the nurse's body.[17] Such traditions permeated Western medieval medical texts; the 'Book on the Conditions of Women', for example, states: 'If a carbuncle appears in the body of the child, let barley water be given to the nurse, and occasionally let her be scarified. Let her eat neither sweet nor salty things' ('Si uero in corpore pueri antrax apparuerit, detur nutrici aqua ordei, et quandoque scarificetur. Nec dulcia nec salsa comedat').[18] These stratagems denote not only caution surrounding the over-zealous medical management of the child's weak body, but also the wet nurse's performance of a wider role: that of the healing surrogate. As an intermediary for the powerful cures thought to be too potent for direct administration to the child, her milk is bestowed with properties beyond nutriment: with transformative potential.

The curative power of breastmilk, both as a vehicle for treatment and as a remedy itself, extends in some medieval medical texts beyond treatment for paediatric illness. Milk also permeates remedies for adult ailments, suggesting a multifunctionality that imbues it with meanings far greater than nourishment alone, and which elevate the lactating mother to the status of esoteric physician. *The Knowing of Woman's Kind in Childing* recommends breastmilk as a cure for excessive heat in the uterus, when it is as hot as burning coals: 'For þat euyll ye muste tak oyle of þe white of xij eggys, saffvrne, mylk of a woman; let menge all to-gethyre & [mynyster] hit with a pessary.'[19] The *Sickness of Women* also includes women's milk in a recipe for a pessary to aid superfluous bleeding as a result of the heat of the uterus:

---

[14] For the MED definition of 'nurse', see Chapter 3 of this study, p. 120, n. 101. Monica Green has advised caution in the use of the term 'nurse' since some modern commentators 'cannot rid themselves of the medical connotations of the term fixed by the development of professional nursing in the nineteenth century'. Green prioritises nurse duties as those of wet-nurses and nannies. See Green, 'Documenting Medieval Women's Medical Practice', in *Practical Medicine from Salerno to the Black Death*, ed. García-Ballester et al., p. 341.

[15] *On the Properties of Things*, p. 304.

[16] Avicenna, *Canon*, adapt. Bahkhtiar, vol. 1, 15.2.4–7, pp. 363–6.

[17] See MacLehose, *A Tender Age*, pp. 24–5.

[18] 'Book on the Conditions of Women', in *The Trotula*, pp. 112–13.

[19] *The Knowing of Woman's Kind in Childing*, p. 96.

Also if hir thynke that it brennyth that comeþ from hir at the prevy membre, take than the muscillage of psilium, of the muscillage of the seedis of quynces and of the gumme of draganti ana –3 1, of wommans mylke –3 6, cast it into prevy membre and this medicyne helith and staunchith al bloode that cometh thurgh hote causes.[20]

The 'Book on the Conditions of Women' similarly prescribes 'the milk of a woman' (lac mulieris) for a pessary to alleviate a womb that is burning with heat.[21] It also recommends 'the milk of another woman' (lac alterius mulieris) to be given as a drink for labouring women who are experiencing delays or who are carrying a dead foetus.[22] The *Sickness of Women* advises that 'wommans mylke and oile toguyder idrunke makith a womman to be delivered of chielde', perhaps partly because of a sympathetic association.[23] The medical indication of human milk thus appears to reside in its cooling, calming nature; milk is able to soothe, subdue, and reduce affliction but also to as an active catalyst for efficacy. The author of the *Sickness of Women* also considers milk an effective treatment for uterine sores that are caused, the text asserts, by excessive heat, 'as comonly it doeth, more than of cold'.[24] However, sores caused by the *cold* are also to be treated by a pessary containing breastmilk: 'medle hem toguyder with wommans mylke and with the juce of plantayne ana 3 2 and s.; whan thei bien wele imedled, do it to the malady in the prevy membre'.[25] Clearly, the curative properties of breastmilk are not restricted to a single effect: its benefits are multifarious and its precise efficacious constituent is ambiguously potent.

More variously, the *Sickness of Women* advises on treatments for the inflammation of the uterus and the abscesses that subsequently develop. To 'make th'emposteme [abscess] ripe', a mixture, including 'wommans mylke', is made to create 'emplastres' (poultices or salves) for external or internal application.[26] *The Knowing of Woman's Kind in Childing* has a comparable recipe for an 'emplaustre' that will ripen 'apostemys [abscesses]', this time applicable to '*man & woman*'.[27] Tree bark is softened and mixed with pork fat, butter, wine, and 'mylk of a woman'.[28] For *in utero* ulceration the 'Book on the Conditions of Women' advises a mixture of deadly nightshade, great plantain, rose oil, and white of egg 'with woman's milk' (cum lacte mulieris) to anaesthetise the stabbing pain of the womb; these ingredients are all noted to be cold in nature ('frigide nature').[29] Whilst the cooling properties of breastmilk feature

---

[20] *Sickness of Women*, pp. 500–1.
[21] 'Book on the Conditions of Women', in *The Trotula*, pp. 88–9.
[22] Ibid., pp. 102–3.
[23] *Sickness of Women*, p. 523.
[24] Ibid., p. 538.
[25] Ibid., p. 539.
[26] *Sickness of Women*, pp. 519–20.
[27] My emphasis. *The Knowing of Women's Kind in Childing*, pp. 108–10.
[28] *The Knowing of Women's Kind in Childing*, p. 110.
[29] 'Book on the Conditions of Women', in *The Trotula*, pp. 92–3.

as a common denominator, the multiple and occasionally contradictory uses of breastmilk for curative purposes imply an inherent potency that remains ambiguous. An apt illustration of this broad efficacy can be found in the 'Book on the Conditions of Women':

> In order to know whether a woman is carrying a male or a female, take water from a spring and let the woman extract two or three drops of blood *or milk* from her right side and let these be dropped in the water. And if they fall to the bottom, she is carrying a male; if they float on top, a female.
>
> [Ad cognoscendum utrum mulier gestet masculum siue feminam, accipe aquam de fonte et mulier extrahat .ii. uel .iii. guttas sanguinis uel lactis de dextro latere et infundantur in aqua, et si fundum petant, masculum gerit; si supernatant, feminam.][30]

The diverse meanings that the medieval world attached to blood and its various manifestations inside and outside the body were explored in the previous chapter. Here, not only is the parturient female's blood made interchangeable with her breastmilk (as we might expect in the medieval context), but the prophetic power it is accorded conveys an esotericism beyond a singular, medical usage. Such miraculous metamorphoses of breastmilk also occur in religious *vitae*. Christina Mirabilis, having been bound and fettered with chains of iron, escapes with God's help and goes into hiding 'in wildernesse priuely with oure Lorde'. Looking on her dry, virgin breast, she 'sawe hit drepe swete milke agaynes alle righte of kynde and nature … And so the virgyne Cristyn was norysched nyne wokes with the mylke of hir owne pappe.'[31] Because Christina sustains herself for nine weeks, her hagiographer, Thomas of Cantimpré, compares her to the Virgin Mary – 'the incomparabil and singler virgyne, Cristes moder' – who feeds Christ from her virgin breasts.[32] Similarly, when Christine is incarcerated once again and unable to eat, 'hire maydenly pappes bigan to sprynge licoure of ful swete oyle, and that toke she and sauerd hir brede with alle and hadde hit for potage and *oynement*'.[33] The concomitance

---

[30] 'The Book on the Conditions of Women', in *The Trotula*, pp. 102–5. This practice is widely copied in medieval recipe collections. In the *Liber de diversis medicinis*, a woman 'þat is with childe [should] mylke a droppe' into the water of a well, and if it 'synke to þe grounde, þan is it taken of a knafe childe &, if it flete a-bown, þan es taken of a mayden childe', p. 56.

[31] Thomas of Cantimpré, '"The Middle English Life of Christina Mirabilis", in *Three Women of Liège*, ed. Brown, pp. 51–84 (pp. 57–8). The legendary Catherine of Alexandria, from whose tomb on Mount Sinai holy oil was carried all over the Western world, was said to have bled milk rather than blood from her severed veins when she was decapitated. Several holy virgins from the Low Countries – Christina the Astonishing, Gertrude van Oosten, Lidwina of Schiedam – 'supposedly nursed their adherents or *cured others with their breast milk*' (my emphasis). See Bynum, *Holy Feast, Holy Fast*, p. 273.

[32] 'The Middle English Life of Christina Mirabilis', in *Three Women of* Liège, ed. Brown, p. 58.

[33] Ibid., p. 64. MED s.v. oinement 1(a) A medicinal salve prepared or used for external application; (b) a specified medicinal ointment. 3(a) An ointment prepared for ceremonial or sacramental purposes; (b) the ointment used to consecrate kings and priests;

between Christina's breasts as sources of food and a healing 'ointment' is clear. Furthermore, after her leg is deliberately broken and a 'leche' (physician) is called, she 'thoghte it vnworthy to haue annothere leche to hire woundes but oure sauyour Jhesu Cryste'. She subsequently escapes, having developed a sudden and miraculous strength absorbed from Christ the Physician. In *The Pore Caitif*, St Agatha (the patron saint of wet nurses) describes receiving a vision of 'goddis massenger', St Paul the Apostle, during her incarceration; he 'cam to hele hir woundis, fleshly medicyn to my bodi,' a tale which connects her severed breasts with healing through divine intervention.[34]

These examples demonstrate, then, that women's milk has a multipurpose and transformational power that not only heals and soothes pain, but also metaphysically communicates the wisdom and intuition associated with motherhood. Through the wet-nursing identifications that Margery Kempe enacts in her post-reproductive state, I therefore suggest that a new development in her spiritual journey occurs via a transition from wet nurse, to healing nurse, to healer. For now that she emulates the Virgin via her literal and surrogate mothering experiences, the maturing Kempe is able to minister to others, offering her healing powers as a physician of both the physical and heavenly worlds. The pain surrogacy in the *Book* underlies Kempe's strategy of making productive use of her prior painful experiences, to visualise Christ's pain in every 'patient' whom she adopts, and to position herself as God's doctoring disciple and ultimate surrogate of divine pain.

Margery Kempe's Medica

While still in Rome, Margery Kempe is called on by her confessor to care for an elderly and infirm woman for 'obediens' and 'penawns', forming a direct reciprocation between the suffering patient and Kempe's tribulatory toil:

> Than þe good preste hir r bad hir be vertu of obediens & also in party of penawns þat sche xulde seruyn an hold woman þat was a poure creatur in Rome. & sche dede so sex wekys. Sche seruyd hir as sche wolde a don owyr Lady. & sche had no bed to lyn in ne no clothys to be cured wyth saf hir owyn mentyl. & þan was sche ful of vermin & suffyrd gret peyn þerwyth. Also sche fet hom watyr & stykkys in hir necke for þe poure woman and beggyd mete and wyn bothyn for hir. And, whan þe pour womans wyn was sowr, þis creatur hir-self drank þat sowr wyn & ȝaf þe powr woman good wyn þat sche had bowt for hir owyn selfe (85–6).

Kempe is careful to emphasise the 'gret peyne' that she experiences in caring for the woman, re-enacting the devotional techniques learned from the 'worshepful wyfys' whose mothering of the Christ-doll was underscored by a

---

consecration with this ointment; (c) the ointment or sacrament of extreme unction; (d) the oil or sacrament of baptism.

[34] *The Pore Caitif*, p. 194.

silent acknowledgement of Mary's maternal sacrifice. In fact, Kempe administers to the elderly woman 'as sche wolde a don owyr Lady', foregrounding her rationale of the task as both divinely aligned and painfully sacrificial. Her recollection of this episode of six weeks fails to mention the physical infirmity or suffering of the poverty-stricken woman, whose situation was bleak enough to warrant priestly intervention. Rather, Kempe is at pains to describe the surrendering of her own comfort: her priestly amanuensis employs the pronoun 'sche' eight times to accentuate her sacrifice of food, wine, and bed, and her humility in begging for food and drink. Indeed, Christ's bearing of the cross is evoked by the sticks that she carries on her shoulders, an image that affirms the penitential aspect of the endeavour and establishes Kempe's nursing role as an explicit facet of her spiritual trajectory. It is perhaps no coincidence that this period of charitable care precedes her marriage to the Godhead in the following chapter, recalled, then, as a vitally sacrificial step on her path to ultimate divine union.

Kempe's activity as self-appointed physician develops as a logical extension of her life experience and growing holiness. When in St Margaret's Church, presumably during her fairly settled years in Lynn after 1418, she discovers a man in distress who is kneeling and wringing his hands in despair. Her concern is evident, as 'sche, parceyuyng hys heuynes, askyd what hym eylyd' (177). The man responds to Kempe as 'dame', illustrating that this episode occurs during her mature years.[35] He describes a postpartum wife who is 'owt hir mende' (177), and who, because of her violent and aggressive behaviour, is manacled by the wrists – a striking parallel to Kempe's own period of postpartum trauma. Kempe's credibility as a spiritual authority is acknowledged by the distraught husband when she offers her services: the man replies, '3a, dame, for Goddys lofe' (178), an unspoken acceptance of her status as a religious woman whose authoritative demeanour now extends to that of a healing agent. In stark contrast to the woman's roars, cries, and the 'smytyn & bityn' that precipitated her shackling, Kempe's entry calms her, ratifying the older woman's presence as comforting, and revealing the afflicted women as having paradoxical insight into Kempe's celestial aura that belies her psychotic symptoms. She tells Kempe, 'For 3e arn ... a ryth good woman & I beheld many fayr awngelys a-bowte 30w, & þerfor, I pray 30w, goth not fro me, for I am gretly comfortyd be 30w' (178). In the presence of other visitors the woman remains frenzied: 'And, whan oþer folke cam to hir, sche cryid & gapyd as sche wolde an etyn hem & seyd þat sche saw many deuelys a-bowtyn hem' (178).[36] The woman's disordered behaviour results in her being removed to the far end of town, like a leper, where she is 'bowyndn handys and feet wyth chenys of yron þat sche xulde smytyn no-body' (178). Displaced and

---

[35] MED s.v. dame: 1. A woman of rank or position, a superior, a mistress, a mother.

[36] Such an agitated reaction to other visitors may be explained by the violation of the lying-in room. See Chapter 2 of this study, pp. 71–2.

fettered, like the young Margery Kempe, her unruly postpartum body is threateningly unpredictable.

In poignant identification, Kempe acts antithetically to the people who remove the woman from their uncomfortable gaze and instead adopts her suffering, visiting twice daily in a compassionate acknowledgement of the authenticity of this new mother's anguish. By the late Middle Ages midwives had acquired a salvific authority which, according to Gibson, 'came close to the power of clergy'.[37] Canon law required midwives to be instructed in the form of infant baptism. Whilst any Christian was theoretically permitted to perform an emergency baptism, midwives were the only laypeople specifically empowered to do so. John Myrc offered instructions for midwives conducting infant baptism, emphasising the importance of uttering the sacred words accurately – 'alle on rowe' – and disallowing any 'wymmenes lore'.[38] Through her prayers and her presence, Kempe therefore validates the woman's pain and, in this midwifery mission, effects a miraculous therapy of life-saving magnitude:[39]

> And þe sayd creatur preyid for þis woman euery day þat God xulde, ȝyf it were hys wille, restoryn hir to hir wittys a-geyn. And owr Lord answeryd in hir sowle & seyd, 'Sche xulde faryn ryth wel'. Þan was sche mor bolde to preyin for hir recuryng [recovery; cure] þan sche was be-forn, & iche day, wepyng & sorwyng, preyid for hir recur tyl God ȝaf hir hir witte & hir mende a-ȝen (178).[40]

Like a medic increasing a patient's dosage, Kempe takes God's reassurance as a catalyst to increase her prayers, amplifying their efficacy with weeping and sorrowing, and acting as a surrogate for the pain that she labours to alleviate.[41] Such is the extent of the woman's recovery that Kempe's priest-scribe heralds it a miracle, revering her healing powers grounds for sanctification.[42] Not only

---

[37] Gibson, 'Scene and Obscene', pp. 15–16.

[38] John Myrc, *Instructions for Parish Priests, edited from Cotton MS. Claudius A II*, ed. Edward Peacock, EETS o.s. 31 (London: Trübner, 1868), p. 5. MED s.v: godsip: 1(a) One's sponsor at baptism or confirmation, a godparent; and 2(a) A close friend, companion, pal. This indicates a cultural connection between midwifery and ministry in medieval culture.

[39] Given the predominant exclusion of men at the birthing site until the sixteenth century and beyond, the Church had little choice but to imbue midwives with this substitute priestly role. See Jean Towler, *Midwives in History and Society* (London: Croom Helm, c. 1986), pp. 24–5.

[40] MED s.v. recūren.

[41] Medical historians debate whether the midwife can be regarded as a medical practitioner, since childbirth is perhaps not a 'condition' to be pathologized. Monica Green notes how male physicians turned to female *obstetrix* as their 'eyes and hands' when conducting intimate examinations. See 'Documenting medieval women's medical practice' in *Practical Medicine*, ed. García-Ballester et al., p. 340, n. 72. Peregrine Horden argues that nurses provided a promotion of the 'balance of the non-naturals', and *were* therefore medical practioners, since medieval medicine focused on prevention rather than cure. See 'A Non-Natural Environment', in *The Medieval Hospital and Medical Practice*, ed. Bowers, p. 139.

[42] For other instances of Kempe's suggested sanctity, see *BMK* pp. 22, 37 and 156. Hope Emily Allen notes that Kempe seems to show hope of being venerated in the Church of St

is the woman reborn into a mind of worship and praise, she is even 'browt to chirche & purifijd as oþer women be', and reintegrated into the community (178). Through its implicit connection to the purification ceremony, Watt suggests that 'in intervening in the life of this very distressed and ill woman, Margery Kempe was emulating the Virgin's care for the sick'.[43] Kempe thus succeeds not only in facilitating a recovery from psychosis to serenity but also in bringing the woman from apparent demonic possession to purification in the Churching ceremony. Coming full circle, she utilises her post-reproductive status to redress the childbirth trauma that she herself once endured. In her new understanding of healing praxes she experientially reproduces in a way that witnesses a fragmented woman become whole, and which situates her not at the margins of the town but in ritual therapy at the church door.[44]

Kempe attaches considerable significance to the Churching ritual, which is reinforced by a vision that she experiences on Purification Day, when the Virgin Mary presented Christ at the temple.[45] She is 'raueschyd' by her perception of this event, witnessing it in such verisimilitude that she imagines herself offering up Christ 'wyth owr Ladys owyn persone' (198) and thus participating intrinsically in the purification of Mary's postpartum body. The intensity of the experience provokes a visceral reaction; Kempe struggles to walk with her candle towards the priest: '[she] went waueryng of eche syde as it had ben a dronkyn woman, wepyng & sobbyng so sor þat vn-ethe sche

---

Margaret's in Lynn. See p. 325, n. 156/26. See also Gail McMurray Gibson, 'St Margery: *The Book of Margery Kempe*', in *Equally in God's Image*, ed. Holloway et al., pp. 144–63; and Katherine Lewis, 'Margery Kempe and Saint Making in Later Medieval England', in *A Companion to The Book of Margery Kempe*, ed. Arnold and Lewis, pp. 195–216.

[43] Diane Watt, 'Mary the Physician', in *Medicine, Religion and Gender in Medieval Culture*, ed. Yoshikawa, pp. 27–44 (p. 39).

[44] It is significant that widows specifically, presumably because of their mature wisdom as *sages-femme*, were empowered by the Church for female medical care. Given that a widow is, by her nature, post-reproductive, due either to age or removal from the debt of matrimony, it is apt that Kempe adopts a midwife role in her own post-reproductive yet fruitful life phase. The Church insisted that physicians first call a priest, but also stipulated that every community should appoint 'at least one widow to assist women who are stricken with illness'. See Towler, *Midwives in History and Society*, pp. 29–30. See also M. Chamberlain, *Old Wives' Tales. Their History, Remedies and Spells* (London: Virago, 1981).

[45] On the Churching ceremony see Sue Niebrzydowski, '*Asperges Me, Domine, hyssopo*: Male Voices, Female Interpretation and the medieval English Purification of Women after Childbirth Ceremony', *Early Music*, 39 (2011), 327–34 (p. 5). Midwives participated in the ceremony 'as keepers of the custom … their prominence at churchings also advertised their skills in the birthing room'. See David Cressy, 'Purification, Thanksgiving and the Churching of Women in Post-Reformation England', *Past and Present* (1993), 106–46 (p. 114). The spiritual danger of childbirth was considerable. Not only was the child considered a product of Original Sin, but it had been nourished in the womb on retained, and thus contaminated, menstrual blood. Women who died in childbirth could not be buried in the church. Postpartum women frequently visited icons and altars of the Virgin and St Anne, offering candles in thanksgiving. See Carole Rawcliffe, 'Women, Religion and Childbirth in Later Medieval England', in *Women and Religion in Medieval England*, ed. Wood, pp. 95–6.

myth stondyn on hir feet' (198). Struggling to bear the anguish, she falls to the ground climactically, the 'feruowr of þe spiryt' so great that it triggers corporeal failure: 'þe body fayld & myth not endur it' (198). Her witnessing of the purification rite resonates so strongly that she can no longer endure the intensity of the experience – to be integrated into a moment of such ceremonial import is to be reminded of the Christian possibility of rebirth, particularly female rebirth: a central pivot on which Kempe's reproductive future rests. She therefore meditates 'many tymes whan sche saw women ben purifyid of her childeryn' (198), transposing the inspirational image of Mary and the Christ Child onto the lay women of her community and thus, in an intercessory act, creating salvific opportunities for all childbearing women to be freed of defilement.[46]

This preoccupation largely explains Kempe's unyielding commitment to healing the fractured postpartum woman, to enable the mother to regain her physical health and therefore gain access to spiritual health through the rite of purification. But her willingness also stems from the visions of herself as handmaiden to the Virgin and to St Anne, which occur in the earliest part of her dictated recollection and beyond, suggesting the centrality of childbirth rituals as vital for her construction of a spiritual and healing self. Kempe sees St Anne 'gret wyth chylde', for instance, and concomitantly prays to be 'hir mayden & hir seruawnt' (18), illustrating an instinctive desire to act as St Anne's midwife and reflecting the medieval reliance on female communities for childbirth procedures. Kempe is present at the birth – '& anon ower Lady was born' – and mystically 'kepe[s]' Mary until she is twelve years old: a privileged position of influence on the future Mother of God (18). The vision develops to show Kempe as Mary's companion in adult life, where they, along with Joseph, visit St John the Baptist's mother, Elizabeth, when St John is born. Characteristically, Kempe begs to administer 'seruyse & plesawns' to St Elizabeth, her caring instincts presumably roused by her visionary witnessing of John's birth. This duty is anticipated strikingly by her decision to take on the journey to Elizabeth 'a potel of pyment & spycys þerto' (18).[47] The honeyed and spiced wine 'pyment' symbolises the comforting therapies of the physician's pack (and spices, as we have seen from the recipe in the Book's manuscript, were used medicinally for their warming properties); moreover,

[46] Kempe's adoration of the Virgin and child is emphasised during her pilgrimage to Aachen when she is around sixty. She sees 'owr Ladys smoke & oþer holy reliqwiis which wer schewyd on Seynt Margaretys Day' (237). The relics were the garment of Our Lady worn at Christ's birth, the swaddling-clothes of Jesus, the cloth which had received the head of John the Baptist, and the waist-cloth Jesus wore on the cross (See BMK, 356, n. 237/34–7). Our Lady's smock was thought to have apotropaic qualities in assisting women in childbirth. Kempe's interest in this relic must have been in relation to the assistance she provided for labouring women.

[47] MED s.v. piment: (a) A sweetened, spiced wine used for refreshment and in medical recipes; a medicinal potion (c) a medicinal ingredient.

a 'potel' – the vessel into which the 'pyment' is poured – contains the specific quantity of two quarts and thus has connotations of medicinal dosage.[48]

Medieval medical texts confirm the commonplace of midwives as an integral part of birthing practices. The 'Book on the Conditions of Women' explains how a midwife should assist with her hands when the birth is difficult, and suggests decoctions and odoriferous spices like those found in Kempe's 'pyment'.[49] It further states that 'It should be noted that there are certain physical remedies whose power is *obscure* to us, which are helpful when done by midwives' (Item notandum est quod sunt quedam phisicalia remedia quorum uirtus est nobis *obscura*, que ab obstetricibus facta profuerunt).[50] Such a notion is reminiscent of the broad potency of breastmilk and its intangible power. Another esoteric object – a magnet – is then recommended for the midwife to hold during the birthing process, deepening the association between the abstruse maternal body and the performative midwife-surrogate. The *Sickness of Women* documents a problematic lack of competent midwives, a shortage perpetuated by the secrecy surrounding female generation: 'Dyvers tymes it hapith of dyvers wymmen a myscheuous grevaunce in travailyng of chield for defaute of goode mydwifes, and that greuaunce kepen prevy and it nedith for to be holpen'.[51] Indeed, 'On Treatments for Women' warns of the danger of *poor* midwifery, stating that problems during childbirth are 'because of the failure of those assisting them: that is to say, this is kept hidden by the women' ('propter defectum astantium, scilicet istud mulieribus fit secretum').[52] Like the wet nurse whose milk is simultaneously nourishing and pathological, the midwife is here considered both integral and threatening to the birthing room – a privileged physician of female secrets, and perilously accountable. *The Knowing of Woman's Kind in Childing* similarly implies suspicion of older midwives, whose actions when severing the umbilical cord should be scrutinised: 'And assentyth nevyre to þe foly of sume olde women þat were wont to kot hym with glas or with a pese of a potte of erthe or with a scharp ston, or all þat ys by foly & wyche-crafte.'[53] The text also warns of old midwives' bad advice to wet nurses: 'And lok ye do not afture svme old women þat gyf here norysse to ete, when here mylk faylyth, þe estrayne of schepe or of kow or of oþer bestys femalys … so hit turnyth to corrupcion & rotyth þe chylde.'[54] Such patriarchal anxieties about the power of midwives and wet nurses, power which excludes and marginalises men from the mystery of birth, is regarded by Nikki Stiller as 'the source of women's latent power and men's latent envy'.

---

[48] MED s.v. potel(le), also pottel: 1 (b) a liquid measure.
[49] 'Book on the Conditions of Women', in *The Trotula*, pp. 100–1.
[50] Ibid., pp. 106–7 (my emphases).
[51] *Sickness of Women*, p. 547.
[52] 'On Treatments for Women', in *The Trotula*, pp. 124–7. On female secrecy, see Monica Green, *Making Women's Medicine Masculine*, especially Ch. 2, pp. 70–117, and Ch. 5, pp. 204–45.
[53] *The Knowing of Woman's Kind in Childing*, p. 72.
[54] Ibid., p. 72.

Pejorative suspicion, she argues, 'stem[s] from reactions to the situation in which the powerful mother-surrogate helps the daughter achieve exclusively feminine ends,' ends through which Margery Kempe finds fruitful opportunity for pain surrogacy in Marian devotion.[55]

Even in a medical hegemony, the midwife remains a crucial surrogate in facilitating a successful birth.[56] The writer of *The Knowing of Woman's Kind in Childing* addresses the reader – the birth assistant – as a partner in their shared objective: 'How ye schall help a woman þat [trauelyth] of chylde'.[57] But it is the advice for a stillborn delivery in *The Knowing of Woman's Kind in Childing* that most acutely illustrates the conflation of midwife and minister, where the birth assistant not only shares in the physical act of her patient's delivery, but also embodies the shared duties of medic and priest in an act of spiritual and surgical hope:

> And yf þe chylde be dede, ȝef here to drynk ysop & hote watere & sone schall sche be delyuerde. Or tak a lytyll scrowe [scroll] & wryt þys with-in: + In nomine Patris et Filij & Spiritus Sancti Amen + Sancta Maria + Sancta Margareta + ogor + sogor + nogo + and *kyt þat scrov in-to small pecys & ȝiffe here to drynk.* Or wrytt in a long escrow all þe psalme of Magnificat anima mea & gyrde hit a-boute here. But wethyth well þat þis ne none oþer kepyth no woman at commenabyll tyme of delyuerance [but as a preparatyue] & þer-for let þe mydwyffe helpe.[58]

The treatise not only stipulates that the written prayer be offered by the birth assistants to the mother as a scriptural medicine to be *ingested* and internalised, but also states, unambiguously, that this preparation is to be administered in accordance with the midwife's physical intervention. The fourteenth-century priest and physician John of Mirfield recorded such practices in the *Breviarium Bartholomei* and stated his disbelief in the use of scripture for 'magical' purposes, which were perceived by the male clergy as verbal or superstitious cures.[59] But Lea Olsan has argued that, to a considerable extent, 'religious rituals were involved in medical care in the fifteenth century'. In one recipe a fully devel-

---

[55] Nikki Stiller, *Eve's Orphans: Mothers and Daughters in Medieval English Literature* (Conneticut and London: Greenwood Press, 1980), pp. 64–6.

[56] Medieval male physicians, despite their theoretical training, had little experience of intimate examinations of female patients, which were normally the preserve of 'a midwife, acting as his intermediary'. See Rawcliffe, 'Women, Childbirth, and Religion', in *Women and Religion in Medieval England*, ed. Wood, p. 95.

[57] *The Knowing of Woman's Kind in Childing*, p. 62.

[58] My emphasis. *The Knowing of Woman's Kind in Childing*, pp. 64–6. The Latin meaning of 'sogor' is the conjugation of 'sugor': to suck, or to take in. The meanings of 'ogor' and 'nogo' appear obscure, which suggests that they function as lyrical, mnemonic, or esoteric words.

[59] See Towler, *Midwives in History and Society*, p. 32. On such clerical concerns, see Catherine Rider, *Magic and Religion in Medieval England* (London: Reaktion Books, 2012), pp. 46–69. See also Don Skemer, *Binding Words: Textual Amulets in the Middle Ages* (Pennsylvania: The Pennsylvania State University Press, 2006).

oped 'mimesis of the Eucharist' employs a mother's milk in place of wine, regarded by Olsan as a sacramental act, albeit one not officially recognised by the Church.[60] Words to be written on the Host in Latin in similar 'recipes' illustrate the place of the Eucharist as a healing object within the household.[61] Indeed, there is some evidence to suggest that the 'eating' of scripture was conceptualised by holy women as a means to experience Christ. Ida of Louvain 'ate' Christ by reciting John 1:14, literally tasting the Word on her tongue and feeling flesh in her mouth, which tasted of 'honey'; this experience is paralleled in her *Vita* to Mary's bearing of Christ in her uterus.[62] The ingestion of scripture – literally eating the 'Word' – and the generation of childbirth thus hold implicit Eucharistic associations. It is not implied in the *Book* that Kempe employed textual amulets in her care of the postpartum woman. However, we *are* made aware of her intensified praying in this episode ('Þan was sche mor bolde to preyin for hir recuryng þan sche was be-forn, & iche day, wepyng & sorwyng, preyid for hir recur' [178]). Now that she has gained the woman's trust and that of her husband as a holy medic, Kempe's prayers demonstrate an amalgamation of medicine and ministering that are concomitant with the social status of the mature, wise midwife, and offer an explanation for why this form of surrogacy so appeals to Kempe in her mid- and older age.

The efficacy of Kempe's healing actions is emphasised throughout the *Book*, where she is also integrated into the holy scenes of her visions. Her role as Mary's handmaid extends to her presence in scenes of Christ's Passion and illustrates the way in which maternalised pain – that is, pain which is predicated on and *known* through the mother's body – is fundamental to Kempe's own pain perception.[63] During the intensely affective Passion visions, discussed at length in Chapter 5, Kempe shares the Virgin's pain on witnessing the scourging of Christ: 'And þan owr Lady & sche hyr vnworthy handmaydyn for þe tyme wept & syhyd ful sor for þe Iewys ferd so fowle & so ven[ym]owslych wyth hir blisful Lord' (190). This union-in-pain between Mary and Kempe, enacted in a communal time and place, foregrounds maternal experience as the principle site in which Kempe can understand and *bear* her, and others', pain. In a subsequent

---

[60] Lea T. Olsan, 'The Language of Charms in a Middle English Recipe Collection', *ANQ: A Quarterly Journal of Short Articles, Notes and Reviews*, 18 (2005), 29–35 (pp. 31–2). See also Olsan, 'Charms and Prayers in Medieval Medical Theory and Practice', *Social History of Medicine*, 16 (2003), 343–66; Peter Murray Jones and Lea T. Olsan, 'Performative Rituals for Conception and Childbirth in England, 900–1500', *Bulletin of the History of Medicine*, 89 (2015), 406–33; and Hilary Powell, 'The "Miracle of Childbirth": The Portrayal of Parturient Women in Medieval Miracle Narratives', *Social History of Medicine*, 25 (2012), 795–811.

[61] See Alessandra Foscati, 'Healing with the Body of Christ. Religion, Medicine and Magic', in *Il 'Corpus Domini': Teologia, Antropologia e Politica*, ed. Laura Andreani and Agostino Paravicini Bagliani (Firenze: Sismel, 2015), pp. 209–26 (pp. 211–12).

[62] Caroline Walker Bynum, 'Women Mystics and Eucharistic Devotion in the Thirteenth Century', *Women's Studies*, 11 (1984), 179–214 (p. 188).

[63] Allen notes how Kempe develops the handmaiden narrative throughout her *Book*, probably inspired by 'The Meditations of St Elizabeth'. *BMK*, p. 265, n 18/31.

vision of a time after the crucifixion Kempe's pain surrogacy is once again manifest when she comforts and cares for the grieving Mary: 'Than þe creatur thowt, whan owr Lady was comyn hom & was leyd down on a bed, þan sche mad for owr Lady a good cawdel & browt it hir to comfortyn hir' (195). In a moment that recalls how the wives in Rome comforted her and laid her on a bed in maternal care, Kempe now re-enacts the nursing tableau through her ongoing and privileged duties as handmaid to the Mother of God. The 'cawdel' that Kempe blends and offers Mary is a fortified drink of spices or a broth, and, like the pyment that she carries in service to the postpartum St Elizabeth, represents a curative offering that reveals her self-conceptualisation as physician and healer.[64] Kempe reinforces this belief when she instructs Mary to accept the mixture, demonstrating her intense desire to cure and the assumed efficacy of her medicine: 'A, blissyd Lady, 3e must nedys comfortyn 30wr-self & cesyn of 30wr sorwyng' (195). In a curative reversal of this image, Henry of Lancaster longs to drink the milk of the Virgin Mary as a healing aid: 'And, most sweet Lady, as it seems to me, I may say that to drink your sweet milk would be good for my wounds, just as those who are wounded drink a little salve.'[65]

Margery Kempe's holy nursing develops from her mystical offerings as the Virgin's handmaiden to her later metamorphosis as Christ's 'keeper' throughout his childhood: 'sche in contemplacyon & in meditacyon had ben hys Modyrs maydyn & holpyn to kepyn hym in hys childhod & so forth in-to þe tyme of hys deth' (203).[66] Indeed, it is Christ himself who authorises her meditative care-giving, since, for it, she will gain 'þe same mede in Heuyn *as thow þu dedist it to myn owyn persone er to my blissyd Modyr*, & I xal thankyn þe þerfor' (203). Substitution, or surrogacy, therefore, has divine validation as an activity of holy merit, and Kempe finds numerous healing strategies, using both earthly and mystical subjects, through which to gain edification and by which to render herself productive.

The Pain of 'Leprous' Affliction

In Chapter 74 of the *Book* Margery Kempe indicates her increased age when she contemplates her death, which she considers overdue: 'heryng hir Messe & reuoluyng in hir mende þe tyme of hir deth, sor syhyng & sorwyng for it was so long delayd' (176). Christ responds by revealing that she will live the precise term of 'Al þis xv 3er', which, given that the earliest possible date of her death is 1438, and assuming that events unfold as Christ says, positions

---

[64] MED s.v. 'caudel' 1(a) A hot fortified drink, esp. one containing spiced wine or ale; also, a broth; (b) a pudding, meat loaf, or the like; (c) a mess.

[65] Henry of Lancaster, *Le livre de seyntz medicines*, trans. Batt p. 190.

[66] Wet nurses were often retained in the households of more wealthy families for an extended period, throughout a child's formative years. See McLaughlin, 'Survivors and Surrogates', in *Medieval Families*, ed. Neel, p. 117.

the chapter at around 1423, when Kempe would be about fifty. Her reaction is one of distress – fifteen years of further life, separate from God, seems to her like a thousand years – but Christ reassures her of his love and renews her meditations on his Passion. This moment is a critical turning point in Kempe's spiritual development, as henceforth she begins to connect the sick and afflicted with Christ's corporeal suffering in a graphic and ocular manner. Now she is unable to endure the sight of a leper or other 'seke man, specialy ʒyf he had any wowndys aperyng on hym' (176). The pain-surrogacy hermeneutic evolves so that, on witnessing lepers or impaired people, Kempe weeps 'as ʒyf sche had sen owr Lord Ihesu Crist wyth hys wowndys bledyng' (176), the lepers now symbolising the tortured Christic body through their substitute and pitiful injuries.[67] Though the sight of lepers had been 'abhomynabyl' to her during her 'ʒerys of worldly prosperite', she now desires to kiss and embrace them for the 'lofe of Ihesu' (176–7), substituting love for hatred and mourning her inability to demonstrate physically this polarised shift in her perception of the afflicted.

The association of leprosy with sin has biblical origin: Moses' sister Mary is punished with leprosy for criticising him (Numbers 12:8–15), and Christ's healing of lepers is recounted many times in the gospels, where the concomitance of bodily contamination and spiritual health is implicit.[68] Medieval writers often saw physical affliction as a positive fortuity, where the sick are regarded as 'chosen' and their souls considered more able to progress heavenwards. Chaucer's Parson asserts that 'peyne is sent by the rightwys sonde of God, and by his sufferance, be it meselrie, or mayhem, or maladie';[69] St Anselm (1033–1109) counselled the dying Bishop of Rochester that 'the progress of the soul grows out of the failure of the flesh';[70] and *The Manere of Good Lyvyng*, a Middle English translation of the late twelfth- or early thirteenth-century treatise the *Liber de modo bene vivendi ad sororoem*, which was often attributed to Bernard of Clairvaux (1090–1153), instructs a community of nuns (probably those at Syon Abbey) that sickness should be embraced as a divine gift. The *Liber* was known as one of Bridget of Sweden's favourite contemplative texts, and she played an important role in spreading its popularity, including at Syon. The text states that 'Suche as be strong and hool it ys profitable for them to be seke, les by the strength of bodely helth they rejoyse

---

[67] The slipperiness of the term 'leper' was initiated by Jerome's translation of the Bible into the Vulgate in AD 383, which created a shift in meaning. The Hebrew word *sāra'ath* (understood in Mosaic Law to indicate imprecise skin conditions such as scaly, scabrous and raw skin), translated into the Greek *lepra*, and then into the Latin *leprosy*. Jerome's description of Christ as a leper, then, was intended to convey the image of Christ's bruises, lesions and damaged flesh. See Carole Rawcliffe, *Leprosy in Medieval England* (Woodbridge: Boydell Press, 2006), p. 73. See also Isaiah 53:4, 'Surely he hath borne our infirmities and carried our sorrows: and we have thought him as a leper, and as one struck by God and afflicted'.

[68] Mary is named Miriam in later biblical translations. Luke 17:12–19, for example, describes ten men who ask Jesus for mercy. On his instruction to go to the priests, they are made 'clean'.

[69] 'The Parson's Tale', in *The Riverside Chaucer*, p. 308, ll. 622–5.

[70] From Rawcliffe, *Leprosy*, p. 55.

more in transitory and worldly thyngys than they ouȝt to doo.' Addressing a 'Reverent suster', it advises 'be ye not hevy in your seknes but thanke God. Wysche ye to have the helth of the soule rather than of the bodye. The diseasis of the bodye be remedyes and medicyns of the soule'.[71] A comparable message is conveyed by the author of the *Ancrene Wisse*, who advises his female ancho-ritic audience that illness is the 'soul's salvation':

Secnesse is a brune hat forte þolien, ah na þing ne clenseð gold as hit deð þe sawle. Secnesse þet Godd send – nawt þet sum lecheð þurgh hire ahne dusischipe – deð þeose six þinges: (i) wescheð þe sunnen þe beoð ear iwrahte (ii) wardeð toȝein þeo þe weren towards (iii) pruueð patience (iii[i]) halt in eadmodnesse (v) muchleð þe mede, [(vi)] eueneð to martir þene þolemode. Þus is secnesse sawlene heale, salue of hir wunden, scheld þet ha ne kecche ma, as Godd sið þet ha schulde ȝef secnesse hit ne lette.

[Illness is a hot fire to bear, but nothing purifies gold as it does the soul. Illness that God sends – not what a woman may come down with through her own foolishness – does these six things: (i) washes away the sins that have already been committed (ii) protects against those that were about to be (iii) tests patience (iv) maintains humility (v) increases the reward (vi) makes whoever bears it patiently equal to a martyr. In this way illness is the soul's salvation, an ointment for its wounds, a shield against its receiving more, as God sees that it would if illness did not prevent it.][72]

In a similar vein the *Cyrurgie of Guy de Chauliac*, in a passage on leprosy, emphasises that it is a mark of election as opposed to a curse: 'this passioun or sekenesse is saluacioun of the soule and nought to say the trouthe, for if leprouse men were reproued, it wer a purgatorie to þe soule'.[73] However, med-ico-religious understandings did not hold sin, or divine election, as the only cause of leprosy. Several natural causes were also posited, including an excess of choler or black bile.[74] Being conceived when one's mother was menstruat-ing was another frequent explanation, as seen in the relentlessly misogynistic treatise *De secretis mulierum*.[75] Kempe's fixation on 'lepers' – in fact, anyone afflicted with skin lesions or marks – is thus explained by their affliction's visual

[71] The XLIII exhortation, *The Manere of Good Lyvyng: A Middle English Translation of Pseudo-Bernard's Liber de mono bene vivendi ad sororem*, ed. Anne E. Mouron (Turnhout: Brepols, 2014), pp. 125–7.

[72] *Ancrene Wisse: A Corrected Edition*, ed. Bella Millett, Part 4, section 7, p. 69. Translation from *Ancrene Wisse: Guide for Anchoresses, a Translation based on Cambridge, Corpus Christi College, MS 402*, Bella Millett (Exeter: University of Exeter Press, 2009), Part 4, section 7, p. 69.

[73] *The Cyrurgie of Guy de Chauliac*, p. 381.

[74] See Rawcliffe, *Leprosy*, p. 51.

[75] *De secretis mulierum*, trans. Lemay, pp. 130–1. See also Rawcliffe, *Leprosy*, pp. 64–103; Luke Demaitre, *Leprosy in Premodern Medicine: A Malady of the Whole Body* (Baltimore: The John Hopkins University Press, 2007), pp. 168–70; and Susan Zimmerman, 'Leprosy in the Medieval Imaginary', *Journal of Medieval and Early Modern Studies*, 38 (2008), 559–87.

identification with Christ's wounds, the substitute closeness that she desires with the Christic body, and her desire to heal their pain (as Christ healed lepers) through a ministry which proposes affliction as divinely elected.

When Kempe's confessor accedes to her kissing leper women but not men, she embarks on a visit to the hospital where her intended act of surrogacy hinges on a performance between the pious 'self' and the contaminated 'other':[76]

> Þan was sche glad, for sche had leue to kyssyn þe seke women & went to a place wher seke women dwellyd whech wer ryth ful of þe sekenes & fel down on hir kneys be-forn hem, preyng hem þat sche myth kyssyn her mowth for þe lofe of Ihesu. & so sche kyssyd þer ij seke women with many an holy thowt & many a deuowt teer, &, whan sche had kyssyd hem & telde hem ful many good wordys & steryd hem to mekenes & pacyens þat þei xulde not grutchyn wyth her sekenes but hyly thankyn God þerfor & þei xulde han gret blysse in Heuyn thorw þe mercy of owr Lord Ihesu Crist ... (177).

That she is allowed this visit directly after experiencing 'gret mornyng & sorwyng for sche myth not kyssyn þe laʒers' (176) illustrates that some of these 'seke women' must have had leprosy. Kempe's insistence on repeatedly kissing them illustrates her desire to access Christ via the surrogate activity of receiving contamination and potential pain.[77] This kissing, 'for þe lofe of Ihesu', represents a reciprocity of healing power whereby Kempe is sanctified through the potential receipt of contamination, the substitution of the women's sickness for Christ's wounds, and her ministry in response to their despair. The risk to the health of women who cared for the sick inevitably reduced their life expectancy through their exposure to infection.[78] But such acts, which defiantly transgress medieval conceptions of female pollution and defilement, were likely inspired by the taboo encounters of other mystical women, about whom Kempe would have been aware.[79] Some Italian saints

---

[76] This was probably the hospital of St Mary Magdalen, founded on the causeway leading to Gaywood in 1145, although it could have been one of four others mentioned by Stephen Guybord of North Lynn in his will of 1432. See *BMK*, p. 332, n. 177/9–10. Lazar hospitals were frequently named after St Mary Magdalen because of the biblical association of sexual promiscuity with leprosy.

[77] Although prolonged contact with the leprous was considered a risk for contagion, fears about contamination were slow to develop, and not universal. 'Contagion', in the medieval context, was understood in humoral terms and was therefore more loosely defined, encompassing notions of pollution, putrefaction, heredity and personal contact. See Carole Rawcliffe, *Leprosy*, pp. 4 and 90–5. See also F.O. Touati, 'Contagion and Leprosy: Myth, Ideas and Evolution in Medieval Minds and Societies', in *Contagion: Perspectives from Premodern Societies*, ed. L.I. Conrad and D. Wujastyk (Aldershot: Ashgate, 2000), pp. 179–201.

[78] See Shulamith Shahar, *Growing Old in the Middle Ages: 'Winter clothes us in shadow and pain'* (London and New York: Routledge, 1997), p. 35.

[79] On kissing lepers, see Catherine Peyroux, 'The Leper's Kiss', in *Monks and Nuns, Saints and Outcasts: Religion in Medieval Society. Essays in Honor of Lester K. Little*, ed. S. Farmer and B.H. Rosenwein (Ithaca, NY: Cornell University Press, 2000), pp. 172–88. See also S. Farmer, 'The Leper in the Master Bedroom: Thinking Through a Thirteenth-

drank pus or scabs from lepers' sores, ingesting disease. The nuns of Töss, Unterlinden, and Ethgelthal prayed to be afflicted with leprosy.[80] Elizabeth of Hungary (1207–31) – another married holy woman – built a hospital in Marburg and spent much of her life nursing the diseased outcasts of society: 'there was a woman with a horrible leprosy whom she bathed and put to bed, cleansing and bandaging her sores, applying remedies, trimming her finger-nails, and kneeling at her feet to loosen her shoes'.[81] In an abject interpretation of care-giving, Angela of Foligno (c. 1248–1309) drank the bathwater of lepers after having washed their feet, in order to attain what Karma Lochrie sees as a 'perverse eucharistic sacrament' that involves 'risks of perversion on the verge of perfection'.[82] While this example reveals extreme somatic control to achieve Christic union, it is clear that Margery Kempe wishes to identify with the other holy women, about whom she was told, who nursed the leprous. Bridget of Sweden soberly nursed sick men's lesions: 'Of hir owne substaunce she repayred in hir countre many desolate hospytalles & as a busy administratrice mercyful & pytuous she visited the nedy syke men that were ther & handeled and wasshyd theyr sores without horror or lothsomnes.'[83] Marie of Oignies (1177–1213) was also known to have cared for lepers: 'they [Marie and her husband, now living chaste] serued sumwhile to summe mesellis [lepers] bisyde Niuelle, in a place that is named Villambrote'.[84]

Though Kempe's communing with 'lepers' is perhaps less foul and exces-sive, her mouth as portal to the body's vulnerable internality nevertheless makes contact with the tainted patients, whose defilement marks a meaningful healing fissure into which she can enter. The motivation of the holy physician is dichotomously selfless/self-centric, as Julie Orlemanski attests: 'While the leprous kiss posed new experiential and intersubjective possibilities in the Middle Ages, these ran up against the asymmetry of its imagining, the solip-sism of its intimacy'.[85] Still, Kempe's 'many good wordys' – emerging from that same, disrupted mouth – are transformational, turning the despairing female patients who 'grutchyn' (complain) into humble receivers of God's

Century Exemplum', in *Framing the Family: Narrative and Representation in the Medieval and Early Modern Periods*, ed. Rosalynn Voaden and Diane Wolfthal (Tempe: Arizona Centre for Medieval and Renaissance Studies, 2005), pp. 79–84.

[80] The nuns of Töss, Unterlinden and Ethgelthal composed biographies in the fourteenth century, which were compiled in the *Nonnenbücher*. See Bynum, *Holy Feast and Holy Fast*, pp. 130–1 and p. 209.

[81] Jacobus de Voragine's 'The Life of Saint Elizabeth', in *The Golden Legend: Readings on the Saints*, ed. William Granger Ryan and Eamon Duffy (Princeton: Princeton University Press, 2012), p. 693 and p. 697. Kempe was read the *Vita* of St Elizabeth of Hungary, as is reported in the *Book*. See Chapter 1 of this study, p. 43, n. 55 and p. 49, n. 80.

[82] Karma Lochrie, *Margery Kempe and Translations of the Flesh*, pp. 42–3.

[83] Thomas Gascoigne, 'Lyfe of seynt Birgette', in *The Myroure of Our Ladye*, p. liii.

[84] 'The Middle English Life of Marie d'Oignies', in *Three Women of Liège*, ed. Brown, p. 90.

[85] Julie Orlemanski, 'How to Kiss a Leper', *Postmedieval: A Journal of Medieval Cultural Studies*, 3 (2012), 142–57 (p. 144).

love, and offering a revision of their situation as imbued with grace and hope.[86] Furthermore, her inclusion strategy, where the women are drawn into God's love not in spite of their affliction but because of it, is reminiscent of her healing of the 'contaminated' postpartum woman, whose final cure was her reintegration into the community that had marginalised her in fear. Despite Kempe's desire to receive the lepers' disease through her kissing mouth, to use the women as conduits through which to demonstrate her Christ-like love of humanity, she nevertheless paradoxically perpetuates the women's otherness by positioning herself as a religious authority, piously ministering to these objects of sin and affliction from the standpoint of healthy elevation.

This is anticipated in Chapter 65 when God reminds Kempe of the charity he has shown her:

> whan þu seest any laȝerys, þu hast gret compassion of hem, ȝeldyng me than-kyngs & presyngys þat I am mor fauorabyl to þe þan I am to hem, and also, dowtyr, for þe gret sorwe þat þu hast for al þis world þat þu mythyst helpyn hem as wel as þu woldist helpyn þi-self boþe gostly & bodily, & forþermore for þe sorwys þat þu hast for þe sowlys in Purgatory þat þu woldist so gladly þat þei wer owt of her peyn þat þei mythyn preysyn me wyth-owtyn end (160).

Christ's words reinforce Kempe's desire to heal pain and suffering, both ghostly and bodily, with the same authenticity as if she were helping herself, and thus also her willingness to act as a substitute for others' pain. However, she is also grateful for the *difference* that she perceives between herself and the lepers, thanking God for his favouring her in place of them. There is a powerful disconnect here that locates Kempe as at once unconditional surrogate and privileged medic. Clearly, Kempe's spiritual maturation now assures her of God's forgiveness and protection from earthly contamination; her actions are, in a way, a test of the divine prophylactic, and see her inclusion into the healing realm in stark contrast to the lepers' exclusion in quarantine, the 'place wher seke women dwellyd'.[87]

To the female lepers whose bodies are so riddled with disease that they are 'ryth ful of þe sekenes', Kempe offers the remedy of redemption, replacing their 'sinful impurity' with the promise of heavenly bliss and, in so doing, a corporeal rebirth. Such reproductivity allows her to maintain a pious vigil over the Christic wounds that she imagines through the leprous women whilst simultaneously effecting the rebirth that those wounds sanctioned. The edifying

---

[86] MED s.v. grucchen: To murmur, grumble; complain.

[87] Although the leprous were cared for in designated *leprosaria,* often on the outskirts of towns, recent archaeological evidence suggests that the leprous were not as marginalized and mistreated as has been suggested. The body of a pilgrim, buried with a scallop shell, was found to be buried alongside lepers' bodies. The shell is a symbol of pilgrimage to the shrine of St James at Santiago de Compostela, Spain, where Margery Kempe is known to have travelled. See Simon Roffey and Phil Marter, 'Treating Leprosy: Inside the Medieval Hospital of St Mary Magdalen, Winchester', *Current Archaeology*, 267 (2012), 12–18.

ocularity of the experience is an ironic one, given that blindness is a common symptom of leprosy.[88] She not only comforts the women, then, through the touching and kissing from which they are otherwise excluded, but also replaces their eyes via the new vision of mystical discernment, bypassing bodily faculty. When one of the sick women is beset with temptations and terror, Kempe substitutes her 'fowle & horibyl thowtys' (177) with her own vision of God and her faith in his healing power. Beyond this surrogate vision, however, is the further paradox of Kempe's willingness to risk the pain and symptoms of the women's sores, and thus the pain of Christ's wounds, through kissing. Other symptoms of leprosy (now known as Hansen's disease) include permanent nerve damage and swelling. This anaesthetises parts of the face or the extremities that have been subject to the injurious bacteria. The dangerous absence of pain – inbuilt as a protective warning signal – from the cuts, sores, and abrasions thus makes their infection more likely, leading to the loss of fingers and toes.[89] Bartholomaeus Anglicus noted how sensation is lost when the body's members are numbed: 'in oþir vttir parties felinge is somdele bynome'.[90] That the 'leper' women have potentially lost the pain-signals that Kempe seeks to substitute renders her pain surrogacy as a more crucial intercession in her development as God's healing disciple. As a surrogate and salvific 'safety net' for the women, Kempe is doubly assured of her own 'safety' in heaven.

According to Michel Foucault, leper houses faded away in the fourteenth century since their 'social exclusion' in fact effected 'spiritual reintegration'; then the 'mad', as 'a sort of great unreason', replaced the leprous as social subjects of otherness and segregation.[91] Such an amalgamation of diseased otherness is evident in the *Book* when one of the sick women in the same hospital is beset by so many temptations that 'sche wist not how sche myth best be gouernyd' (177). This woman's mental affliction is so ungovernable – deranged, even – that she anticipates diabolic annihilation:

> Sche was so labowryd wyth hir gostly enmy þat sche durst not blissyn hir ne do no worschep to God for dreed þat þe Deuyl xuld a slayn hir. And sche was labowryd wyth many fowle & horibyl thowtys, many mo þan sche cowde tellyn. &, as sche seyd, sche was a mayde. Þerfor þe sayd creatur went to hir many tymys to comfortyn hir & preyd for hir, also ful specialy þat God xulde strength hir a-geyn hir enmye, & it is to beleuyn þat he dede so, blissyd mote he ben (177).

Kempe's paradigmatic inclusion therapy of kissing leper women is now transferred as a remedy for the diabolic torment of this woman. The 'fowle & horibyl thowtys' that overcome her disordered mind are unspeakable, excluding her as an aberration, unauthorised to be blessed or to worship

---

[88] See Rawcliffe, *Leprosy*, p. 3. See also Demaitre, *Leprosy in Premodern Medicine*, p. 220.
[89] Rawcliffe, *Leprosy*, p. 2. Demaitre, ibid.
[90] *On the Properties of Things*, p. 424.
[91] Michel Foucault, *Madness and Civilisation* (London and New York: Routledge, 1961), pp. 4–24.

God. Though her distress evokes Kempe's postpartum trauma at the beginning of the *Book*, when she 'lost reson & her wyttes a long tyme' (2), the cause is antithetic: while Kempe was wracked with the guilt of unconfessed concupiscence, this woman is 'a mayde'. Her frenzy is therefore a polarised transformation from purity to possession, and Kempe's labour as a healer must be as bold as the metamorphosis is extreme. Her ensuing synthesis of comfort and prayer focuses prophylactically on the construction of a protective field against evil, and the cure is efficacious once more. The experiential undoing of Kempe's own childbirth trauma, being out of her 'mende', has provided an esoteric medico-religious training that enables her prayers to be tailored through an intuitive pain surrogacy. Unlike the other hospital 'kepars', who have abandoned the woman to her own distracted wits, Kempe is unafraid of the pain, because it has also been hers.

* * *

That Book II begins with the story of Margery Kempe's adult son situates the episode as a significant structural and symbolic moment on her trajectory towards holy *medicina*. Medieval conduct-book literature impressed the expectation that mothers should guide their children in the epistemics of morality, added to which Kempe's post-reproductive life stage and spiritual maturation compel her to cure her son of his sinful lifestyle.[92] The story of Bridget of Sweden's prodigal son, Karl, whose soul Bridget saved through her tears, would have been well known, and Kempe is imitatively driven to draw her son from the 'wretchyd & vnstabyl worlde' – to persuade him to focus less on his business pursuits and instead follow Christ – if 'hir power myth a teynyd þerto' (221).[93] The semantic emphasis of *Kempe's* transformative power, as opposed to divine intervention, evidences a new authority, stressed also by the 'many tymys' that she meets with him: a persistence that in fact catalyses a temporary disintegration of the mother–son relationship. Her prescription for her son is that he should remain chaste until marriage, and it is a sanctified cure for worldliness since, if he fails, she prays that God will 'chastise' him and 'ponysch' him for it (222). The threat of divine retribution brought about by Kempe's intercession evokes a curse-like subtext and could be viewed, as McAvoy has suggested, 'as a holy mother ... abusing her privileged power in a quasi-diabolical way'.[94] Indeed, Barbara Newman

---

[92] On domestic ideals in the *Book* see Hwanhee Park, 'Domestic Ideals and Devotional Authority in *The Book of Margery Kempe*', *The Journal of Medieval Religious Cultures*, 1, 40 (2014), 1–19. Kempe's attempts to draw her son away from worldly matters (before he goes overseas) occurs soon after her conversion, when she was in her early to mid forties: 'It befel sone aftyr þat þe creatur be-forn-wretyn had forsakyn þe occupasyon of þe worlde & was joynyd in hir mende to God as meche as frelte wolde suffyr', is immediately followed by 'The seyd creatur had a sone ... whom sche desyrd to a drawyn owte of þe perellys of þis wretchyd & vnstabyl worlde' (221).

[93] See Clarissa Atkinson, *The Oldest Vocation* (Ithaca: Cornell University Press, 1991), pp. 177–9.

[94] McAvoy, *Authority and the Female Body*, p. 43.

regards the event as an invocation of 'the rhetoric of child sacrifice: so great is her devotion that she would sooner curse her own son with leprosy than risk the damnation of his soul'.[95] Rather, I argue that this episode is an instance of Kempe's using her middle-aged, surrogate healing praxes, predicated on curative powers ordained by God, to act as a substitute physician, and that this potential *ponyschment* is in fact conceived of as salvific therapy.

After his mother's sharp words of correction, the son travels overseas until his profligate lifestyle forces him to return, complete with facial lesions:

> throw euyl entisyng of oþer personys & foly of hys owyn gouernawnce, he fel in-to þe synne of letchery. Sone aftyr hys colowr chawngyd, hys face wex ful of whelys & bloberys as it had ben a lepyr. Þan he cam hom a-geyn in-to Lynne to hys maistyr wyth whech he had ben dwelling be-for-tyme. Hys maistyr put hym owt of hys seruyse for no defawte he fond wyth hym, but perauentur supposyng he had ben a laȝer as it schewyd be hys visage (222).

The phonetic juxtaposition of 'letchery' and 'lepyr' emphasises their cultural assimilation. A medical diagnosis of leprosy is absent, replaced instead with the suggestion of its *appearance* or representation. The son is 'as it had ben' a leper, the employer 'supposyng' leprosy from the external facial evidence. Multifarious afflictions were associated with skin disorders in the medieval imaginary, including venereal disease.[96] The public shame of a 'leprous' face is encapsulated by the medical writer Jordanus de Turre (fl. 1310–35), who describes 'the roundness of the eyeballs, which seem to be starting from their sockets, so that a leper's face is horrible to see; its natural expression being distorted, it is a terrible sight'.[97] The conflation of leprosy and sexual incontinence in the Middle Ages would presumably have worried the son's employer in that disfiguration was concomitant with poor moral conduct, which might damage his business. Such cultural assumptions had even infiltrated medical texts like that of Gilbertus Anglicus, who asserts that 'Lepers search for sexual pleasure more than usual and more than they should; they are ardent in the act, yet find themselves weaker than usual.'[98]

It is easy to see, then, how the 'whelys & bloberys' that cover Kempe's son's face might be construed by the community at Lynn, to which he returns, as a symbol of iniquity and shame. However, when he goes about the town proclaiming 'wher hym liked' that this punishment from God was, 'as he supposyd', brought about by his mother, certain neighbours' interpretations locate Kempe as an evil perpetrator.[99] The locals' condemnation of Kempe's teaching as wicked is not unfamiliar. Defamatory hearsay was ventriloquised

---

[95] Newman, *Virile Woman*, p. 92.
[96] See Rawcliffe, *Leprosy*, pp. 72–3; and Demaitre, *Leprosy in Premodern Medicine*, pp. 198–239.
[97] From Wallis, *Medieval Medicine*, p. 343.
[98] Ibid., p. 341.
[99] A shift in diagnostic practice was necessitated by the disease of leprosy since the application of humoral theory in practice was problematic. Doctors had to treat leprosy as a specific entity, separate from the patient. See Wallis, *Medieval Medicine*, p. 339. This

by the Archbishop of York when he confronted her in his chapel at Cawood, saying 'I am euyl enformyd of þe; I her seyn þu art a ryth wikked woman' (125). Similarly, the York anchoress, who had previously shown Kempe great kindness, at one point turns against her and 'wolde not receyuen hir, for sche had herd telde so mech euyl telde of hir' (119).[100] In the face of this this latest enmity, however, Kempe's spiritual progress is clearly evident; accused of having 'takyn veniawns on hir owyn childe' (222), she takes little heed, remaining resolute and insisting that her son comes to seek grace and forgiveness himself. Indeed, Olga Burakov Mongan rightly suggests that slander – synonymous with blasphemy in medieval culture – actively enables Kempe to achieve sanctification and 'constitutes part of her highly affective *imitatio Christi*'.[101] Kempe's steadfastness illustrates a conviction in her holy path and the strength of her providential faith. For just as she displays a diagnostic certainty in praying for her son's divine punishment, so she reasons that that son, afflicted with facial lesions so abhorrent that they effect his instant dismissal from employment, should return to her in an act of free will: a desire for healing salvation.[102]

Medieval medical treatments for leprosy were organised around the central topos that it was, in fact, an incurable disease. Writers such as Aretaeus affirmed this by suggesting that leprosy entailed an 'inevitable demise', and Jacques de Vitry (c. 1160–1240) admitted reluctance and ignorance when addressing an audience in a leprosarium chapel, stating that 'we cannot, or we do not want to, or we do not know how to heal your illness'.[103] In concurrence, recent archaeological work has shown little skeletal evidence for radical medical intervention in patients with leprosy. The regimes at leper hospitals appear to have been based on diet, bed rest, frequent washing, and 'spiritual intensive care', whilst entering a hospital involved a 'quasi-monastic life of obedience, chastity and humility'.[104] However, the cultural value of female blood as therapeutic for lepers is evident in several sources, and marks a conceptual tension with the simultaneous understanding of menstruating women as *causative* of some cases of leprosy. Hildegard of Bingen recommends the use of menstrual blood in a curative bath:

---

shift suggests that it was easy to ascribe a visually horrifying disease such as leprosy to an external cause; namely, a curse, or moral depravity.

[100] On defamation, see Brian VanGinhoven, 'Margery Kempe and the Legal Status of Defamation', *The Journal of Medieval Religious Cultures*, 40 (2014), 20–43.

[101] Olga Burakov Mongan, 'Slanderers and Saints: The Function of Slander in *The Book of Margery Kempe*', p. 36.

[102] The son's employment is likely to have been an apprenticeship, his leprous appearance implying a 'lack of control'. See Daniel F. Pigg, 'Margery Kempe and Her Son: Representing the Discourse of Family', in *Childhood in the Middle Ages: The Results of a Paradigm Shift in the History of Mentality*, ed. Albrecht Classen (Berlin and New York: de Gruyter, 2005), pp. 329–39 (p. 336).

[103] Demaitre, *Leprosy in Premodern Medicine*, pp. 244–6.

[104] See Christopher Catling, 'The Archaeology of Leprosy and the Black Death', *Current Archaeology*, 236 (2009), 22–9.

If a person becomes leprous from lust or intemperance, he should cook agri-
mony, and a third part hyssop, and twice as much asarum as there is of the other
two in a cauldron. He should make a bath from these, and mix in menstrual
blood, as much as he can get, and get into the bath.

[Si autem homo di libidine aut incontinentia leprosus efficitur, agrimonium, et
secundum ejus tertiam partem hysopum, et aseri bis tantum ut istorum duorum
est, in caldario coquat, et ex his balneum faciat, et menstruum sanguinem,
quantum habere poterit, admisceat, et balneo se imponat.][105]

That menstrual blood – a substance of toxicity and danger in the medieval sexual
dialectic – is here employed as a therapeutic substance recalls the multivalency
of blood that was examined in the preceding chapter. In the thirteenth-century
Queste del saint graal the virgin sister of the grail knight, Perceval, allows her
blood to be drained to cure a leprous lady (the sister's virginity being the vital
quality that ensures the efficacy of the cure); in this example, the 'purity' of
female blood is the locus of its potency.[106] In the medieval poem *Amis and
Amiloun*, Amiloun contracts leprosy but is healed by an angelic vision which
tells him that the cure is the blood of his friend Amis's children.[107] The ontology
of blood in the medieval imaginary is, then, at once polluting, sinful, fertile,
curative, and, chiefly, powerful; blood is capable of causing, and curing, leprosy.

Since Margery Kempe has neither virgin nor menstrual blood at this menopausal life stage, and so has lost the bloody codification of purity and pollution,
she is, I argue, freer to act as a healer of her son's affliction, caused, as she
assumes, by his sexual *incontinentia*. When, therefore, the son fails to find
another remedy ('bote') for his sickness, his homecoming is marked by the
trauma of his infirmity and his faith that his mother will be an efficacious healer:

So at last, whan he sey non oþer bote, he cam to hys modyr, telling hir of
hys mysgouernawns, promittyng he xulde ben obedient to God & to hir &
to a-mende hys defawte thorw þe help of God echewyng al mysgouernawns
fro þat tyme for-ward vp-on hys power. He preyid hys modyr of hir blissyng,
& specialy he preyd hir to prey for hym þat owr Lord of hys hy mercy wolde
forȝeuyn hym þat he had trespasyd & takyn a-wey þat gret sekenes for whech
men fleddyn hys company & hys felaschep as for a lepyr. For he supposyd be hir
preyerys owr Lord sent hym þat ponischyng, & þerfor he trustyd be hir preyerys
to be deliueryd þer-of ȝyf sche wolde of hir charite preyin for hym (222–3).

105 PL, vol. 197, Hildegardis, '*Physica*: cujus titulus ex cod. ms.: Subtilitatem Diversarum
Naturarum Creaturam', in *Opera Omnia*, ed. Jacques-Paul Migne, Cap. CIV, col. 1176.
Translation from *Hildegard von Bingen's Physica: The Complete English Translation of Her
Classic Work on Health and Healing*, trans. Priscilla Throop (Rochester: Healing Arts
Press, 1998), p. 61.
106 On this, see Peggy McCracken, *The Curse of Eve, the Wound of the Hero: Blood, Gender,
and Medieval Literature* (Philadelphia: University of Pennsylvania Press, 2003), pp. 2–3
and p. 120, n. 2.
107 *Amis and Amiloun*, ed. M. Leach, EETS o.s. 203 (London: Oxford University Press,
1937, 2001 reprint).

Just as the postpartum woman is appeased by Kempe's blessed presence, so her son now seeks his mother's prayerful healing as quasi-priest in a moment of confession and desperation. His sickness and suffering, the latter made acute by the public revulsion that excludes him from company and from employment, represent both the evidence and the cure, as his mother's power as a divine physician must be held in faith if his future is to be salvaged. And she willingly intervenes, now compassionate towards the suffering of her progeny, and activates the hermeneutic of pain surrogacy that is at her ready disposal:

> Þan sche, hauyng trust of hys a-mendyng & compassyon of hys infirmyte, wyth scharp wordys of correpcyon promysyd to fulfillyn hys entent ȝyf God wolde grawntyn it. Whan sche cam to hir meditacyon, not forȝetyng þe frute of hir wombe, [sche] askyd forȝeuenes of hys synne & relesyng of þe sekenes þat owr Lord had ȝouyn hym ȝyf it wer hys plesawns & profite to hys sowle. So longe sche preyid þat he was clene delyueryd of þe sekenes and leuyd many ȝerys aftyr (223).

Kempe's cure is twofold as she utilises the 'sharp words' that befit a chastising mother and also the accelerated, remedial prayer that, in its persistent efficacy, relieves the affliction and sees the son delivered to purity and to health.

This eventual coming to her son's aid not only evidences the necessity to Kempe's pain surrogacy of genuine compassion for the suffering of the 'other', but also the caveat that it is God's will that provides the curative authority.[108] Despite her non-reproductive status, she facilitates a transformational rebirth of the 'frute of hir wombe' by offering herself as a maternal intercessor, capable of relieving pain if that be God's wish.[109] That same rebirth is compounded when the son marries and fathers a child – the only grandchild whom Kempe mentions in her *Book* – thus coming full circle from his mother's original injunction that he should be chaste until marriage.[110] In fulfilling the Christian edict of marital procreation, his mother's fecund *medicina* is reproduced in paradigmatic multiplicity. Indeed, in light of the evidence for this son's being the first amanuensis of the *Book*, and therefore undertaking a holy endeavour of his own, the transition from pain-racked 'leper' to edified surrogate for his mother's dictation constructs a complex layering of curative productivity.[111]

---

[108] Hildegard of Bingen also emphasises Christ as the ultimate physician when recommending a different treatment for leprosy which will heal the affliction 'unless God does not wish it'. Hildegard von Bingen, *Physica*, ed. Throop, p. 108.

[109] Karen A. Winstead has noted the strategic parallelism between the openings of Books I and II. Where Christ is instrumental in Kempe's recovery and conversion at the start of Book I, so she 'plays the role *vis à vis* her son' at the start of Book II, thus assuming Christ's role. See Winstead, 'The Conversion of Margery Kempe's Son', *English Language Notes*, 32 (1994), 9–13.

[110] *BMK*, p. 223.

[111] On the evidence for Kempe's son as scribe, see Sobecki, '"The writyng of this tretys"'; Samuel Fanous, 'Measuring the Pilgrim's Progress: Internal Emphases in *The Book of Margery Kempe*', in *Writing Religious Women*, ed. Renevey and Whitehead, pp. 157–74 (p. 158); Nicholas Watson, 'The Making of *The Book of Margery Kempe*', in *Voices in Dialogue*, ed. Olson and Kerby-Fulton (pp. 398–9); and Ruth Evans, 'The *Book of*

Paralleling the holistic ebb and flow of Galenic medicine, Margery Kempe tends to her son's body and soul in a single action; his cure is complete when, several years later, he returns to Lynn once again, 'al chongyd in hys aray & hys condicyonis' (223). His gratitude for his mother's intervention is unwavering, and his spiritual progress apparent – Kempe notices how 'sadde' he appears, and how 'reuerent to-owr-Lord-ward' (224). Now more aged, she finds it timely to disclose to him her own revelatory experience, to instruct him as mother to child but also as holy physic to patient: 'sche openyd hir hert to hym, schewyng hym & enformyng how owr Lord had drawyn hir thorw hys mercy & be what menys, also how meche grace he had schewyd for hir, þe whech he seyd he was vnworthy to heryn' (224). As a final therapy, then, Kempe's testimony propels her son onto a literally holy path. He makes pil-grimages in his mother's footsteps to Rome and beyond, signifying the repro-duction of spiritual progression and Kempe's evolving status as a medicating minister. Karen Winstead has argued that 'the conversion of Margery Kempe's son has none of the extreme consequences of Margery's own conversion'.[112] However, given the impact of the *Book*'s religious, historical, and literary ramifications (and notwithstanding its subsequent redrafting), the son's pro-motion to witness and scribe-recorder of Kempe's revelations, I think, locates this event as a indispensable facet in the text's testimony to salvation and to production. This scribal intercession is symbolic of a generative cycle where the transgression-conversion-surrogate template is duplicated from mother to son in a fitting moment of textual as well as spiritual reproduction. On the son's final return to Lynn from Danzig, Kempe is approximately fifty-eight years old, and thus her ageing, healing, and the writing of the first draft of the *Book* powerfully converge.[113]

Transitional Pain: From Wife to Widow

When John Kempe falls down the stairs and sustains life-threatening injuries to his head, which was 'greuowsly brokyn & bresyd', the period of his sickness is so extended that 'men wend þat he xulde a be deed' (179). In a reciprocal retribution, the neighbours who discover John 'half on lyfe' and covered in blood demand that Kempe should be hanged if he dies; she has reneged on her wifely duties because she has not 'kept hym' (179) and should therefore be sent to death with the man to whom she is matrimonially tied. Such a shared

---

Margery Kempe', in *A Companion to Medieval English Literature and Culture*, c. 1350–c. 1500, ed. Peter Brown (Oxford: Blackwell, 2007), pp. 507–21 (p. 511).

[112] Winstead, 'The Conversion of Margery Kempe's Son', p. 11.

[113] Allen suggests the year of the son's death to be in 1431 (*BMK*, p. *l*). Sebastian Sobecki has discovered a letter prepared in Danzig for one John Kempe on 12 June 1431, to take leave to help recover debts from England. This enables us to fairly accurately date Margery Kempe's age at this point. See Sobecki, '"The writyng of this tretys"', pp. 5–6.

terminus – or 'death surrogacy', a hermeneutic that I develop in Chapter 5 – is testament both to the social expectation that a wife must care for her husband without fail, and to the belief that her life is interchangeable with his to the ultimate degree. Kempe's role as healer in this episode, therefore, not only involves John's palliative care over many years but also represents a period of urgency in which she must save herself as well as her patient. She knows only too well the heavy weight of social and ecclesiastical admonition: threats to her life have been made with terrifying reality previously in the *Book*.[114] The nursing of her now-elderly husband thus affords her an opportunity to negotiate her life in the wake of his, and to find hope within the pain, on the cusp of liberating widowhood.

The *Book* stresses the socio-spiritual motivation behind Kempe's absence from the home in which John was injured. Their vow of chastity had pre-cipitated a physical separation – to 'enchewyn alle perellys þei dwellyd & soiowryd in diuers placys wher no suspicyon xulde ben had of her incon-tinens' – because an initial period of cohabitation had resulted in slanderous gossip about their supposed infraction of the vow (179). But there is also a further reason for her geographical remove: 'þat sche xulde not be lettyd fro hir contemplacyon' (180). This spiritual focus jars with the doctrinal contract of dutiful marriage and leaves Kempe with a slippery route to negotiate, since she is now located at a dangerous impasse where her elected vow com-promises her ability to meet her domestic obligations. The text repeats, in frightening emphasis, that 'þe pepil seyd, ȝyf he deyid, it was worthy þat sche xulde answeryn for hys deth' (180).

The public outcry at Kempe's perceived repudiation of her wifely duties stems from a vast discourse about the *mulier bona* – or, its inversion, the wicked wife – in the Middle Ages. As Sue Niebrzydowski has shown, 'Canon and secular law, the marriage liturgy, medical treatises on the female body, sermons, manuals of spiritual instruction, biblical paradigms, conduct books and misogamous writings all endeavour to define and regulate being a wife.'[115] In 'The Wife of Bath's Prologue', Jankyn reads nightly from his book of 'wikked wyves', whose selection of misogynistic stories about non-virtuous wives sends Alisoun into a paroxysm of rage. After lambasting her husband, she tears pages from the book and eventually (after sustaining a near-fatal

---

[114] At Canterbury, Kempe is accused of Lollardy by the monks, who cry out, 'Þow xalt be brent, fals lollare. Her is a cartful of thornys redy for þe & a tonne to bren þe wyth'. The people from the town cry: 'Tak & bren hir'. Ironically, it is John's protection that she eventually seeks (*BMK*, 28–9). For a discussion of this event, see Tara Williams, '"As thu wer a wedow": Margery Kempe's Wifehood and Widowhood', *Exemplaria*, 21:4 (2009), 345–62. In Chapter 53, Kempe is arrested and accused of Lollardy once more. As she is escorted through Hessle, men and women come out on the streets and cry, 'Brennyth þis fals heretyk' (129).

[115] Sue Niebrzydowski, *Bonoure and Buxom*, pp. 13–14. See also Anna Dronzek, 'Gender Roles and the Marriage Market in Fifteenth-Century England: Ideals and Practices', in *Love, Marriage, and Family Ties*, ed. Davis et al., pp. 63–76.

blow to the head in punishment) annihilates the libellous text by 'ma[king] hym brenne his book anon right tho'.[116] Though the male authority in marriage that is prescribed by conduct literature is perpetuated by Jankyn's act of domestic violence, Alisoun's destruction of the book by which she is so affronted and by which her husband's habits are governed is a rare challenge to the textualisation of wifehood that resists the individuation that women like Margery Kempe strove to forge. Furthermore, the textual construction of Alisoun and Jankyn itself underscores a literary multilayering which reveals Kempe's neighbours' threats as products of a culturally enforced code of marital observance. The good wife was expected to perform several services within the household, including 'car[ing] for the sick'.[117] The poet Marbode, Bishop of Rennes, wrote in the late eleventh century, 'For who would assume the care of a nurse, if not a woman? Without her no one born could prolong his life.'[118] A medieval lyric entitled 'In Praise of Women' similarly extols the virtues of the dutiful wife: 'A woman is a worthy wyght, / she seruyth a man both daye and nyght, / therto she puttyth all her mygth, / And yet she hathe bot care and woo.'[119] That last example illustrates what Niebrzydowski sees as a movement towards acknowledging wives' excellence in nursing, healing, and running households.[120] However, it also illustrates that the wife's duty to her husband is perpetual – 'both daye and nyght' – and shows the relentlessness of that endeavour in spite of the woman's own tribulations.

Kempe's proficiency as a physician is required, therefore, in order to recover two lives. When she confesses her concern to God that this nursing devotion will divert her energies from prayer and contemplation, she is assured of the surrogacy of the endeavour, as her tending to John's pain will be *for* the love of God:

> Dowtyr, þu xalt haue þi bone, for he xal leuyn & I haue wrowt a gret myrakyl for þe þat he was not ded. And I bydde þe take hym hom & kepe hym *for my lofe* … þu xalt haue as meche mede for to kepyn hym & helpyn hym in hys need at hom as ȝyf þu wer in chirche to makyn þi preyerys (180).

The holy value of nursing her husband in his infirmity is thus reinforced by its status as divine service, upholding the Augustinian rule that 'marriage provides a natural society between the sexes that is not dissolved by sterility or when the couple is past their reproductive years'.[121] Christ repeats that Kempe's

---

[116] 'The Wife of Bath's Prologue' (ll. 685–816), in *The Riverside Chaucer*, pp. 114–16.

[117] See David Herlihy, *Medieval Households* (Cambridge, Mass.: Harvard University Press, 1985), p. 116. See also Felicity Riddy, '"Burgeis" domesticity in late-medieval England', in *Medieval Domesticity: Home, Housing and Household in Medieval England*, ed. Maryanne Kowaleski and P.J.P. Goldberg (Cambridge: Cambridge University Press, 2008), pp. 259–76.

[118] From Herlihy, *Medieval Households*, p. 116.

[119] From Niebrzydowski, *Bonoure and Buxum*, p. 22.

[120] Ibid.

[121] Augustine stipulates that even after a vow of chastity, a dutiful tie between the couple

pledge will hypostatise 'þe lofe of me' and situates her forthcoming sacrifice as a correlative gift to John in humble gratitude for his gift to her of chastity and acceptance: 'for he hath sumtyme fulfillyd þi wil & my wil boþe and he hath mad þi body fre to me þat þu xuldist seruyn me & leuyn chast & clene, and þerfor I wil þat þu be fre to helpyn hym at hys nede in my name' (180). But though John's life has been saved, his condition is grim and Kempe's nursing task is correspondingly arduous. Her suffering during their sexual marriage, as we have seen, was alleviated by John's eventually agreeing to swear to a vow of chastity. Now, his pain must be adopted by Kempe in return as she substitutes his suffering for her own and reproduces the painful cycle of marital reciprocity and debt that she must withstand until the closure of that marriage in death. Unlike the leper women whose affliction she embraced in an active identification with other holy women who sought similar encounters, this undertaking is conceptualised as a punishment, albeit one which she gladly accepts as tending to her spiritual profit. She feels the heavy penalty of her marriage, both in the returned favour of John's vow of chastity and in the recollection of the fleshly lust which precipitated the vow in the first place:

> Þan sche toke hom hir husbond to hir & kept hym ʒerys aftyr as long as he leuyd & had ful mech labowr wyth hym, for in hys last days he turnyd childisch a-ʒen & lakkyd reson þat he cowd not don hys owyn esement to gon to a sege, er ellys he wolde not, but as a childe voydyd his natural digestyon in hys lynyn clothys þer he sat be þe fyre er at þe tabil, wheþyr it wer, he wolde sparyn no place. And þerfor was hir labowr meche þe mor in waschyng & wryngyng & hir costage in fyryng & lettyd hir ful meche fro hir contemplacyon þat many tymys sche xuld an yrkyd hir labowr saf sche bethowt hir how sche in hir ʒong age had ful many delectabyl thowtys, fleschly lustys, & inordinate louys to hys persone. & þerfor sche was glad to be ponischyd wyth þe same persone & toke it mech þe mor esily & seruyd hym & helpyd hym, as hir thowt, as sche wolde a don Crist hym-self (180–1).

In an account that is punctuated many more with the details of domestic work than the *Book* usually allows, Kempe juxtaposes fetching and carrying, washing and cleaning, with horror at the sexuality of her younger years, now recalled to memory as the re-encounters John's body in old age. The mundanity of her role as carer figures as a suitable penance for her antecedent, lustful marriage and as a symbol of the menial female-centric housework that she, as a bourgeois citizen and emerging holy woman of God, has hitherto escaped. Beyond the practicalities of her labours, Kempe's therapeutic sacrifice goes further as John's condition worsens and his mental deterioration and physical incontinence manifest as symptoms of a growing *childischness*.[122]

---

remains: 'the order of charity still flourishes between husband and wife'. From Elliott, *Spiritual Marriage*, p. 47.

[122] Sue Niebrzydowski remarks that Kempe 'remained John's wife, in all ways except sexual, until his death in c. 1431', while Sarah Salih argues that Kempe is interested in housewifery, including the care of her infirm husband, only 'when it can be shown to

This domestic nursing endeavour is far removed from the mystical marriages that have already marked Kempe's transition from earthly wife to heavenly bride. As was discussed in Chapter 2, she was mystically married to the Godhead in the Apostle's Church in Rome on St John Lateran's Day.[123] Her marriage to the Manhood is recalled in the very next chapter as a revelation that literalises the replacement of John with Christ in the marriage bed and which positions the Christic body as her new spouse, using the semiotics of physical conjugality:

> For it is conuenyent þe wyf to be homly wyth hir husbond … Ryght so mot it be twyx þe & me, for I take non hed what þu hast be but what þu woldist be. And oftyntymes haue I telde þe þat I haue clene foȝoue þe alle thy synnes. Þerfor most I nedys be homly wyth þe & lyn in þi bed wyth þe. Dowtyr, thow desyrest gretly to se me, & þu mayst boldly, whan þu art in þi bed, take me to þe as for þi weddyd husbond, as thy derworthy derlyng, & as for thy swete sone, for I wyl be louyd as a sone schuld be louyd wyth þe modyr & wil þat þu loue me, dowtyr, as a *good [wife]* owyth to loue hir husbonde. & þerfor þu mayst boldly take me in þe armys of þi sowle & kyssen my mowth, myn hed, & my fete as sweetly as thow wylt (90).

That Christ tells Kempe that she should take him in 'þe arms of [her] sowle' is a declaration of their mystical union but one which is simultaneously located in the domestic site of the marriage bed. Moreover, it is the hypostatisation of Kempe's wifehood as, through her spiritual wedlock, John is replaced in the marriage bed by her divine spouse, whose 'homly' language intertwines a mystical encounter with a conflation of various familial bonds. Here, she is a wife, a mother, and a daughter to Christ, evidencing what Barbara Newman terms the 'incest taboo' of the holy family, where mother-bride and father-husband become amalgamated in late medieval iconography, to fantastical ends.[124] Kempe thus imagines herself as part of that holy family in an ontological leap, but also as a corporeal 'good wife', lying with Christ in *swete* union and replacing in her marriage bed one husband with another. Yet she still cares for the infirm John, since that care has been divinely sanctioned as a direct substitution for the love of her new, divine bridegroom, and since care for John will be rewarded in heaven as might care for Christ's own body:

> And also, dowtyr, whan þu dost any seruyse to þe & to þin husbond in mete or drynke er any oþer thyng þat is nedful to ȝow, to þi gostly fadirs, er to any oþer þat þu receyuyst in my name, þu xalt han þe same mede in Heuyn as thow þu dedist it to myn owyn persone er to my blissyd Modyr, & I xal thankyn þe þerfor (203).

---

have spiritual significance'. See Niebryzdowski, *Bonoure and Buxum*, p. 129; and Sarah Salih, 'At home; out of the house', in *The Cambridge Companion to Medieval Women's Writing*, ed. Dinshaw and Wallace, pp. 124–40 (p. 124).

[123] See Chapter 35 of the *Book*. On Kempe's marriage to the Godhead and her holy dalliance, see Laura Kalas Williams, 'The Swetenesse of Confection'.

[124] See Barbara Newman, 'Intimate Pieties: Holy Trinity and Holy Family in the late Middle Ages', *Religion and Literature*, 31 (1999), 77–101 (pp. 78–80).

Thus, we witness first the replacement of John for Christ, and then of Christ for John, in a placing and re-placing of the husband-subject according to physical need and spiritual necessity. Kempe's wifeliness, therefore, is predicated on divine ordination and not on the edicts of the conduct book or the socio-communal machine. Though Christ has replaced John in the marriage bed, John is now replaced into her care, in God's place, in a multivalent surrogacy hermeneutic. Kempe's duties as physician and giver of palliative care are performed with the same adaptation in wifehood with which she approaches all the other female-centric roles that she simultaneously embraces and rejects, and which enable her trajectory towards eschatological perfection.

That John is thought to have died in the summer or early autumn of 1431, when Kempe was approximately fifty-eight years old, and that she mentions caring for him for 'ȝerys aftyr as long as he leuyd' (180–1), indicates that these long years of nursing corresponded with her menopausal and post-menopausal life stages.[125] The suffering that she is 'ponischyd wyth' in this protracted task nevertheless bears generative fruit in its surrogate productivity: her *medicina* is 'in [Christ's] name' (180). The climactic fecundity of this palliative sacrifice, though, is the gift of widowhood that is born from John's death, a dichotomous event that brings to a close a seemingly companionate marriage and yet heralds a new – and, we might assume, silently longed-for – phase in Kempe's life journey. Widowhood is a state for which Kempe has been preparing, and has been prepared for, during decades of contemplation. By revelation she is informed that 'þe state of maydenhode be mor parfyte & mor holy þan þe state of wedewhode, & þe state of wedewhode mor parfyte þan þe state of wedlake' (49), affirming the transition from wife to widow as unambiguously advantageous. Widows were accorded a measure of legal independence on a par with men in private law – a legal concomitance with the medico-biological masculinisation of the post-menopausal woman. Several life options were available to widows, including continuing husbands' commercial enterprises, owning property, or becoming a vowess (a state that Margery Kempe never achieved).[126] But Kempe has been suspended in an existence of quasi-widowhood for some time, told by Christ that 'þu hast þi wil of chastite as þu wer a wedow, thyn husbond leuyng in good hele' (161). This intangible – or surrogate – widowhood, despite its optimism, is no

[125] Allen notes that since Kempe's daughter-in-law spent eighteen months of widowhood in Lynn and embarked from Ipswich for her return to Germany in April 1433, the son and father must have died in the second half of 1431. See *BMK*, p. 342, n. 225/13–14.
[126] See Barbara Hanawalt, 'Widows', in *The Cambridge Companion to Medieval Women's Writing*, ed. Dinshaw and Wallace, pp. 58–69. See also Joel Rosenthal, 'Other Victims: Peeresses as War Widows, 1450–1500', in *Upon My Husband's Death: Widows in the Literature and Histories of Medieval Europe*, ed. Louise Mirrer (Ann Arbor: University of Michigan Press, 1992), pp. 131–52; 'Fifteenth-Century Widows and Widowhood: Bereavement, Reintegration, and Life Choices', in *Wife and Widow in Medieval England*, ed. Sue Sheridan Walker (Ann Arbor: University of Michigan Press: 1993), pp. 33–58; and Marie-Françoise Alamichel, *Widows in Anglo-Saxon and Medieval Britain* (Bern: Peter Lang, 2008).

substitute, however, for the concrete state in which she now rests, liberated finally to forge a singularly spiritual career and to return Christ, for the final time, to the marital bedchamber. John's demise is reiterated in Book II, when his death is noted as following shortly after their son's, whose own spiritual transfiguration forms a key episode in Kempe's healing chronicle: 'In schort tyme aftyr, þe fadyr of þe sayd persone folowyd þe sone þe wey whech euery man must gon' (225). The somewhat ill-defined states of wife and widow in the *Book* are regarded by Tara Williams as a harnessing of its achronicity that Kempe plays upon, since John's death, mentioned twice (in Chapter 76 of Book I and Chapter 2 of Book II), denotes a 'textual resurrection' that enables her to 'leverage the benefits of each [wife and widow] more directly'.[127] Yet, whilst the performativity of quasi-widowhood is certainly a central *modus operandi* in her spiritual career, the very definitive event of John's death, heralding literal widowhood, is a deictic devotional turning point. The lived experience of *þis creatur* is, I argue, primary to her textual progeny, and the actualised moment of widowhood a transformational apotheosis.

In this way, the deaths of Margery Kempe's husband and son in quick succession not only catalyse the more 'parfyte' state of widowhood and spiritual transcendence, but also signal the practical corollary of domestic emancipation. Immediately after the inscribed confirmation of John's death, it is noted that 'Than leuyd stille þe modyr of þe sayd persone, of whom þis tretys specyaly makyth mencyon' (225). Apart from the daughter-in-law who remains with Kempe for eighteen months ('sche þat was hys wife, a Dewche woman' [225]), there is no mention of any other offspring or extended family who might influence her future path.[128] Kempe is now situated in isolation – it is she alone who 'leuyd stille' – she is the final legacy of a family that has disappeared, at least from the text. Widowhood, therefore, also symbolises Kempe's own healing as she is cured of the marriage that represented a persistent barrier to the holy life for which she strove. Relieved of the punitive labour of caring for John, and of the pain of the marital state, the paradox of the husband's death for the wife's restoration becomes a telling metaphor for Kempe's reproductive 'death' as a surrogate healer of pain. Having practised her devotional medicine and substitutional receipt of others' earthly pain, she is able now to more fully contemplate the acroamatic suffering of Christ's Passion and the sins of the world, for which she has been appointed as adoptive intercessor.[129]

[127] Williams, 'As thu wer a wedow', pp. 352–3. On Kempe's authorial control, see Watson, 'The Making of *The Book of Margery Kempe*', in *Voices in Dialogue*, ed. Olson and Kerby-Fulton (pp. 397–400); and Staley, 'The Trope of the Scribe and the Question of Literary Authority'.

[128] We know of Kempe's granddaughter, but she still resides in 'Pruce' with the friends of her daughter-in-law (*BMK*, p. 225).

[129] Kempe asks God to forgive the sins of mankind on several occasions, placing her own need second to the more spiritually pressing issue of worldly damnation. For example, 'Sche seyd, "I aske ryth nowt Lord, but þat þu mayst wel 3euyn me, & þat is mercy

As she has been told, 'forbearing' (or forgoing) God brings pain, whilst joy is borne from *feeling* him.[130] This is a danger that Christ repeats in striking emphasis: 'wetyn what peyn it is for to forbere me, & how swet it is for to fele me … And þu maist not, dowtyr, forberyn me oo day *wyth-owtyn gret peyn*' (205). The remedy for Kempe's own suffering, therefore, is a perpetual state of oneness with, or *feeling* of, God, like that achieved in the intimacy of the Christic marriage bed, and which can now, in earthly widowhood, be expressed in mystical totalisation. Such *oneing* resonates with Julian of Norwich's vision of the Passion, which evoked such a shared pain as to prompt *henosis* (mystical oneness) with Christ and his *even cristen*: 'Here I sawe a grete aninge [oneing] betwyx Criste and us. For whan he was in paine, we ware in paine, and alle creatures that might suffer paine sufferde with him.'[131] For Julian, the passage towards union with the Divine is a pain surrogacy that eliminates the borders of self and other and creates an acute amalgamation of experience, not just between herself and Christ but with 'us' all: all Christians in the 'body' of his Church. Now initiated through the painful transitions of her earthly roles, and having proven her efficacy as God's appointed physician, Kempe's knowledge of the pain of the world will provide the key to her own 'anchorhold' of contemplation, in stark contrast to the keys to the 'botery' which marked both the occupation of her young married life and the juncture between sickness and health.[132] At the age of fifty-eight, emancipated from the lacuna of wifehood in which she was suspended for nearly four decades, she is now free to *feel* God through the willing embrace of Christ's tortured flesh.

---

whech I aske for þe pepil synnys. Þu seyst oftyn-tymes in þe 3er to me þat þu hast for3ouyn me my synnes. Þerfor I aske now mercy for þe synne of þe pepil, as I wolde don for myn owyn, for, Lord, þu art alle charite, & charite browt þe in-to þis wretchyd worlde & cawsyd þe to suffyr ful harde peynys for owr synnys'" (141). Further instances of such spiritual intercession can be located on pp. 20, 48, 140, 142, 204, 208, 251.

[130] MED s.v. forbēren (v.); also forbēr, forbār(e: 4(a) To forego, relinquish, give up, part with, or lose (something); to become separated from.

[131] Julian of Norwich, 'A Vision Showed to a Devout Woman', in *The Writings of Julian of Norwich*, ed. Watson and Jenkins, p. 85. *Henosis* is from Ancient Greek (ἕνωσις), and means 'mystical oneness', 'union', or 'unity'.

[132] After her recovery from postpartum illness, Kempe requests the 'keys of þe botery' (8), symbolising her return to health and the duties of the female householder.

5

The Passion of Death Surrogacy

The late fourteenth-century religious handbook *The Pore Caitif* encapsulates the deep connection between the blackness of mourning and the green regeneration of flourishing by advising the pious to wear an entwined garland on the head of their souls: 'And so beringe bifore crist ʒoure garlond, þat corown bitokeneþ: with *knottis of mournyng* for synne as of *blak* silk & *with grene wouun togidir*.'[1] This symbolic image, redolent with notions of the black bile of melancholia, mysticism, generation and fecundity that are central to this study, epitomises the symbiosis of Margery Kempe's pain with Christ's. The visions of the crucifixion that are recalled in the *Book* are more than temporal moments of excruciating rapture, however, since they are relived, reanimated, and reintegrated in her soul time and again as opportunities for Christic union. As she is told by revelation, 'I haue oftyn-tymes seyd to þe þat I schuld be newe crucified in þe' (85) – a divine promise that Christ's body will be perpetually crucified and situated within her own in a timeless ecstasy of pain and desire.

The Passion visions function in the *Book* as ultimate exemplars of suffering, developing the pain-surrogacy hermeneutic to its logical conclusion – that is – Kempe's willingness to become a death surrogate for Christ. Indeed, her envisioning of the Virgin Mary offering her own life for Christ's ('I wolde, Sone, þat I myth suffir deth for þe so þat þu xuldist not deyin' [187]) gestures towards the spiritual currency of such a sacrifice, a willingness to *suffir* annihilation in order to retain God incarnate. Such ascetic profit becomes more explicit when, early in the *Book*, it is recounted that Christ mystically conceives Kempe as a fleshly sacrifice to be consumed and martyred in an example of quasi-Eucharistic substitution: 'Þow xalt ben etyn & knawyn of þe pepul of þe world as any raton knawyth þe stokfysch' (17). Kempe therefore reveals her conceptualisation as a willing sacrificial lamb early in her recollections, deliberately foregrounding her embodiment in vulnerable human flesh at the same time as insisting on the amalgamation of Christ's painful torture with her own, and thereby both humanising and transcending her spiritual trajectory. In exploring what I argue to be a preoccupation with her own death, the deathbed vigils that she undertakes in the parish, her patent understanding of the physiology of death signs and prognostication, and her faith

---

[1] My emphasis. 'Þe Myrour off chastite' in *The Pore Caitif*, p. 197.

in her own posthumous existence, this chapter uncovers the centrality of the semiosis of death and dying for Kempe's eschatological progress. The intense verisimilitude of her visions of Christ's Passion escalate to a liminal state of altered consciousness not unlike the mystical deaths experienced by other female visionaries of the Middle Ages, and evidence Kempe's fundamental dependency on the surrogacy template.

Writing about the living mystic as 'between two deaths', Dyan Elliott argues that the visions and miracles of living saints are congruous with a death of sorts, bringing new meaning to the phrase 'dead to the world'.[2] She posits that the 'passing of the orthodox martyr corresponded to the rise of the living saint', often bearing somatic signs of injury or decay that denoted a bodily state that hovered between the corporeal and the spiritual worlds. Mystics such as Lydwine of Schiedam (1380–1433), whose living, disintegrating body was rotten and infested with maggots, and Vanna of Orvieto (c. 1264–1306), who, during rapture, would seem so death-like that flies settled on her half-open eyes, demonstrated physical afflictions or lifeless behaviours during rapture that were interpreted as liminal in their life-death state and were thus either reified as holy or interrogated for heterodoxy.[3] Jacques de Vitry and Thomas of Cantimpré had both identified a 'grey zone between two deaths on behalf of their holy clients'.[4] The liminality of female mystics-in-rapture prompted various response strategies from the Church, which sought to interrogate the validity of such insensible behaviour, sometimes using painfully cruel tests.[5] Such tortures and inquisitions reveal not only the Church's apparent need to prove or disprove spiritual discernment – *Discretio spirituum* – but also its hegemonic fear of the esoteric female mystical body, rapt in the spirit.[6] Indeed, the very image of clerics interrupting, invading, and hurting the woman-in-rapture signifies a paradoxical desire to make publicly legible what is inherently inner, much like the impatience of Margery Kempe's onlookers as she weeps and writhes in lamentation. Such events, however, offer an opportunity for the mystic-in-pain to reorient pain as a locus of sanctification and transcendence, as Marla Carlson has explored, seeing a 'loophole through which women using pain as a means to alter consciousness create a way to speak within regimes that would silence them'.[7] If visionary experience is an already altered state of consciousness, the intense pain of a quasi-death offers Margery Kempe access to another space between 'two deaths' in which she transcends traditional iterations of affective piety.

The mystical death experienced by Catherine of Siena (c. 1347–1380) illuminates such an altered consciousness. Catherine recounts several death-like

---

[2] Dyan Elliott, *Proving Woman*, pp. 180–230 (pp. 180–93).
[3] Ibid., p.183 and p. 189.
[4] Ibid., p. 181.
[5] Ibid., pp. 184–5.
[6] On *Discretio spirituum* see Nancy Caciola, *Discerning Spirits: Divine and Demonic Possession in the Middle Ages* (Ithaca: Cornell University Press, 2003).
[7] Marla Carlson, *Performing Bodies in Pain: Medieval and Post-Modern Martyrs, Mystics, and Artists* (New York: Palgrave Macmillan, 2010), p. 79.

episodes in the 1378 *Il dialogo della divina provvidenza*, including an experience of prayer resembling death: she had been 'feeling a disposition coming, like the one she had felt at the time of death', where her soul and body felt altogether separate; 'this was in a new way, as if the memory, intellect, and will had nothing to do with my body'.[8] Catherine later dictates a full out-of-body experience that her confessor, Raymond of Capua, would later clarify as a mystical death. She describes being 'immediately thrown down. And as I was thrown down, it seemed to me as if the soul had left the body … I did not seem to be in the body, but I saw my body as if I were someone else.' She recounts that she was inanimate for 'a very long time, so long that the *famiglia* cried over me as if I had died'.[9] In the *Legenda major* Raymond of Capua seeks Catherine's canonisation in part by elaborating on this mystical death as an early turning point in her sanctified life; in describing this temporary physical annihilation, Raymond is able to imply that Catherine was thereafter dead to herself and completely possessed by God. Catherine, he notes, was divinely sanctioned to suffer more and more of Christ's Passion, before her heart was literally wrenched in two: 'there was created in her heart such a violence of charity and love that her heart was not capable of remaining whole without being entirely broken in two'.[10] This event was witnessed by the women of the neighbourhood and lasted for four hours. Later Catherine revealed to Raymond that her soul had indeed 'been separated from her body and that she could still feel physically the pain of her broken heart'.[11] Kempe's visions of the Passion represent, I contend, a similar experiential altered state of consciousness and pseudo-death, where her mystical responses as a simultaneous surrogate and disciple signal an intensity and desperation that are unequalled elsewhere in the *Book*. In meditating on Christ's tortured body and wounds, Kempe is dismantled, too, running wildly and prostrating herself as if her heart too, like Catherine's, is broken.

According to Karen Scott, Raymond of Capua 'shaped Catherine's life according to a theological scheme of general spiritual stages, in which the soul's progressively greater openness to God brings her closer and closer to death; then she experiences a mystical death manifesting conclusively her death to self and her life in Christ'.[12] This notion of death as an active event was precipitated by Augustine's idea of an eighth age, conceived because Christ had risen on

---

[8] From Karen Scott, 'Mystical Death, Bodily Death: Catherine of Siena and Raymond of Capua on the Mystic's Encounter with God', in *Gendered Voices: Medieval Saints and Their Interpreters*, ed. Catherine Mooney (Philadelphia: University of Pennsylvania Press, 1995), pp. 136–67 (p. 152). Catherine of Siena's *Il Dialogo* was translated into Middle English for the Syon nuns in the early fifteenth century, and later printed as *The Orcherd of Syon* by Wynkyn de Worde in 1519. Her *Vita* was also known and owned in various religious houses. See C. Annette Grisé, 'Catherine of Siena', in *The History of British Writing, 700–1500*, ed. Liz Herbert McAvoy and Diane Watt (Basingstoke and New York: Palgrave Macmillan, 2011), pp. 216–22.

[9] Scott, 'Mystical Death, Bodily Death', p. 159.

[10] Ibid., p.165.

[11] Ibid.

[12] Ibid., p. 163.

the day after the Sabbath: the eighth day. This stage, 'outside of time', was developed in his *Of True Religion* (390 AD), where he distinguishes between the earthly man and the *novus homo*, reborn within, in a series of seven *spirituales aetates*. The seventh stage involved spiritual growth – an age unconstrained by time – identified by Augustine as one of eternal rest and perpetual beatitude.[13] In the central Middle Ages, Thomas of Cantimpré proposed a schema of the Seven Ages of Man which incorporated death as the distinct seventh stage of life – that is, a corporeal age.[14] Similarly, Bartholomaeus Anglicus identified death as synchronically an 'age', an end, and a beginning. Despite the 'euelys' of elderly decrepitude, it is also 'goode', and linguistically charged as a transitional continuum, couched in the present continuous tense: the 'ende of wrecchidnes and of woo, and bigynnynge of welþe of ioye, and *passinge* out of perile and *comynge* in prise, parfitnes in medeful dedis, and disposicioun *to be* parfite'.[15] The medieval conceptualisation of death is regarded by Patrick Geary as 'a transition, a change in status, but not an end. The dead were present among the living through liturgical commemoration, in dreams and visions, and in their physical remains, especially the tombs and relics of the saints'.[16] From the deathbed activities of last rites, communion and extreme unction, and the full Christian burial – all of which symbolise the 'good death' to which all medieval Christians aspired – to the putrefaction of the corpse in the tomb, death represented a continued process, deserving of its own clear stage in the life cycle.[17] The medieval insistence on a personalised death-experience 'valorized individual experience' as well as bodily suffering, according to Caroline Walker Bynum; redemption was founded on a 'psychosomatic unity, a person, fully individual both in its physicality and its consciousness'.[18] Whilst the moment of literal death was thus as significant for the soul as it was for the body in temporal synchronicity and with eternal ramifications, the phenomenon of mystical death might also be suggested to adhere to such existential philosophies as those of Augustine, where a climactic, spiritual event moves the religious visionary 'out of time' itself.

I wish to argue that the significance of death and dying for Margery Kempe's self-consciousness, her privileged role as a death prophet, and her

---

[13] Elizabeth Sears, *The Ages of Man*, p. 57.

[14] Thomas Cantimpratensis, *Liber de natura rerum* (Berlin: Walter De Gruyter, 1973), I, LXXXIV, p. 82.

[15] My emphasis. *On the Properties of Things*, vol. 1., pp. 292–3.

[16] Patrick Geary, *Living with the Dead in the Middle Ages* (Ithaca: Cornell University Press, 1994), pp. 2–3. See also *Memory and Commemoration in Medieval England*, ed. Clive Burgess and Caroline M. Barron (Donington: Tyas, 2010).

[17] Most Christians believed that putrefaction in the grave was not the end of the human body, as it would be reborn at the end of time, at the Last Judgement, when body and soul would finally reunite. This event is viewed by Katharine Park as an eighth stage of human existence, in extension to Thomas of Cantimpré's seven-stage model. See Park, 'Birth and Death', in *A Cultural History of the Human Body*, ed. Kalof, p. 36.

[18] Caroline Walker Bynum, 'Death and Resurrection in the Middle Ages: Some Modern Implications', *Proceedings of the American Philosophical Society*, 142 (1998), 589–96 (p. 594).

intense meditations on Christ's Passion denote a spiritual maturation and desire to become the ultimate surrogate for the death of Christ himself. The chronological positioning of the Passion visions in Kempe's specific life-course is, of course, hard to determine, and this chapter thus deliberately lifts the temporal lens of this book to demonstrate an alternative type of growth. But while the chronological occurrence of the visions is notoriously fluid in the *Book*, and whilst she mentions in Chapter 85 that 'þes maner of visyons & felyngys' (208) occur soon after her conversion, there is ambiguity in the phrase 'þes maner' which suggests that such intense visions of Christ's Passion are just as likely to have occurred later in her spiritual journey as earlier.[19] Certainly, the Passion visions are located towards the end of Book I, and they have a distinctively climactic feel: the climax, in fact, of the first draft of the text. And although Kempe makes efforts to delineate her spiritual progression from her devotion to the Manhood to the Godhead, there is in fact little evidence to suggest that she deviates from the Christocentric focus to which she has always tended.[20] When *en route* to Aachen, for instance, she mentions to her guide that she 'wepe[s] whan I se þe Sacrament & whan I thynke on owr Lordys Passyon' (236); this demonstrates that she continues to meditate on Christ's Passion during her older age. There is also, moreover, a persistent implication in the text that such visions represent a devotional zenith. The exegesis of these visions in the overarching context of Kempe's age of spiritual maturation therefore seems apt. Since the final amanuensis revises Book I in 1436, when Kempe is sixty-three years old, and since we are told that those revisions took place under Kempe's authorial supervision ('sche sum-tyme helping where ony difficulte was' [5]) – she being concerned less with the 'ordyr' of events than with writing only 'þat sche knew rygth wel for very trewth' (5) – the incisive verisimilitude of the Passion-vision accounts illustrates their reliving and reimagining during a phase of holy advancement, effecting their textual and phenomenological resurrection.[21]

Margery Kempe's intercessory role in matters of death and dying is in fact introduced early in the *Book*. Chapter 22 is dedicated to relaying Kempe's prophetic powers as she is increasingly sent divine word about the prospects of the sick and of those in Purgatory. These examples function in an antithetic mode to the strategies of Catherine of Siena's hagiographer, however, as

[19] Kempe envisions Christ standing over her one day, as if in 'very flesch & bon'. Subsequently, 'thorw þes gostly sytys hir affecyon was al drawyn in-to þe manhood of Crist & in-to þe mynde of hys Passyon' (208).

[20] '... owr Lord of hys hy mercy drow hir affeccyon in-to hys Godhed, & þat was mor feruent in lofe & desyr & mor sotyl in vndirstondyng þan was þe Manhod' (209). I am grateful to Barry Windeatt for sharing with me his thoughts about the chronology of the Passion visions.

[21] See Roger Ellis, 'Margery Kempe's Scribe and the Miraculous Books', in *Langland, the Mystics, and the Medieval English Religious Tradition: Essays in Honour of S.S. Hussey*, ed. Helen Phillips (Cambridge: D.S. Brewer, 1990); and Watson, 'The Making of *The Book of Margery Kempe*', in *Voices in Dialogue*, ed. Olson and Kerby-Fulton.

here narrative brevity takes precedence over the accumulation of evidence of beatified activity: Kempe makes clear that 'Many mo swech reuelacyons þis creatur had in felyng; hem alle for to wryten it xuld be lettyng perauentur of mor profyte. Þes be wretyn for to schewyn þe homlynes & þe goodlynes of owyr merciful Lord Crist Ihesu & for no commendacyon of þe creatur' (54). She is aware, no doubt, of the inherent danger in intimating a saintly predisposition. These revelations also appear to represent an inchoate stage in her spirituality; she is burdened by the 'gret peyne & ponyschyng' of the discernments, especially those which reveal acquaintances who will 'be dammyd' (54), and she struggles to interpret them, gaining relief only when their truth is unravelled in contemplation. Increasingly, then, she is transformed as God's privileged death prophet and mystically told the fate of many people in the parish, granted the deific knowledge of life and death and the spiritual tools to perform a '*discretio* litmus test' that enables her to judge the efficacy of her revelations as time passes:

> As þis creatur was in a church of Seynt Margarete in þe qwer wher a cors was present, & he þat was husbond of þe same cors whyl sche leuyd was þer in good hele for to offeryn hir Messe-peny aftyr þe custom of þe place, owyr Lord seyd to þe forseyd creatur, 'Lo, dowtyr, þe sowle of þis cors is in Purgatory, & he þat was hir husband is now in good hele, & 3et he xal be ded in schort tyme'. & so it be-fel as sche felt be reuelacyon (53).

In developing her appointment as a prophet of death, prays to God on behalf of the dying, her privileged understanding and transition from enlightened holy woman to operational healer revealed by the requests of others: 'Thys creaturys gostly fader cam to hir, mevyng hir to prey for a woman whech lay in poynt of deth to mannys syghte. & a-non owyr Lord seyd sche xuld levyn & faryn wel, & so sche dede' (54). Several similar examples appear in the chapter, although not all prove her intercessory success, as the case of the *litster* (dyer) suggests: 'An-oþer good man whech was a lyster lay seke also, &, whan þis creatur preyd for hym, it was answeryd to hir mende þat he xulde languryn a whyle & sythen he xuld ben ded wyth þat same sekenesse. & so he was in schort tyme aftyr' (54). While Kempe's therapeutic prayers are not adequate in this instance, she is nevertheless privy to divine prescience of the man's demise, drawing her closer to an understanding of the fragile liminality of the life/death hinterland, and offering her an insight into her own mortal precipice.

An extension of these prophetic events occurs later in the *Book* when Kempe reveals how her growing holiness prompts her fellow parishioners to seek out her comfort on their deathbeds:

> Also þe sayd creatur was desiryd of mech pepil to be wyth hem at her deying & to prey for hem, for, þow þei louyd not hir wepyng ne hir crying in her lyfe-tyme, þei de[sir]ryd þat sche xulde bothyn wepyn & cryin whan þei xulde deyin, & so sche dede. Whan sche sey folke be a-noyntyd, sche had many holy thowtys, many holy meditacyons, &, 3yf sche saw hem deyin, hir thowt

sche saw owr Lord deyin & sum-tyme owr Lady, as owr God wolde illumyn
hir gostly syth of vndirstondyng. Þan xulde sche cryin, wepyn, & sobbyn ful
wonderfully as sche had be-heldyn owr Lord in hys deying er owr Lady in hir
deying (172–3).

Notwithstanding the satirical potential in the Lynn residents' wish to reappro-
priate Kempe's bothersome crying performances and to utilise their ebullience
for their own dramatic end (quite literally), she evidently complies willingly,
and regularly attends deathbed vigils. That '*mech* pepil' request her service, and
the phrase '*Whan* sche sey folke be a-noyntyd', suggest a plurality of activity, perhaps because her prophetic sensibilities had become well known, or
because her devout local presence prompts growing trust in her wisdom and
power to soothe. To witness the deaths of individuals time and again provides
Kempe with an elected familiarity with the ultimate transition from this world
to the next, greater even than the average medieval person, whose contact
with death was ordinarily frequent.[22] And as Peregrine Horden has argued,
'Spiritual medicine is genuinely medicinal, not just in theological but also
in medical terms. It is another kind of medicine without doctors. Anything
that promotes medicine for the soul – sacraments, devotional images and the
like – can be seen as altering the accidents of the soul.'[23]

The 'wepyn & cryin' offered by Margery Kempe as a deathbed oblation is
connected to the cultural gravity of the *ars moriendi* tradition (the art of dying
well), which Amy Appleford has shown to have been important in the process
of laicisation after the Great Schism of 1376. Whilst sacraments such as the
Eucharist and confession required the involvement of a priest, 'good deaths'
did not: according to a range of deathbed manuals, 'laymen could and should
attend the deathbeds of other laymen'.[24] Texts such as *The Book of the Craft of
Dying* offered instructions for the deathbed custodian on dying well, and the
interrogations, obsecrations, and prayers to address to the dying person.[25] An
important aspect of deathbed activity was the support of the dying person's
neighbours, or *even cristen*, whose 'role as witnesses', as Appleford attests, 'was
understood to have both personal and communal values and who had always
directly participated in the ritual at various levels'.[26] The greater officiating
role of the lay householder that was promoted in texts such as the *Visitation
of the Sick* (c. 1380) may be consequent of the dearth of priests after the Black

---

[22] See Pamela Nightingale, 'Some New Evidence of Crises and Trends of Mortality in Late Medieval England'.
[23] Peregrine Horden, 'A Non-Natural Environment', in *The Medieval Hospital and Medical Practice* ed. Bowers, pp. 133–45 (p. 142).
[24] Amy Appleford, *Learning to Die in London, 1380–1540* (Philadelphia: University of Pennsylvania Press, 2015), p. 11. See also *Death in the Middle Ages and Early Modern Times: The Material and Spiritual Conditions of the Culture of Death*, ed. Albrecht Classen (Berlin: De Gruyter, 2016).
[25] See *The Book of the Craft of Dying: And other Early English Tracts Concerning Death*, ed. Frances M.M. Comper (New York: Arno Press, 1977).
[26] Appleford, *Learning to Die in London*, p. 25.

Death, but there was personal edification, also, to be gained from visiting the sick and dying; such visits were a work of mercy necessary for one's own salvation as well as that of the afflicted.[27] The equality of all Christians in the face of death, and thus the import of death-attendant praxes, is also embraced in Julian of Norwich's *Revelations*, in which she ontologically unites herself with her community and the existential nexus of all Christians: 'Alle that I saye of myself, I meene in the persone of alle mine evencristen.'[28] Julian herself is anointed for death on the fourth night of a bodily sickness so acute that she and 'they that were with me' perceived the outward signs of dying, indicating that she was attended at this time by others.[29] It is notable, therefore, that Kempe's own visit to Julian's cell in Norwich, probably in 1413, and which included much 'holy dalyawns' over several days, would almost inevitably have included Julian's recounting the edifying story of her grave illness and near-death as part of the 'good cownsel' that she gave; reason perhaps also for her prayers that Kempe should be granted 'perseuerawns' and 'pacyens' (43).[30] Indeed, Julian explicitly advises Kempe that she should fulfil God's will, so long as it is to the 'profyte of hir *euyn-cristen* (42). Kempe's understanding of spiritual medicine is therefore inextricably subsumed within a paradigm of suffering, mortality, resilience, and Christian community, her own fleshly experience of pain symbiotic with Christ's pain on the cross and its concomitant sacrifice for humanity's salvation.

Meditation / Medication

Margery Kempe's growing knowledge of pain, made violently and kinetically animate in the Passion visions, is heightened following her return to Lynn in 1418 after a trip to London to acquire a letter and seal from the Archbishop of Canterbury. This return marks the beginning of about a decade of chronic illness, when Margery Kempe succumbs to 'many gret & diuers sekenes' (137). She is, then, forty-five years old at its onset and somewhere in her mid-fifties at her recovery, and the sickness is so severe that she, like Julian, is anointed for death:[31]

---

[27] On the manuscript versions of the *Visitation of the Sick* and their wide pastoral usage see Appleford, *Learning to Die*, pp. 23–6.

[28] Julian of Norwich, 'A Vision Showed to a Devout Woman', in *The Writings of Julian of Norwich*, ed. Watson and Jenkins, p. 73. See also Amy Appleford, 'The 'Comene Course of Prayer': Julian of Norwich and Late Medieval Death Culture', *Journal of English and Germanic Philology*, 107:2 (2008), 190–214.

[29] Julian of Norwich, 'A Revelation of Love', in *The Writings of Julian of Norwich*, ed. Watson and Jenkins, pp. 129–31.

[30] On the dating of this visit see Windeatt, *BMK*, p. vii.

[31] Hope Emily Allen notes that the period of her illness was likely to be 'considerably more than eight years long', and her recovery therefore beyond the year of 1426, when she was fifty-three. See *BMK*, p. 318, n. 137/19–22.

She had þe flyx [flux] a long tyme tyl sche was anoyntyd, wenyng to a be deed. Sche was so febyl þat sche myth not heldyn a spon in hir hand. Þan owr Lord Ihesu Crist spak to hir in hir sowle & seyd þat sche xulde not dey ȝet. Þan sche recuryd aȝen a lytyl while. And a-non aftyr sche had a gret sekenes in hir heuyd and sithyn in hir bakke þat sche feryd to a lost hir witte þer-thorw. Aftyrwarde, whan sche was recuryd of alle þes sekenessys, in schort tyme folwyd an-oþer sekenes which was sett in hir ryth syde, duryng þe terme of viij ȝer, saf viij wokys, be diuers tymes. Sumtyme sche had it onys in a weke contunyng sumtyme xxx owrys, sumtyme xx, sumtyme x, sumtyme viij, sumtyme iiij, & sumtyme ij, so hard & so scharp þat sche must voydyn þat was in hir stomak as bittyr as it had ben galle, neyþyr etyng ne drynkyng whil þe sekenes enduryd but euyr gronyng tyl it was gon (137).

The illness of flux – a condition mentioned in the first line of the annotated recipe on fol. 142v of the manuscript – causes Kempe so much distress that she anticipates death.[32] Though she does in fact recover, she then endures a further affliction to her head and back, causing such psychological distraction that she 'lost hir witte þer-thorw' – a painful cognizance that resonates with the early post-partum sickness that saw her go 'owt of hir mende' (7) more than twenty years earlier. Having recovered once again, returning from the brink of annihilation for at least the fourth time in her life, she succumbs to a further illness in her right side, which lasts for eight years.[33] That the final sickness in her right side marks the onset of the eight-year period indicates that the entire duration of illness is far longer; until she perhaps approaches her seventh decade. So intense is this intermittent pain that she vomits, groans, and fasts in a form of semi-existence, defined by the agony and existing, suspended, within the pain. The meticulous, mathematical notation of the number of hours of pain that consume her reveals a conscious demarcation of her existence within, or outside, the torment.

The prolonged, incapacitating pain in Kempe's right side could have been caused by a number of physiological conditions, including disorders more commonly experienced in mature women, such as fibroids, cysts, prolapse of the uterus, diverticulitis, kidney infections or stones, diseases of the gallblad-der, liver disease, or hepatitis. Medieval medical texts for women's health offer some explanations and treatments for conditions linked to female affliction, not least the 'suffocated womb', when the uterus was thought to become dis-placed and move upwards in the body as a quasi-animated entity, seeking heat from other internal organs ('whan þe matrice rysyth out of hys ryȝht plase & goyth ouer-hy').[34] The 'Book on the Conditions of Women' states that the condition causes syncope and pain, is characterised by gritted teeth and a dou-

[32] On the possibility that flux is mentioned in the recipe on the final folio of the manu-script, see Introduction, p. 1, n. 1.
[33] Kempe fears death during the delivery of her first child, summoning a confessor, as was explored in Chapter 2 of this study. She is hit by a falling beam and stone in St Margaret's Church in Chapter 9 of the *Book*, perceiving that she was dead for a little while. Two further instances when physical or mental annihilation are anticipated are evident in the present passage.
[34] *The Knowing of Woman's Kind in Childing*, p. 50.

bling up of the body, and is most common in celibate and non-menstruating women, namely virgins and widows:

> This happens to those women who do not use men, especially to widows who were accustomed to carnal commerce. It regularly comes upon virgins, too, when they reach the age of marriage and are not able to use men and when the semen abounds in them a lot, which Nature wishes to draw out by means of the male. From this superabundant and corrupt semen, a certain cold fumosity is released.

> [Contingit autem hoc eis que uiris non utuntur, maxime uiduis que consueuerunt uti carnali commercio. Virginibus etiam solet euenire cum ad annos nubiles peruenerunt et uiris uti non possunt, et cum in eis multum habundet sperma, quod per masculum natura uellet educere, ex hoc semine superhabundante et corrupto quedam fumositas frigida dissoluitur.][35]

The older woman in a post-menopause and celibate state is, then, more susceptible to the socio-somatic disorder of uterine suffocation. Characteristically, *De secretis mulierum* audaciously advises widows and vowesses to abandon the righteous ethics of their chastity for remedial pragmatism: 'And so it is good that such women, whatever they may be, whether young or old, often use men, so that such matter might be expelled' ('Et ideo bonum est quod tales mulieres, quæcunque fuerint, sive juvenes, sive antiquæ, sæpe viris utantur ut materia talis expellatur').[36] Since Margery Kempe's vow of chastity would preclude her from this 'cure', the spiritual medicament that the Passion visions offer her are ever more central for her psychosomatic wholeness.[37] The precipitation of the uterus, or uterine prolapse, is also associated with older women or those who do not menstruate. Pertinently, it causes pain in the side: 'The precipitacioun of the matrice is another sikenes whan the matrice fallith from hir kyndely place. And that may be in ij maners: other aside or ellis donwarde. If it fallith aside, men may it knowe bi the greuaunce of the side.'[38]

With the cause of Margery Kempe's illness undetermined, her perception of its pain is measured by its parallels to Christ's Passion as she connects her suffering intimately with his. In her prayers, she acknowledges the inferiority of her pain, yet confesses her inability to endure, or bear, it:

> A, blysful Lord, why woldist þu be-comyn man & suffyr so meche peyne for my synnes & for alle mennys synnes þat xal be sauyd, & we arn so vnkynde, Lord, to þe, & I, most vnworthy, *can not suffyr þis lityl peyne?* A, Lord, for thy gret peyn haue mercy on my lityl peyne; for þe gret peyne þat þu suffredyst ȝef me not so meche as I am worthy, for *I may not beryn so meche* as I am worthy. And, ȝyf þu wilte, Lord, þat I ber it, sende me pacyens, for ellys *I may not suffyr it* (137).

---

[35] 'Book on the Conditions of Women', in *The Trotula*, pp. 84–5.
[36] *De secretis mulierum*, trans. Lemay, p. 132. Albertus Magnus, *De secretis mulierum*, p. 112.
[37] For the treatment of suffocation, Johannes Platearius' *Practica* recommends remarriage for widows. Other medical texts recommend masturbation. See Green, *The Trotula*, p. 219, n. 114.
[38] *Sickness of Women*, pp. 507–8.

The juxtaposition of 'lityl' and 'gret' in this passage exposes Kempe's sense of her human inadequacy against Christ's awesome endurance. Her call for God's mercy, or at least for the ability to bear the suffering – 'sende me pacyens' – echoes Julian of Norwich's prayer that she should be granted that patience. Conceptualising her own pain in terms of its relation to the Passion, she takes its meaning from Christ's pain in sharp relief. This suffering-narrative is relived later in the episode, when Kempe's contemplations of the Passion during times of sickness prove analgesic. The contemplative displacement of her pain to Christ's removes all feeling and absents the conscious self, the eventual and total removal of her pain thus predicated directly upon the bodily suffering of Christ:

> Sumtyme, not-wythstondyng þe sayd creatur had gret bodily sekenes, ʒet þe Passyon of owr merciful Lord Crist Ihesu wrowt so in hir sowle þat for þe tyme *sche felt not hir owyn sekenes* but wept & sobbyd in þe mend of owr Lordys Passyon as thow sche sey hym wyth hir bodily eye suffering peyne & passyon be-forn hir. Sithyn, whan viij ʒer wer passyd, hir sekenes scapyd þat it cam not weke be weke as it dede be-forn, but þan encresyd hir cryes & hir wepyngys (138).

The preposition 'sithyn' denotes a direct connection between Kempe's meditations on the Passion and her subsequent renewal and recovery from sickness.[39] Such meditations symbolise not merely an absolute cure for her illness, but a *panacea totalis*: a treatment with which she will self-medicate as her spiritual journey unfolds. The Passion visions, then, hold increasing significance as Margery Kempe's earthly body weakens in synchrony with the intensification of her receptive, mystical body.

The visions' import is heightened by Kempe's evident physiological understanding of the *signa mortifera*, or signs of death; these were commonly known in the Middle Ages, largely due to the collection, editing, and wide circulation of texts by Hippocrates and Galen by monastic scribes and compilers.[40] The primary medical text on prognostication was the Hippocratic treatise *Prognostics*, translated from Greek into Latin in southern Italy in the fifth or sixth century, and which popularised the notion of the 'Hippocratic face'. Short treatises based on translations of the *Prognosis*, named the *articella*, were produced at the medical school at Salerno from the eleventh century and thereafter formed the centre of curricula in the central and late Middle Ages.[41] The Middle English translation

---

[39] MED s.v. sithyn [sitthen]: Continually from (a specified time or event); ever since.

[40] For an index of all known references to Signs of Death in medical and scientific texts, see the eVK2 database (2014): An expanded and revised version of Linda Ehrsam Voigts and Patricia Deery Kurtz, *Scientific and Medical Writings in Old and Middle English: An Electronic Reference* CD (Ann Arbor: University of Michigan Press, 2000), available at <http://cctr1.umkc.edu/search>.

[41] See Frederick S. Paxton, '*Signa Mortifera*: Death and Prognostication in Early Medieval Monastic Medicine', *Bulletin of the History of Medicine*, 67 (1993), 631–50 (pp. 632–3). On prognostication in university teaching see Luke Demaitre, 'The Art and Science of Prognostication in Early University Medicine', *Bulletin of the History of Medicine*, 77 (2003), 765–88.

of a Latin commentary on the *Prognostics* – the first substantial instance of a
Hippocratic text in the English vernacular – advises that some of the outward
signs of death are that 'his nose be sharp or his nosethrilles sharp, holow eyed,
playn tymples, colde eeres and streighte, and the pulpis of hem turned inward,
and the skyn which is vpon the forhed drie, hard, and straight, and the colour of
the face al grene or blac'.[42] The text emphasises the importance of the tightening
and contracting of the skin and features, with the 'holowe eyed' as the most
deadly sign as it indicates 'sharp fevers [that cause] consumpcioun of moisture
of the lacerates conteyneng the eyen'.[43] The eyes appear frequently as signs
of approaching death, sometimes bulging and avoiding the light, sometimes
becoming black.[44] Likewise if the 'eyeliddis' are 'intorned' and only the 'white
of the eyen in sleep appieryng', and the person 'seeth nat and so of other', then,
especially if combined with the failure of hearing and smell, death is 'in the
yaatis and at the dore'.[45]

In addition, the colour of the dying person's face was regarded as significant, especially if it was 'grene or blac or pale or leedissh of colour'. The
worst alteration was 'to blac, forwhi it is made of superfluite ovircomyng
of cold vpon the bloode': an image strikingly evocative of the black bile of
melancholia and, as I have argued, concomitant with mystical perspicacity.[46]
The *Cyrurgie of Guy de Chauliac* makes a similar observation – 'Blak colour
and grene, asky and of dyuers coloures is euel, and it bytokeneth rotynge of
þe humoures'; unless purgation occurs, 'her state is perilous'.[47] Such creeping
blackness is also evident in Glasgow University Library, MS Hunter 513, a
mid-fifteenth-century medical manuscript which notes that if the patient's
urine is 'blake and medelyd wyth blode þe viii day he schall dye'. Furthermore,
'yf the seke Caste blood and there waxe blacke spottes þoroughe owte his
body … he dyethe for sothe'.[48]

The popular *Liber de diversis medicinis* lists signs from changing eyes to a
sharpened nose, coldness, a red forehead, and rattling breath:

[42] 'Commentary on the Hippocratic *Prognostics*, Part I', in *Sex, Aging, and Death in a Medieval Medical Compendium*, vol. 1, ed. Tavormina, pp. 373–434 (p. 397). The usage of the term 'sharp' occurs frequently, sometimes indicating the acuteness of the sickness, and sometimes suggesting a contracting of the flesh. MED s.v. sharp: 4(a) Of physical pain, sickness, hunger, etc., acute, intense, severe; ~ fever, a high fever.
[43] 'Commentary on the Hippocratic *Prognostics*', in *Sex, Aging, and Death*, ed. Tavormina, p. 397. MED s.v. lacertes: muscles.
[44] Ibid., pp. 398–404.
[45] Ibid., p. 406.
[46] Ibid., p. 401.
[47] *The Cyrurgie of Guy de Chauliac*, p. 545.
[48] The 'Treatise on the Signs of Death' in Glasgow University Library, MS Hunter 513, fols 105r–107v (fol. 106v). Digitised in *The Málaga Corpus of Late Middle English Scientific Prose*, transcribed and described by Teresa Marqués Aguado. At <http://hunter.uma.es/> [accessed 17 March 2018]

When his browes heldes down, the left eghe es mare þan þe reghte eghe, the nose ende waxes sharpe, his eres waxes calde, his eghne waxes holle, the chyn falls, his eghne & his mouthe are opyn when he slepes bot he be wonut þer-to, her ere lappes waxes hethy, his fete waxes calde, þe wambe falles a-waye, if he pull þe strase or þe clathes, if he pyk at his nose thirlles, his forheuede waxes rede, ȝong man ay wakande, alde man ay slepande, his ij membres caldes agayn es kynde & hides þam, if he rotell, thiese are þe takynynges of dede.[49]

The ubiquity of these medically accepted signs of death is evidenced by their appearance in other texts, such as medieval lyrics.[50] In fact, the *signa mortifera* demonstrate aptly the medico-religious culture of the Middle Ages, seen, for example, in a version of the *Fasciculus morum* (1313–17) from an early fifteenth-century collection of mystical verse and prose. The text conflates medical and religious practice via structural parallelism, as each physiological sign of death is directly connected to Latin rubrics that advise which religious act should occur in response to that symptom:

When þi hede quakes	Memento
And þi lyppis Blakes	Confessio
When þi brest pantes	Contricio
When þy wynde wantes	Satisfaccio
When þi lymys ryveleth	libera me domine
When þi nose keleþ	þen miserere
When þyn eyȝen holeweth	Nosce te ipsum
ffor þan deth foleweth	veni ad Iudicium[51]

Indeed, the signs of death were also mentioned in the prose sermons of Bromyard, Wimbledon, and Myrc, further illustrating the permeation of medical knowledge into religious texts. They also featured directly in parish life in the form of ritual booklets and handbooks for parish priests, who required sufficient medical understanding of *signa mortifera* to allow them to recognise when a parishioner required the vital deathbed liturgy and rites. Lay parishioners like Margery Kempe would have therefore gathered knowledge about dying both corporeally, by witnessing the decline of the *even cristen* over whose bodies they kept vigil, and textually, where such physical signs were reiterated by preachers in religious services.[52]

---

[49] The *Liber de diversis medicinis*, ed. Ogden, p. 58. MED s.v. rotelen: To make a rattling sound in breathing.

[50] See, for example, IMEV 3998 in *The Digital Index of Middle English Verse*, ed. Linne R. Mooney, Daniel W. Mosser, and Elizabeth Solopova, <http://dimev.net/>. See also Rosemary Woolf, 'Lyrics on Death', in *Middle English Lyrics*, ed. Luria and Hoffman, pp. 290–308.

[51] IMEV 4035. Longleat MS 29, from Rossell Hope Robbins, 'Signs of Death in Middle English', *Mediaeval Studies*, 32 (1970), 282–98 (p. 293).

[52] See Robbins, 'Signs of Death in Middle English', pp. 296–7; Alan J. Fletcher, 'The Lyric in the Sermon', in *A Companion to the Middle English Lyric*, ed. Thomas G. Duncan (Cambridge: D.S. Brewer, 2005), pp. 189–209; Fletcher, *Late Medieval Popular Preaching in Britain and Ireland: Texts, Studies, and Interpretations* (Turnhout: Brepols, 2009); and Julia Boffey, 'Some Middle English Sermon Verse and Its Transmission in Manuscript

But Kempe's imbrication in the medico-cultural milieu of death and dying, and in the surrogacy matrix for which I have argued, plays out most strikingly in the *Liber de diversis medicinis*, which recommends women's milk as a prognostic for determining impending death in a patient. The surrogacy hermeneutic thus operates right up until the end of life itself, the multipliable and esoteric properties of breastmilk now symbolising new life in death: 'For to wiete if a seke man or a woman sall lyfe or dy', the physician should 'Tak þe seke mans pys & late a woman mylke þer-on &, if þe mylk falle to þe grounde, he sall dy &, if it flete, he sal lyfe.'[53] Alternatively, 'Tak his water & menge it with a womans mylke þat hase a knaue childe &, if þat gange to-gedir, he sal lyfe &, if þay depart, he sall dy.'[54] That the maternal body is invested with such symbolic value for the entire duration of the human life cycle not only reinforces the power of substitutional or surrogate activity, but also elucidates Margery Kempe's deep desire to operate as a surrogate at the polarities of the life spectrum. Through the ubiquitous iconography of the Virgin nursing the Christ Child, and the concomitant notion of the dying Christic body providing eternal sustenance for the world, it is little wonder that the metaphor of the mother's milk holds such resonance in medieval culture, and for Margery Kempe, in determining the existence or extinguishing of human life itself.

Dead to the World

Margery Kempe's preoccupation with her own death is visible throughout the *Book*, but most acutely emerges in response to her contemplation of Christ's dying body. Such meditations on the image of the crucifixion were conventional aspects of Eucharistic devotion and an important part of deathbed rituals. Julian of Norwich, for instance, experienced an intense reaction to the crucifix during her near-death encounter.[55] In a similar way, directly after her intercessory prayers cause the fire in Lynn in 1420 to be quenched, Kempe escapes to the prior's cloister (where she will not be vilified for her cries) and experiences a 'gret mende of þe Passyon of owr Lord Ihesu Crist & of hys precyows wowndys' (164). In pained response, she loses control of her body, unable to

---

and Print', in *Preaching the Word in Manuscript and Print in Late Medieval England: Essays in Honour of Susan Powell*, ed. Martha W. Driver and Veronica O'Mara (Turnhout, Brepols, 2013), pp. 259–75. For an index of verse in Middle English sermons see *A Repertorium of Middle English Prose Sermons*, ed. Veronica O'Mara and Suzanne Paul (Turnhout: Brepols, 2007), IV, 2894–5.

[53] The *Liber de diversis medicinis*, p. 58.

[54] Ibid.

[55] See 'A Revelation of Love', in *The Writings of Julian of Norwich*, ed. Watson and Jenkins, pp. 129–35. See also R.N. Swanson, 'Passion and Practice: The Social and Ecclesiastical Implications of Passion Devotion in the Late Middle Ages', in *The Broken Body*, ed. MacDonald et al., pp. 1–30; and Vincent Gillespie, 'Strange Images of Death: The Passion in Later Medieval English Devotional and Mystical Writing', esp. pp. 131–43.

restrain herself, crying, 'Take a-wey þis peyne fro me, for I may not beryn it. *Þi Passyon wil sle me*' (164). As a textual foreshadowing of the further, intensely experienced Passion visions, she also prophesies her own death through the inextricability of Christ's crucifixion from her own suffering, and her conceptualisation of his death as equivalent to her own. The future simple tense of 'Þi Passyon wil sle me' straightforwardly signals her certainty of this terminus in a binary that communicates not only Kempe's current unbearable pain, but also the future repetition of such experience. Its repetitive frequency is in fact catalogued with comparably dichotomous precision and infiniteness: 'Swech gostly syghtys had sche euery Palme Sonday & euery Good Fryday, & in many oþer wise boþe many ȝerys to-gedyr' (190). Kempe's conception of the Passion as the source of her multiple deaths evokes the mystical state of Catherine of Siena's being 'between two deaths', since she knows that she will die over and over again. These replicated, perpetual deaths are testament not only to the indelible inscription of Christ's life and death inside her soul ('I schuld be newe crucified in þe'), but also to the inadequacy of her life-sacrifice as payment of a debt that she considers impossible to fulfil: 'Þerfor, Lord, þei I wer slayn an hundryd sithys [times] on a day, ȝyf it wer possibyl, for thy loue, ȝet cowde I neuyr ȝeldyn [pay back] þe þe goodness þat þu hast schewyd to me' (184). Margery Kempe must, then, die forevermore.

The vision recounted in Chapter 79 is predicated on Kempe's maternal identification with the Virgin Mary and the cues that she takes from the Virgin's desperate sorrowing. Before Christ has been arrested, Mary offers her own life for his: 'I wolde, Sone, þat I myth suffir deth *for þe* so þat þu xuldist not deyin' (187).[56] The centrality of the mother-figure to the crucifixion is brought into sharp focus through Christ's words of comfort, which align the maternal role as giver of flesh and substance (in medieval medical theory, in contrast to the paternal contribution of the child's 'spirit') with the concomitant destruction of that flesh, according to God's will: 'Modyr, I pray ȝow blissyth me & late me go do my Fadrys wille, for þerfor I cam in-to þis worlde & toke flesch & blood of ȝow' (188). Furthermore, the dichotomy of Christ's birth with God's plan for his demise is hinged on the term 'þerfor', implying, in medieval understanding, a consequential benefit to humankind, reliant, as it is, on the maternal body.[57] The Virgin atones for her complicity in her son's destiny by falling to the ground, 'lying stille as sche had ben ded', in a substitutional death redolent with a surrogacy hermeneutic (189). Mary's lamentation over her dead son was depicted variously in Pietà images, mystery plays, and literature in the later Middle Ages as part of the burgeoning cult of the *Mater Dolorosa*

---

[56] MED s.v. shulen (form 'xuldist'). This term, when used as a modal auxiliary, has several denotations including (1) to owe (2) to remedy (3) to express what is right / a duty / a moral obligation / a commandment. The Virgin's desperation to be Christ's death surrogate is thus predicated on multifarious dutiful, spiritual and efficacious motivations.

[57] MED s.v.: ther-for(e): (1) With ref. to a person, a body, or an institution presented as the beneficiary of some action: for the benefit of him, it, or that, on his or its behalf.

(depicted on this book's front cover).[58] Indeed, Margery Kempe experiences an ecstatic rapture inspired by a Pietà in Norwich – 'a fayr ymage of owr Lady clepyd a pyte' – and falls to the ground 'as þei sche xulde a deyd' (148).[59] Female affective devotional responses were also likely to be inspired by Passion treatises such as *Quis dabit capiti meo aquam* by Ogier Locedio (d. 1214), one of the most widely circulated devotional texts in the later Middle Ages and apparently addressed to women. In one passage, Mary laments Christ, wishing to join him on the cross. In another she is described as *emortua mater* (dead mother): 'Dying she lived; and living, she died. Nor could she die, who was a living dead person' ('Viuebat moriens, et viuens moriebatur. Nec potuit mori, que viuens mortua fuit').[60] In the devotional guidebook the *Meditationes vitae Christi*, translated by Nicholas Love as *The Mirror of the Blessed Life of Jesus Christ*, Christ emphasises his symbiosis with Mary as he cries, 'I sholde onely be crucified & not shee. But loo now she hangeþ on the crosse with me.'[61] When the soldier spears Christ's side, Mary 'felle done in swowhen half dede'.[62] Described by Michael Sargent as 'the most important literary version of the life of Christ in English before modern times', it is inconceivable that Kempe was not read this text by her confessors.[63] The liminality of Mary's living death in these examples reaffirms the motherhood matrix as fully implicated in both the enactment and lamentation of the crucifixion, a torturous state of existence in which the mother figures as a synchronic giver and receiver of pain, whilst at the same time an essential component for the fruition of human salvation.

As Kempe witnesses the parting exchange between Christ and his mother in this vision, her own integration within the scene unfolds. Immediately falling at Christ's feet in *imitatio Mariae*, she also offers her own life, imagining an existence without him as a fate worse than death: 'I had wel leuar þat þu woldist sle me þan latyn me abydyn in þe worlde wyth-owtyn þe' (189). Here, as she requests an active death in the form of being killed, as opposed to the passive *suffering* of death that the Virgin offers, she supersedes Mary

[58] On the iconography of the Virgin see Naoë Kukita Yoshikawa, 'The Role of the Virgin Mary and the Structure of Meditation in *The Book of Margery Kempe*', in *The Medieval Mystical Tradition in England: July 1991*, ed. Glasscoe, pp. 169–92. See also Alexandra Barratt, 'Spiritual Virgin to Virgin Mother: Confessions of Margery Kempe', *Paregon*, 17 (1999), 9–44; and Barratt, '*Stabant matres dolorosae*: Women as Readers and Writers of Passion Prayers, Meditations and Visions', in *The Broken Body*, ed. MacDonald et al., pp. 55–71. See also Karma Lochrie, *Translations of the Flesh*, pp. 167–202; Liz Herbert McAvoy, *Authority and the Female Body*, pp. 39–50; Marina Warner, *Alone of all Her Sex*, pp. 206–23; and Miri Rubin, *Mother of God*, pp. 243–8.

[59] See Laura Varnam, 'The Crucifix, the Pietà, and the Female Mystic: Devotional Objects and Performative Identity in the Book of Margery Kempe', *Journal of Medieval Religious Cultures*, 41 (2015), 208–37.

[60] London, British Library, MS. Cotton Vespasian E.i, fol. 200r. From Thomas H. Bestul, *Texts of the Passion: Latin Devotional Literature and Medieval Society* (Philadelphia: University of Pennsylvania Press, 1996), pp. 127–31.

[61] Nicholas Love, *The Mirror of the Blessed Life of Jesus Christ*, Cap. xliij, p. 176.

[62] *Mirror*, Cap. xlv, p.180.

[63] *Mirror*, p. ix.

in the dramatic potential of the scene, underscoring her understanding that, ultimately, she *will be* slain for Christ's Passion. Her consequent 'sorwe & gret peyn' are evident as the Jews' torture of the Christic body begins before the helpless gaze of the Virgin and Kempe – her 'vnworthy handmaydyn for þe tyme' (190). As Christ's body is bound to a pillar and beaten, buffeted and struck with whips and scourges, Margery Kempe and the Virgin weep in painful identification, emblematic of a pain surrogacy entrenched in an ethics of maternity, where Kempe must endure the multiple suffering of both Christ and his mother. Her endurance of anguish is, furthermore, divinely ordained, as God imparts his will that she must be an acroamatic and kinaesthetic symbol of his grace:

> Sum-tyme I ȝeue þe gret cryis and roryngys for to makyn þe pepil a-ferd wyth þe grace þat I putte in þe in-to a tokyn þat I wil þat my Modrys sorwe be knowyn by þe þat men & women myth haue þe mo compassyon of hir sorwe þat sche suffyrd for me (183).

Not only is Kempe given deific licence to *know* the Virgin's grief, and to perform it as a surrogate, but her roars and shrieks in response to the vision denote an inscription of Christ's suffering in privileged embodiment of spectator and spectacle converged.[64] In this way, Kempe's thunderous response to the scourging of Christ and the agony of Mary – her violent amplification of grief a pseudo-usurpation of the Christic mother – is a means through which she can partake in the event as it inevitably materialises, experiencing the Passion performatively, just as she would have witnessed in mystery plays.[65] Such potential complicity problematises the event because of the liminality of the spectator as a possible co-persecutor, as Marla Carlson has considered.[66] But though Kempe's re-enactment effectively reanimates unspeakable pain, it nevertheless ensures her place in the ordered narrative of Christ's crucifixion and the concomitant salvation of humankind.[67] The popular series of devotional prayers memorialising the Passion, *The Fifteen Oes*, traditionally attributed to Bridget of Sweden and doubtless known to Kempe, explicate the way in which Christ's wounds can become inscribed in the body of their 'reader', who thus becomes complicit in his crucifixion:

---

[64] On performative mysticism and the Passion, see Carolyn Muessig, 'Performance of the Passion: The Enactment of Devotion in the later Middle Ages', in *Visualising Medieval Performance*, ed. Gertsman, pp. 129–42.

[65] Allen notes that Kempe had 'almost certainly' been to the York plays in June 1413, and there had also been plays in Lynn in 1385 and in 1409–10. See *BMK*, p. 333, n. 187/19. Claire Sponsler argues for the influence of the cycle plays on Kempe's emotive gestures in 'Drama and Piety: Margery Kempe', in *A Companion to The Book of Margery Kempe*, ed. Arnold and Lewis, pp. 129–44.

[66] See Carlson, *Performing Bodies in Pain*, pp. 92–3.

[67] Kempe's Passion meditations indicate the influence of mystics such as Richard Rolle and Elizabeth of Spalbeck. See Alexandra Barratt, '*Stabant matres dolorosae*', in *The Broken Body*, ed. MacDonald et al., pp. 64–6.

O Blessed myrrour of trouth, token of Unyte, & louesoom bonde of charite; Have mynde of thyne Innumerable peynes and woundes; Wyth the whiche fro the toppe of thy hede to the sole of thy fote thou were wounded. And of the wycked Jewes thou were all to torne and rente. And all thy body thou suffredeste to be rede wyth thy moost clene blessed blode, The whiche grete sorrow Jhesu in thy clene virgynall body thou suffredest. What myghtest thou do more for us than thou dydst. Therfore benygne Jhesu for the mynde of this passion wryte al thy woundes in myn herte wyth thy precyous blode that I may both rede in theym thy drede and thy loue And that I may contynue in praysing & in thankynge the to my liues ende. Amen. Pater nostre. Aue maria.[68]

No doubt a prayer particularly precious to Kempe because of its Brigittine connection, its call for Jesus to 'wryte al thy woundes in myn herte wyth thy precyous blode' echoes the physiological inscription of Christ's promise to Kempe that he will be 'newe crucified' in her (85).[69] Through the dramaturgy of Kempe's visions of the Passion, then, she is further authorised to imbue the very process and rupturing of the crucified Christ into her body and her text, preparing the way for her passage towards her mortal end and the 'good death' to which Christians aspired.

Chapter 80 opens with graphic imagery of torture. In what must resonate for Kempe as a reliving of her own binding and imprisonment during her postpartum episode, she envisions Christ as bound to a pillar once again, his hands tied above his head:

And þan sche sey sextene men wyth sextene scorgys, & eche scorge had viij babelys of leed on þe ende, & euery babyl was ful of scharp prekelys as it had ben þe rowelys of a spor. & þo men wyth þe scorgys madyn comenawnt þat ich of hem xulde ȝeuyn owr Lord xl strokys. Whan sche saw þis petows syght, sche wept & cryid ryth lowed as ȝyf sche xulde a brostyn for sorwe & peyne (191).

Her attempt to calculate the number of strikes delivered and therefore the number of wounds created by these multiple weapons – a popular medieval devotion – indicates her desire to reveal the extent of Christ's injuries and the inconceivable level of pain inflicted. Christ's wounds are, according to Christine Cooper-Rompato in this example, 'largely immeasurable', the resistance of

---

[68] 'O Jhesu endless swetnes of louying soules …', *The Fifteen Oes* no.12 (Westminster: William Caxton, 1491), Bibliographic identifier 20195. In EEBO, part of Jisc Historic Books <https://data.historicaltexts.jisc.ac.uk/view?pubId=eebo-99836861e&terms=Caxton%20The%20Fifteen%20Oes>; images 5 and 6 [accessed 1 January 2019].
[69] Some scholars have argued that the *Oes* were composed by the Brigittines at Syon Abbey. On the authorship, see Rebecca Krug, 'The Fifteen Oes', in *Cultures of Piety: Medieval English Devotional Literature in Translation*, ed. Anne Clark Bartlett and Thomas H. Bestul (Ithaca and London: Cornell University Press, 1999), pp. 107–12. See also Claes Gejrot, 'The *Fifteen Oes*: Latin and Vernacular Versions. With an Edition of the Latin Text', in *The Translation of the Works of St Birgitta of Sweden into the Medieval European Vernaculars*, ed. Bridget Morris and Veronica O'Mara (Turnhout: Brepols, 2000), pp. 213–38. Gejrot argues that whilst the attribution of the text to Bridget has been largely discredited, she was still considered to be the author by the fifteenth-century readership of the prayers.

enumeration intended to encourage 'extended contemplation of Christ's ulti-mate sacrifice'.[70] Kempe's cumulative recording of the piercing, rupturing, and breaking of Christ's body evokes the broken heart of Catherine of Siena, and her own somatic fragmentation. Exploding and bursting forth with emotion, she weeps so boisterously that it is 'as ȝyf sche xulde a brostyn for sorwe & peyne' (191).[71] The ocular vividness of her contemplation continues via descriptions of Christ's body unmade, as he is skinned, drained, and punctured:

And þan sche sey þe Iewys wyth gret violens rendyn of [from] owr Lordys precyows body a cloth of sylke, þe which was cleuyn & hardyd so sadly & streitly to owr Lordys body wyth hys precyows blood þat it drow a-wey al þe hyde & al þe skyn of hys blissyd body & renewyd hys precious wowndys & mad þe blod to renne down al a-bowtyn on euery syde. Þan þat precyows body aperyd to hir syght as rawe as a thyng þat wer newe flayn owt of þe skyn, ful petows & rewful to be-holdyn. And so had sche a new sorwe þar sche wept & cryid ryth sor. & a-non aftyr sche beheld how þe cruel Iewys leyden hys precyows body to þe Crosse & sithyn tokyn a long nayle, a row [rough] & a boistews, & sett to hys on hand & wyth gret violens & cruelness þei dreuyn it thorw hys hande. Hys blisful Modyr beheldyng & þis creatur how hys precyows body schrynkyd & drow to-gedyr wyth alle senwys & veynys in þat precyows body for peyne þat it suffyrd & felt, þei sorwyd and mornyd & syhyd ful sor. Than sey sche wyth hyr gostly eye how þe Iewys festenyd ropis on þe oþer hand, for þe senwys & veynys wer so schrynkyn wyth peyne þat it myth not come to þe hole þat þei had morkyn þerfor, & drowyn þeron to makyn it mete wyth þe hole. & so her peyne & hir sorwe euyr encresyd (191–2).

Like a skinned animal ready for consumption, Christ's raw and mutilated body, his wounds renewed and multiplied by the tearing of the cloth, causes Kempe a 'new sorwe': her weeping is 'sor' (sore). That Christ's 'senwys & veynys wer so schrynkyn wyth peyne' reveals Kempe's understanding of medical knowledge and witnessing of dying bodies, the 'sharp' contracting and drying of the skin indicating signs of death. As she recounts each act of violence and its subsequent damage to the Christic body, she intersperses her own agonised reaction, juxtaposing the pained, crucified Christ with her surrogate suffering. When Christ's hand is drawn excruciatingly to the hole on the cross, so her 'peyne & hir sorwe euyr encresyd', resonating with the *Meditationes vitae Christi* when Christ's body is stretched in order to reach nail holes made too far apart.[72] The sense of painful progression, the deadly torture of the Christic body envisioned graphically and simultaneously to her own agony, highlights how Kempe wishes to die *with* Christ in a slow and

[70] Christine Cooper-Rompato, 'Numeracy and Number in *The Book of Margery Kempe*', in *The Medieval Mystical Tradition in England: Exeter Symposium VIII, Papers read at Charney Manor, July 2011*, ed. E.A. Jones (Cambridge: D.S. Brewer, 2013), pp. 59–73 (p. 71).
[71] Cf. p. 175, n. 56 in this chapter on meanings of 'xulde' (shulen): here indicating an emphatic inevitability.
[72] Bestul, *Texts of the Passion*, p. 44.

torturous unfolding of the destiny in which she feels embroiled. But, more-over, her cries to the Jews to 'Sle me raþar & late hym gon' (192) articulate a superlative willingness for death surrogacy, her torment so visible and physical that the parishioners in the church in which she is enraptured 'wondryd on hir body' (192). Her own corporeality, then, merges with Christ's in an out-of-body experience where she is at once embodied and disembodied; an altered consciousness that wills her own mortal sacrifice, her body mirroring the 'schaky[ing] & schoder[ing]' of Christ's as it writhes in near-death. As Kempe describes Christ's 'precyows wowndys ronnyn down wyth reuerys of blood on euery syde' (192), she is anxious to parallel this with her own pain and seepage, as she has 'mor wepyng & sorwyng': his blood for her tears (193). This reworked pattern of her reciprocation and reply to Christ's suffering body continues throughout the episode, a dialogic exchange of Christic pain and mystical affectivity which implicates her into the scene as an active death surrogate. Never diluting the methodical torture of Christ's flesh, Kempe's account insists on a textual immediacy that allows her to re-live, or *re-die*, each time she recollects the vision, just as she presumably hopes her readers will as they encounter the infinite potential of these visions as subjects for meditation. As she dies with Christ with every blow and incision that he endures, she fulfils the prophecy that his 'Passyon wil sle [her]' (164), joining the other holy women whose liminal existence leaves them 'dead to the world', and closer to God in the next life than in this one.

The emphasis on Christ's body drained of blood (which 'renne down al a-bowtyn on euery syde', 192), and on Kempe's body drained of tears, cor-responds with the late medieval contemplation of Christ's complete exsan-guination, shown in the *Book* through an emphasis on his shrivelled veins: 'hys precyows body schrynkyd & drow to-gedyr wyth alle senwys [sinews] & veynys in þat precyows body for peyne þat it suffyrd & felt' (192). Though Christ's body is portrayed as fully emptied in medieval cultural depictions, Caroline Walker Bynum notes that 'the blood that flowed was understood to be alive'.[73] Theologians argued that the 'gushing forth of water and blood in "living" streams' was a special 'second miracle', which proved that Christ's death was voluntary and life-giving, because blood in dead bodies coagulates and is stagnant.[74] The Monk of Evesham (fl. late twelfth century) claimed to see, in a vision of the Passion, 'blood flowing from the side of the image on the cross, as it does from the veins of a living man when he is cut for blood-letting'.[75] This conceptual amalgamation with the medical procedure of phlebotomy illustrates how exsanguination in the medieval imaginary was not always associated with the loss of life, as it could also be linked to the purgative function of medical procedures. The Monk of Evesham example, equated Christ's blood loss with the purgation that corresponded to health and to

[73] Bynum, *Wonderful Blood*, p. 166.
[74] Ibid., p. 167.
[75] Ibid.

healing, just as the crucifixion symbolises the universal healing of all Christians on earth.[76] Yet whilst that purgation of blood might be an efficacious activity, it simultaneously results in a loss of moisture that characterises somatic deterioration and a drawing towards death. Julian of Norwich describes the dying Christ medically in her own vision of the Passion: a face that was 'drye and blodeles', changing in colour from fresh and fair to brown and black, 'into drye dying', and where 'Blodlessehed [bloodlessness] and paine dried within'.[77] However, Julian is clear that Christ retains 'a moister' in his 'swete flesh', combining the scientific understanding of life-giving moisture and the theology of his transcended humanity. Indeed, she scrutinises the changing colours of his face, the 'spreding of the forehede' and the 'nose [which] clongen togeder and dried', listing the *signa mortifera* as a physiological facet of the later affective turn in medieval piety which focused on the intense viscerality of Christ's suffering.[78] It is perhaps unsurprising, then, that when in 1436, at the age of sixty-three, Margery Kempe oversees the transcription and revision of Book I (the original copy being almost illegible), she ensures that that it concludes with the climactic accounts of the Passion visions. The sensations of exsanguination and dryness are, I suggest, concomitantly gendered and linked to the physiological state of the mature female body, an equivalence that Kempe utilises as an opportunity to achieve *imitatio* of the dying, drying, Christ.

The moment of Christ's actual death is reported in the episode with shocking brevity: '& þerwyth he deyid' (193). In antithesis, Margery Kempe becomes uncontrollably animated. While Mary lies in desolate prostration, 'as sche had ben ded' (193), Kempe runs 'al a-bowte þe place as it had ben a mad woman, crying & roryng' (193), agitated by a potential twofold loss. Though she utters soothing words to the Virgin-in-stasis, emphasising how her son is now out of pain, her own frenzy depicts a bursting paroxysm of grief born from the loss of the Christ whose body she was told would 'be newe crucified in [her]' (85). But the cessation of Christ's pain also intensifies a maternal union between Kempe and Mary – these two holy mothers – as Kempe acts as surrogate for the Virgin's suffering: 'ȝowr sorwe is my sorwe' (193). Such a pain surrogacy fulfils Simeon's prophecy to Mary that 'thy own soul a sword shall pierce' (Luke 2:35), a topos replayed habitually in medieval culture; on medieval lyric, for example, laments: 'My child is outlawed for thy sinne; / My childe is bete for thy trespasse; / Yet prikketh mine hert that so ny [near] my kinne / Shuld be diseased [distressed]'.[79] As Simeon's revelation comes to pass,

---

76 On anchoritic bloodletting see McAvoy, 'Bathing in Blood', in *Medicine, Religion and Gender in Medieval Culture*, ed. Yoshikawa, pp. 85–102.

77 'A Revelation of Love', in *The Writings of Julian of Norwich*, ed. Watson and Jenkins, p. 179. See also Vincent Gillespie, 'The Colours of Contemplation: Less Light on Julian of Norwich', in *The Medieval Mystical Tradition in England*, ed. Jones, pp. 7–28.

78 *A Revelation of Love*, ch. 7, p. 145, and ch. 16, p. 179. See, for example, Sarah McNamer, *Affective Meditation and the Invention of Medieval Compassion*.

79 'In a tabernacle of a toure', IMEV 1460, also no. 196, in *Middle English Lyrics*, ed. Luria and Hoffman, pp. 187–9.

the sword's work is complete only after the subsequent piercing of Christ's own side by the soldiers, when Mary's figurative rupture becomes her son's literal one.[80] As his fractured body is brought down from the cross, Mary 'wept so plentyuowsly ouyr hys blissyd face þat sche wesch a-wey þe blod of hys face wyth þe terys of her eyne' (193). In an inversion of the maternal body, Mary's gestational blood transfigures into tears, literally washing away Christ's spilled, life-giving blood and re-enacting the ceremony of Purification after childbirth, which is notably recounted just two chapters later and which inspires a similar affective response in Margery Kempe.

As Kempe witnesses the failure of Christ's body, the *Book* merges the physical and metaphysical as she watches the reverent actions of Mary Magdalene and the Virgin's sister kissing Christ's hands and feet, and bemoans her own marginality, 'gretly desyryng to an had þe precyows body be hir-self a-lone' (194). Her atavistic reaction to grief gives way to the non-verbal as she runs frantically to and fro as if she were a woman 'wyth-owtyn reson', disoriented and weeping so greatly that 'hir thowt þat sche wolde a deyid', death seeming to be the only possible outcome of a vision which has destroyed the borders of self and space (194). Later, when Christ is finally buried, she wishes to 'a-byden stille be þe graue of owr Lord', so unwilling to be separated that she desires their joint burial: 'Hir thowt sche wolde neuyr a partyd þens but desiryd to a deyd þer & ben berijd wyth owr Lord' (194). As Christ's bride, Kempe enacts a mystical vigil over the grave, like the deathbed vigils of her parish life, longing to be reunited and entombed with her divine spouse, enjoined in corporeal death as well as in eternity; it is, as Bynum puts it, 'an effort to plumb the depths of Christ's humanity at the moment of his most insistent and terrifying humanness – the moment of his dying'.[81] But while, as Gillespie has argued, 'the death of the self' is a necessary spiritual epiphany *en route* to 'the dead stillness of contemplative attention to God', Kempe's driving need for immolation in lamentation for the Manhood does not easily reveal such a transition.[82] Instead, it evokes the mystical conversation between Christ and his mother, relayed by Vanna of Orvieto to her prioress, following the revelation of her own impending death: '"Mother I am dead". And the other, pierced through, answered: "Woe is me, daughter, what are you saying?" The Virgin answered: "Mother, I am entirely dead."'[83] To all intents and purposes, Margery Kempe, suspended here at Christ's graveside, is also 'entirely dead'.

---

[80] 'But one of the soldiers with a spear opened his side, and immediately there came out blood and water' (John, 19:34).

[81] Bynum, *Fragmentation*, p. 131. Kempe may have been familiar with the story of Saphir, who was buried next to her husband Ananias (Acts 5:1–10). Charles J. Reid suggests that husbands and wives were sometimes expected to be buried together in the Middle Ages, in *Power over the Body, Equality in the Family: Rights and Domestic Relations in Medieval Canon Law* (Michigan and Cambridge: William. B. Eerdmans Publishing, 2005), p. 133.

[82] Gillespie, 'Dead Still / Still Dead', p. 66.

[83] Giacomo Scalza, 'The Life of Vanna d'Orvieto', from Elliott, *Proving Woman*, p. 180.

6

Senescent Reproduction:
Writing Anamnestic Pain

This final chapter considers Margery Kempe's old age as a framework for the casting of her entire project, the spiritualisation of her pain, and the *Book* as itself the ultimate surrogate production. As a retrospective, the pain narrative of Kempe's life is an anamnestic production in the context of her increased authority as an 'elder' in the world, therefore the dual forces of old age and the understanding of suffering are necessarily imbricated in the act of writing. Indeed, as Mary Carruthers has argued, 'medieval culture was primarily memorial' and, as a result, 'a book itself is a mnemonic'.[1] In finally inscribing her life and learning to the manuscript page some twenty years after her conversion, Margery Kempe recalls the memory of her pains – more recently experienced in the events of Book II than Book I – from the perspective of old age. From this position, her choices of narrative content are thus meaningful in terms not just of the dictation of her more recent *experientia*, but also the reflectivity upon the other events narrated in Books I and II. Furthermore, as I explore here, and, as the ageing Christine de Pizan (c. 1364–c. 1430) testifies in *The Treasure of the City of Ladies*, 'there is no worse disease than old age'.[2] Senescence, then, might also be regarded as a natural opportunity for what I have termed *aged asceticism*, since the culturally abject, ageing body, is, to an extent, diseased-by-default.

There exists much valuable scholarship about the authorship and authority of Kempe's *Book*, but little on the significance of the production of the text during her old age.[3] The very timing of the *Book*'s first embryonic advent in her elderly years is divinely dictated, since, years before, 'sche was comawndyd in hir sowle þat sche schuld not wrytyn so soone' (3). Only twenty years later, when Christ 'comawnded hyr & chargyd hir þat sche xuld don wryten hyr felyngys & reuelacyons & þe forme of her leuyng þat hys goodnesse myth be knowyn to alle þe world' (3–4), does she employ the services of her first amanuensis (generally thought to be the son who had

[1] Mary Carruthers, *The Book of Memory: A Study of Memory in Medieval Culture*, 2nd edn (Cambridge: Cambridge University Press, 2008), pp. 9–10.
[2] Christine de Pizan, *The Treasure of the City of Ladies, or The Book of the Three Virtues*, trans. Sarah Lawson (Harmondsworth: Penguin, 1985), p. 166.
[3] Exceptions are, for example, Liz Herbert McAvoy in '"[A] péler of holy church"', in *Prime of Their Lives*, ed. Mulder-Bakker, pp. 17–38; and David Wallace, *Strong Women*, p. 85.

been living in Danzig).[4] After his death a priest encounters the text, but has difficulty deciphering its hybrid linguistic form; however, he is eventually so moved by Kempe's story that he commences the transcription of Book I in 'þe 3er of owr Lord a m. cccc.xxxvj [1436]' (6), when Kempe is about sixty-three years old. On finishing, he commences the writing of Book II, in 'þe yer of owr Lord m. cccc.xxxviij [1438]', when Kempe is about sixty-five (221).[5] The events of Book I are thus recounted with the increased wisdom of age and are revised by a priest (probably her confessor, Robert Spryngolde), while those in Book II – which certainly exhibits a different narrative texture from Book I – are dictated with closer proximity to the episodes of her later life and therefore have a tone of increased temporal authenticity. There is, then, less memorial reliance in Book II than in Book I, which, when finally textualised, was distanced by 'xx 3er & mor' from its first revelation (3). I want to suggest, then, that we might grasp more urgently the *voice* of Margery Kempe in Book II, especially since, while there is certainly a subtext of 'saintly box-ticking' at play, the conflation of age, experience, and narrative immediacy brings a particular form of truth to the reader.[6] It is, after all, her very *life* which has been divinely authorised to embody the mystical reception of God's spoken Word into textual word as a powerful model of female holiness, that 'life' now ripe for didactic dissemination to the world.

Older age, as the lives and writings of such holy women as Elizabeth of Hungary, Julian of Norwich, Marie of Oignies, and Bridget of Sweden attest, is a forceful facilitator for the authorised female voice, but paradoxically only after the atrophy of their sexual and reproductive existence renders them somehow less female. In focusing on Margery Kempe the 'elder' (and I employ the term with deliberate recourse to its life-course and ecclesiastical significations), and the locus of that aged body as a site of tension between medieval constructions of the simultaneously repellent yet wise old woman, I argue that it is *through* Kempe's old age that we might know her best. The edifying, senescent pain that replaces the bodily penance of her younger life,

---

[4] See Sebastian Sobecki, '"The writyng of this tretys:"'; and Roger Ellis, 'Margery Kempe's Scribe and the Miraculous Books', in *Langland, the Mystics, and the Medieval English Religious Tradition*, ed. Phillips.

[5] Arnold Sanders speculates that Kempe became minimally literate in the vernacular shortly before the composition of Book II because she wrote letters to her son in Germany in c. 1431 in 'Illiterate Memory and Spiritual Experience: Margery Kempe, the Liturgy, and the "Woman in the Crowd"', in *Mindful Spirit in Late Medieval Literature: Essays in Honor of Elizabeth D. Kirk*, ed. Bonnie Wheeler (Basingstoke: Palgrave Macmillan, 2006), pp. 237–48. See also Josephine Tarvers, 'The Alleged Illiteracy of Margery Kempe: A Reconsideration of the Evidence', *Medieval Perspectives*, XI (1996), 113–24.

[6] Some critics have argued that Book II is little more than a travelogue; a point with which I take issue. See for example, Lynn Staley, 'Margery Kempe', in *The Book of Margery Kempe: A New Translation, Contexts, Criticism*, trans. and ed. Lynn Staley (New York: Norton, 2001), p. xv. See also Lia Ross, 'The Revealing Peregrinations of Margery Kempe', in *Travel, Time, and Space in the Middle Ages and Early Modern Time*, ed. Albrect Classen (Boston and Berlin: De Gruyter, 2018), pp. 359–78 (p. 368).

the ascetic value of elderly pilgrimage, and the fertile teachings that position her as mother to the world open up new routes for surrogacy – reproductivity, even – in an age when they might otherwise be closed.

Pathologising the Old Woman

Margery Kempe's widowhood at the age of fifty-eight, considered in Chapter 4, marked the closure of a critical life stage.[7] The period of grief and double bereavement, and the necessary readjustment provoked by her son and husband dying within a 'schort tyme' (225) of each other, is a transition through which the pain of loss must be reconciled with the fissure of opportunity that such a loss generates. Ambivalence towards new widowhood was perhaps culturally expected, as Joel Rosenthal notes: '[a husband's] death was accepted with resignation, if not with cheer, and her grief was expected to be measured'.[8] But this liberation from the confines of marriage, at the age of fifty-eight, coincides broadly with the medieval understanding of the onset of 'old age', which was considered to be around the age of sixty, thus substituting one form of somatic tribulation for another.[9] Margery Kempe lived in the direct aftermath of the plague and its aftershock, so we might infer that the advanced age of 'iij score 3er' (234) signifies a fortunate passage into senescence in itself. Indeed, the extent to which one felt 'aged' was dependent on contemporary life expectancies: Robert Magnan has suggested the relative unlikelihood of actually reaching the age of sixty-five or above during the period 1276 to 1450.[10]

Old age was nevertheless commonly regarded in the Middle Ages to be between the ages of sixty and seventy.[11] Augustine had considered sixty as the onset.[12] Aldebrandin of Siena thought *senium* (extreme old age) to be from sixty until death, and Vincent of Beauvais modelled a scheme that held the *aetas minuendi* (stage of enfeeblement) to be from sixty until the end of life.[13] Bartholomaeus Anglicus held that the age of *senectus* (old age, as opposed to

---

[7] On this dating see Chapter 4 of this study, p. 158.

[8] Joel T. Rosenthal, 'Fifteenth-Century Widows and Widowhood: Bereavement, Reintegration, and Life Choices', in *Wife and Widow in Medieval England*, ed. Sue Sheridan Walker (Ann Arbor: University of Michigan Press, 1993), p. 48.

[9] Shulamith Shahar, *Growing Old in the Middle Ages*, pp. 12–28. Different medieval writers suggested slightly differing age taxonomies.

[10] 'Out of 1000 people born during this period, an average of 350 reached age 40, 200 or so reached 50, perhaps 90 attained aged 65, and a dozen would live to be 80 or older'. See Magnan, 'Sex and Senescence in Medieval Literature', in *Aging in Literature*, ed. Porter, p. 15.

[11] Shulamith Shahar, 'Who were Old in the Middle Ages?', *Social History of Medicine*, 6 (1993), 313–34; and J.A. Burrow, *The Ages of Man: A Study in Medieval Writing and Thought*.

[12] Shahar, 'Who were Old in the Middle Ages?', p. 315.

[13] Ibid., p. 318.

extreme old age), for some 'endiþ in þe 70 ȝere, and some wolen mene þat it endiþ in none certeyne nombre of ȝeres', while *senium* is 'þe laste age'.[14] The Middle English Gilbertus Anglicus states that 'Elde lastiþ fro fyfty ȝere or sixty tyl on-to þe lyuys ende'.[15] The medico-cultural understanding of what was considered 'old' in the Middle Ages, therefore, would have meant that Kempe felt herself to be at the end of her life when she embarked on her final journeys during her early sixties: sensing 'borrowed time', perhaps, and the concomitant drive to maximise any remaining spiritual capital. Senescence, however, was also imbued with a proclivity to melancholy. Bartholomaeus notes how the blood 'waxiþ coolde', and 'elde ben elenge [wretched] and sorweful'.[16] Gilbertus Anglicus states that 'Malencolie is wount to be plenteuouse in leene old folks in coold and driȝe tymes.'[17] The reductiveness of such medical examples, bypassing the increased imaginative faculties of the melancholic that were discussed in Chapter 1, takes as a given the inherent misery of elderly melancholia. I gesture instead towards Margery Kempe's own melancholic predisposition, perhaps exacerbated in her elderly years, as, rather, an opening up of new potentialities for mystical enlightenment.

Still, medieval representations of old women, or *vetulae*, are typically misogynous imaginings of aged, poisonous 'hags', as this oft-cited example from *De secretis mulierum* illustrates:

> It should be noted that old women who still have their monthly flow, and some who do not menstruate, poison the eyes of children lying in their cradles by their glance ... For the reason why old women who do not menstruate infect children is because the retention of the menses brings about an abundance of evil humours and because old women are deficient in natural heat.

> [Est autem notandum, quod mulieres antiquæ, in quibus menstrua fluunt, & quædam in quibus menstrua sunt retenta, si inspiciunt pueros in cunis jacentes, intoxicant oculos eorum visu ... Causa autem quare antiquæ mulieres, quibus non fluunt menstrua, inficient pueros, est quod retentio menstruorum facit abundantiam malorum humorum, & quia antiquæ mulieres sunt deficientes in calore naturali.][18]

The notion of old women's eyes as sources of pathologising evil – or 'fascination' – was an ancient idea, originating in the works of Pliny, Saint Paul's letter to the Galatians, and, later, Thomas Aquinas, and it permeated medical treatises from the fourteenth century.[19] It developed from an asexual

---

[14] *On the Properties of Things*, p. 292.
[15] *System of Physic*, p. 44.
[16] *On the Properties of Things*, p. 293. MED s.v. elenge: 1(a) wretched, miserable, unhappy, sad.
[17] *System of Physic*, p. 50.
[18] *De secretis mulierum*, trans. Lemay, p. 129. Albertus Magnus, *De secretis mulierum*, p. 109.
[19] See Fernando Salmón and Montserrat Cabré, 'Fascinating Women: The Evil Eye in Medical Scholasticism', in *Medicine from the Black Death to the French Disease*, ed. Roger French, Jon Arrizabalaga, Andrew Cunningham, and Luis Garcia (Aldershot: Ashgate, 1998), pp. 53–84.

framework to a gendered one whereby old women, through their retained menses and cold, increasingly dry constitutions, became the logical exempla of the evil eye at work. These medicalised ideas are also apparent in religious handbooks like the *Ancrene Wisse*, which portrays the seven deadly sins as dangerous, married 'hags', advising its anchoritic audience to beware of the sexual temptation to which even they could succumb:

> Nv ȝe habbeð ane dale iherd, mine leoue sustren, of þeo þe me cleopeð þe seoue moder-sunnen ant of hare teames, ant of hwucche meosters þes ilke men seruið i þe feondes curt þe habbeð iwiuet o þeose seouen haggen, ant hwi ha beoð swiðe to heatien ant to schunien.

> [Now you have heard one part, my dear sisters, about what are called the seven mother-sins, and about their offspring, and about what functions are served in the devil's court by those men who have married those seven hags, and why they are very much to be hated and avoided.][20]

Even the female enclosed are at risk of succumbing to their innate sexual insatiability via these 'hags', who personify everything that is grotesque and wicked about old women. Indeed, literary representations often portray elderly women as preoccupied with sexual matters, acting as go-betweens in the sexual relations of others, like La Vieille, in the *Roman de la rose* – that 'dirty, stinking, foul old woman … who is making me waste away' – and the unapologetically sexual Wife of Bath, whose *auctoritee* is an affront to her husband.[21] The trope of the old, objectified woman is reiterated in the pseudo-Aristotelian *Secretum secretorum*, which describes winter as 'an olde woman, greueed and decreped in age, lakking clothes, neygh to deth': naked and physically infirm, she is the epitome of elderly feminine abjection.[22] Such seeming incongruity of the sexualised old woman is regarded by Gretchen Mieszkowski as indicating a 'deep fear of women's sexual power': reduced in literature to her ageing, inferior corporeality, the old woman's threatening wisdom and generative knowing could be contained, at least inside the book.[23]

---

[20] MED s.v. hagge: An ugly old woman; witch, hag. *Ancrene Wisse: A Corrected Edition*, vol. 1, part 4, section 36, ed. Millett, p. 83. Translation from *Ancrene Wisse: A Guide for Anchoresses, a Translation*, ed. Millet, p. 83.

[21] *The Romance of the Rose*, Guillaume de Lorris and Jean de Meun, trans. Charles Dahlberg, 3rd edn (Princeton: Princeton University Press, 1995), ch. 4, ll. 4110–12, p. 91. See Lorraine K. Stock, 'Just how loathly is the "wyf"? Deconstructing Chaucer's "hag" in *The Wife of Bath's Tale*', in *Magistra Doctissima: Essays in Honor of Bonnie Wheeler*, ed. Dorsey Armstrong, Ann W. Astell, and Howell Chickering (Kalamazoo: Medieval Institute Publications, 2013), pp. 34–42; and Susan Carter, 'A hymenation of hags', in *The English "Loathly Lady" Tales: Boundaries, Traditions, Motifs*, ed. Elizabeth Passmore and Susan Carter (Kalamazoo: Medieval Institute Publications, 2007), pp. 83–99.

[22] 'The Secrete of Secretes' (Ashmole Version), in *Secretum Secretorum: Nine English Versions*, ed. M.A. Manzalaoui, EETS o.s. 276 (Oxford: Oxford University Press, 1977), p. 58.

[23] Gretchen Mieszkowski, 'Old Age and Medieval Misogyny: The Old Woman', in *Old Age in the Middle Ages and the Renaissance*, ed. Classen, pp. 299–319 (p. 309). See also

Older women's discourse, too, was potentially dangerous if it deviated from the tenets of 1 Timothy.[24] The Church Fathers thus promulgated the use of the term 'oldwomanish' to denote worthless and irrational thought, an insult coined by Augustine as 'anicularia phantasmata' (oldwomanish phantasms), and without doubt the antithesis of Margery Kempe and other holy women's esoteric perspicacity and salvific remembrances.[25]

The cultural prejudice against old women and their disease-loaded bodies is also evident in medical and scientific treatises. That Avicenna had written that the old are cold and dry because of 'the long time having elapsed since they originally developed from the blood, semen and ethereal vital force' implies an acceleration of female ageing, since women's production of menstrual blood additionally ceases to regenerate after menopause.[26] Some scholarship on medieval longevity suggests that improvements in the medieval diet from the later Middle Ages meant that women suffered from less anaemia (a condition exacerbated by menstruation) and therefore their life expectancy came to equal that of men. Dietary improvements included a greater proportion of meat and fish (the latter increasingly popular due to Church stipulations over fasting from meat on Fridays in particular).[27] However, since Margery Kempe undertook frequent fasts, and relinquished meat for some time, any broadly social dietary improvements might have passed her by.[28] She may have suffered the after-effects of long-term anaemia following her menstrual span, and also osteoporosis: chronic conditions that were likely an integral and accepted facet of daily life for medieval ageing women.

Other pathologies associated with the older woman, such as uterine precipitation, or prolapse, are described with the somewhat dismissive subtext of elderly incurability in medical texts. The 'Book on the Conditions of Women' explains prolapse of the uterus as exacerbated by the cold: 'A weakening and chilling of this kind happens from cold air entering in from below through the orifices of

---

Herbert C. Covey, 'Perceptions and Attitudes towards Sexuality of the Elderly during the Middle Ages', *The Gerontologist*, 29 (1989), 93–100, pp. 96–7.

[24] 'Not to give heed to fables and endless genealogies: which furnish questions rather than the edification of God, which is in faith'. 1 Timothy 1:4. See Jan M. Ziolkowski, 'The Obscenities of Old Women: Vetularity and Vernacularity', in *Obscenity: Social Control and Artistic Creation in the European Middle Ages*, ed. Jan M. Ziolkowski (Leiden and Boston: Brill, 1998), pp. 73–89 (p. 86).

[25] See Jan Ziolkowski, 'Old Wives' Tales: Classicism and Anti-Classicism from Apuleius to Chaucer', *The Journal of Medieval Latin*, 12 (2002), 90–113 (p. 102). In such literature old women are uneducated, illogical, tale-telling and, importantly, non-reproductive, becoming paradoxically disempowered and feared.

[26] Avicenna, *Canon*, vol. 1, adapt. Bakhtiar, p. 30.

[27] See Vern Bullough and Cameron Campbell, 'Female Longevity and Diet in the Middle Ages', *Speculum*, 55, 2 (1980), 317–25. Deborah Youngs contests this point, suggesting that complications in childbirth, amongst other factors, evidences a higher rate of female mortality compared to men during the adult years. See Youngs, *The Life Cycle in Western Europe*, pp. 28–9.

[28] In Book I, Chapter 5, Jesus tells Kempe to forsake 'þe etyng of flesch' (17). We are told of Christ's relinquishment of this imperative in Chapter 66.

the womb, and sometimes if uncovered she has exposed herself to cold air, or sat upon a cold stone' ('Huiusmodi autem remollicio et frigidatio contingit ex frigido aere per orificia matricis subintrante, et quandoque si detecta dirrecte se opposuerit aeri frigido, uel super lapidem frigidum sederit').[29] Indeed, Kempe's pilgrimages to northern Europe during her sixties, in some hardship as her body began to fail, would inevitably involve walking in the cold and resting on chilled walls, rendering her vulnerable pilgrim body susceptible to such disorder. The *Sickness of Women* dismisses uterine prolapse in the elderly as simply incurable. Whilst some women 'may be holpen' by the use of ointments, fumigations, the physical reinsertion of the womb, and genital *plastres*, the *old* woman's body is beyond repair: 'Also it is to wite þat þe coming out of þe matrice in an olde woman is vncurable.'[30] That such a statement is left unqualified illustrates the medical acceptance that the old female body is more prone to affliction, and that attempts at remedy are futile. This is reiterated later in the text concerning cancers and ulcers of the uterus:

> Cancryng [cancers] and festres [festering] of the matrice comen of old woundes of the matrice that wore nat wele helid, but that maner of sikenes we wil speke but litil of, for phisiciens sayn that cancres that bien hidde, it is better that thei bien vncurid than cured or heled.[31]

The advice to leave hidden cancers uncured indicates, unsurprisingly, medical suspicion of the 'secrets' of womanly flesh, and especially of the 'old' uterine injuries that the 'physiciens' would prefer to avoid in the aged, less valued, female body. The treatise's recommendation of a therapeutic ointment, instead, is intended to soothe – perhaps to quieten – its cancer-plagued subjects from their 'icchyng [itching] also and blaynes [blisters] that bien in the matrice', rather than to attempt a remedy.

Even urinary incontinence – common in older women who have born children, and Kempe, of course, bore fourteen – is addressed in 'On Treatments for Women', though its mention is cursory.[32] Such conditions that denote the inevitability and incurability of somatic decline uphold Robert Magnan's assertion that 'old age is both an end and a beginning, but little else, a time of regrets and preparation, but not enjoyment'.[33] These old-age afflictions presuppose a pain imperative of punitive suffering and bleak irrevocability, and the texts reveal a cultural impatience with the lack of productive capacity in those considered elderly. Indeed, Bartholomaeus Anglicus not only lists the morbidly degenerate signs of ageing entropy, but also notes a social distaste for the stricken old person:

---

[29] The 'Book on the Conditions of Women', in *The Trotula*, pp. 86–7.
[30] *Sickness of Women*, p. 548.
[31] Ibid., p. 539.
[32] See 'On Treatments for Women', in *The Trotula*, pp. 136–7.
[33] Robert Magnan, 'Sex and Senescence', in *Aging in Literature*, ed. Porter, p. 26.

For in þis elde kynde hete quenchiþ, þe vertu of gouernaunce and of re[u] leynge failiþ, humour is dissolued and wasted, myȝt and strengþ passith and faileþ, fleisch and fairnes is consumpt and spendiþ, þe skyn riueliþ, þe sinewis schrinken, þe body bendiþ and crokeþ, fourme and schap is ilost, fairnes of þe body brouȝt to nouȝt. Alle þis failiþ in e[l]de. *Alle men dispisen þe olde man and ben heuy and wery of him.*[34]

Margery Kempe undeniably suffers the spite of her fellow travellers and failing corporeal strength during her later pilgrimages. However, where some medical and scientific treatises might construct the elderly as inutile victims of the slow decline towards 'þe ȝatis of deeþ', I wish to argue for the phenomenon of *aged asceticism*, where the vicissitudes of old age are imbued with a unique opportunity for redemption as a result of the suffering imperative – the being 'diseased-by-default' – of the declining body.[35] This is an opportunity most acutely mined in the accounts of Book II, not only for their locus in the phase of Kempe's old age, but also in their more immediate dictation as recent experiences of memorialised pain. In this way Kempe's lifetime of learning and holy instruction is brought to bear on the later events of her life, when the edifying incorporation of orthodox teaching coincides with the individual experience of the tribulations of senescence in anamnestic productivity. Many years of salvific encounter have thus come to teleological fruition. She receives counsel from Julian of Norwich about her gift of tears and concomitant social ostracisation in Norwich in 1413 (42–3). She is read the *Revelations* of Bridget of Sweden (143) and meets with Bridget's own maiden in Rome in 1414 (95). The corpus of her own reading, via her confessor's narration, spans some seven or eight years, and includes the Bible and its theological commentaries, Walter Hilton's *Scale of Perfection*, Bonaventura's *Stimulus amoris*, and Richard Rolle's *Incendium amoris* (143). Her priest-scribe reads the *vitae* of Marie of Oignies (1177–1213) and Elizabeth of Hungary (1207–31), whose mysticism and affective piety convince him of Kempe's authenticity, and would almost certainly have relayed them to her, particularly since Margery Kempe appears to experience the same form of spirituality as Marie (152–4). As opposed to a gradual, acquiescent decrepitude, then, Margery Kempe defies the socio-medical pathologisation of the old woman in myriad ways: she travels on pilgrimage, she resists the repression of female discourse by teaching the Word of God, and she utilises her senescent pains as a way of co-suffering with Christ. Crucially, she transmogrifies the social paranoia about old women's 'evil eyes', substituting malevolent ocularity with the divine privilege of mystical vision. And she writes her *Book*, in a senescent production that both memorialises and recaptures the lifelong wisdom that is not pathological but rather the opposite, an act of eschatological creation.

---

[34] My emphasis. *On the Properties of Things*, p. 293.
[35] Quotation from *On the Properties of Things*, p. 293.

Reproductive Senescence

With structural import, near the very start of Book II, the reader is told of the birth of Margery Kempe's grandchild (perhaps, but not necessarily, her first): 'hys [Kempe's son's] wife had a childe, a fayr mayde-child' (223). Aware of her increasing years, Kempe is anxious to see her family, who live in Germany, before she dies ('sche xulde seen hem alle er þan sche deyid' [223]), despite the physical challenge of crossing the sea, the travail of which she had deemed hitherto prohibitive, 'neuyr purposing to passyn þe see whil sche leuyd' (223). She achieves her aim, and her evolving status as sagacious matriarch is later compounded by her daughter-in-law's references to her as 'eldmodyr' (225), a term of address that seals her elevation to the position of respected and authoritative (grand)mother-figure, and is aligned also with Kempe's metaphysical growth at this life stage.[36]

While some female mystics like Margery Kempe adapted their mature biology through the utilisation of surrogate strategies of nursing, caring, and mystical fecundity, there remained a paradigmatic exclusion from the idealised model of the Virgin Mary that old, holy women were forced to endure and to resist. The *vetulae* were far, far removed from the ubiquitous iconography of a young, breastfeeding Virgin Mary in the Middle Ages. As Shahar suggests, 'The old woman whose milk has dried cannot personify Mary the Holy Mother, who suckles her child – the symbol of good and mercy.'[37] Yet the aged woman – post childbearing – also had a vital social role in contributing to the pastoral care of her family and community, as St Paul had outlined:

> The aged women … in holy attire, not false accusers, not given to much wine, teaching well: That they may teach the young women to be wise, to love their husbands, to love their children, To be discreet, chaste, sober, having a care of the house, gentle, obedient to their husbands, that the word of God be not blasphemed (Titus 2:2–5).

Paul's tenet gestures towards an alternative role for Christian women, who in their older years may enter a phase of teaching and instruction as wise, mature women who bear a valuable, efficacious didacticism. While this direction is partly at odds with his ruling in the Epistle to Timothy – 'I suffer not a woman to teach' – the distinction resides in the opposing contexts of public and private spaces: the aged woman is permitted to teach feminine and domestic

---

[36] MED s.v. elde-moder: 1(a) Grandmother (2) mother-in-law (3) the earth as the 'mother' of mankind. As well as the first denotation being the mature role of the grandmother, the prefix *elde* denotes clear gerontological meanings. E.g. MED s.v. elde: 1(a) maturity; adulthood (3) a period of life in which one is naturally or conventionally qualified for some function or activity. The term *eldmodyr* thus imbues senescent connotations as well as domestic ones and is a mode of address that encompasses not only a familial relationship but which also acknowledges women's status and age.

[37] Shahar, *Growing Old*, p. 49.

virtues in a domestic setting, but not, apparently, to teach in the formal sense or to suppose authority over men.[38]

This transfigured productivity is borne out linguistically by the *Sickness of Women*, which explicates the nomenclature of the female reproductive system by aligning the terms *marice* and *moder* as synonymous: 'the matrice that is clepid the moder and norice [nourisher] to the cheildren right conceived in hem. Þe matrice is a skynne that the child is enclosed in his moder wombe and many of the sikenessis that wymmen han comen of the greuaunces of this moder that we clepen the matrice.'[39] The naming of the uterus in terms of the woman's social *and* biological functions evidences their cultural assimilation, suggesting that mothering is a transferable activity that can operate both intra-bodily and extra-bodily. Older women thus have integral functions as caregivers beyond their immediate, biological capacity. Furthermore, enhanced by the *eldmodyr* appellation that Kempe is assigned in her later years, there appears to be a place for the post-reproductive, old woman in medieval society whereby her literal mothering shifts into a wise *grand*mother's didacticism and sagacious pastoral care. As Anneke B. Mulder-Bakker has noted, there exists no menopause in the animal world, nor in the male of the human species. Through a Darwinist lens, old women must therefore offer a second productive function.[40] Indeed, Sarah Blaffer-Hrdy has argued for 'the grandmother's clock hypothesis': that the human race has evolved into an intelligent species because of the grandmother's role in the raising of offspring. By gathering food or supporting the care of the young, the grandmother's labours mean that human infants can remain helpless for longer. For Blaffer-Hrdy 'the long postmenopausal stint is, in fact, an integral part of the human organism's *reproductive plan*'.[41] The *oma erecta* ('grandmother erecta') is not a figure of withering senescence, but one whose contribution to her community is both vital and life-affirming, and, as Mulder-Bakker shows, is also historically granted a spiritual function:[42]

[38] 'I suffer not a woman to teach, nor to use authority over the man: but to be in silence' (1 Timothy 2:12). There is debate over the authorship of I Timothy. See 'Introduction', in *The Blackwell Companion to The New Testament*, ed. David E. Aune (Malden, MA: Wiley-Blackwell, 2010), pp. 1–14.

[39] *Sickness of Women*, p. 486. MED s.v. marice: the uterus; moder; from the time of conception. Cf. Latin mater / matrix. Green notes that both 'mother' and 'matrice' would continue to be used to refer to the uterus well into the nineteenth century. *Sickness of Women*, p. 481, n. 69.

[40] Mulder-Bakker, *The Prime of Their Lives*, p. xii.

[41] Sarah Blaffer-Hrdy, *Mother Nature: Maternal Instincts and the Shaping of the Species* (London: Vintage, 2000), p. 285. See also Kirkwood and Shanley, 'The connections between general and reproductive senescence and the evolutionary basis of menopause'; and A. Friederike Kachel, L.S. Premo and Jean-Jacques Hublin, 'Grandmothering and natural selection revisited', *Proceedings: Biological Sciences*, 278 (2011), 1939–41.

[42] From Mulder-Bakker, p. xii.

Pre-conquest English society knew older matrons as the counterparts of the male priests. They were called *nonna*, after the Roman word for 'grandmother'. We discover here a spiritualised transformation of the biological grandmother. In later centuries the *nonna* evolved into the *nonna* we know, that is the nun in a cloister.[43]

This category of medieval women is termed by Mulder-Bakker as 'Wise Old Women': women who flourish in their senescence by teaching, writing, and authorising, in stark contrast to the denigratory constructions of the old woman that populate so many medieval medical and religious texts.[44] Such a woman, whose didactic potentiality resists the pejorative proscriptions of ancient thought might be considered, in Alastair Minnis's terms, as an *auctrice*.[45]

In *Le livre de l'advision Christine*, Christine de Pizan recognises in herself an ageing wisdom brought about, importantly, by existential retrospection:

> At the time when I had naturally arrived at an age that brings with it a certain degree of understanding, looking back at my past adventures and ahead to the end of things … I embarked on the path to which nature and the stars inclined me, that is, the love of learning.[46]

Likewise, the Dame de la Tour in Christine's *Le livre du duc des vrais amans* (1403–5) is not fully legitimised but, as Albrecht Classen concludes, 'Old age … proves to be instrumental in giving advice and suggesting directions to be taken by young people'.[47] Christine views ageing partly as an intellectual pursuit, characterised by the learning that she was able to undertake once she had become widowed, and by the sagacity born from extended life experience. More positive representations of woman in medieval texts are, according to Lucie Doležalová, found largely when an aspect of her entirety is modified: her sexuality, the extent of her agedness, or her individuality (i.e., she is employed simply as a symbol of something else); Doležalová cites the typology of 'saint grandmothers' who are never depicted as old.[48]

---

[43] Mulder-Bakker, 'The Age of Discretion', in *The Prime of Their Lives*, p. 24.

[44] Mulder-Bakker, *The Prime of Their Lives*, p. xiv.

[45] MED s.v. auctrice: A woman whose opinion is accepted as authoritative. See Alastair Minnis, 'The Wisdom of Old Women: Alisoun of Bath as *Auctrice*', in *Writings on Love in the English Middle Ages*, ed. Helen Cooney (New York: Palgrave Macmillan, 2006), pp. 99–114.

[46] From Renate Blumenfeld-Kosinski, 'The Compensations of Aging: Sexuality and Writing in Christine de Pizan, with an Epilogue on Colette', in *The Prime of Their Lives*, ed. Mulder-Bakker, pp. 2–16 (p. 11).

[47] 'Introduction', *Old Age in the Middle Ages and the Renaissance*, ed. Classen, pp. 1–84 (p. 24).

[48] Lucie Doležalová, '*Nemini vetula placet?* In search of the Positive Representation of Old Women in the Middle Ages', *Alterskulturen des Mittelalters und der frühen Neuzeit: internationaler Kongress, Krems an der Donau, 16. Bis 18. Oktober 2006*, ed. Elisabeth Vavra (Wien: Verlag der Österreichischen Akademie der Wissenschaften, 2008), pp. 175–82 (pp. 176–7).

However, the aged body brings a unique opportunity for atonement, as through somatic suffering the pious can draw closer to God in the aged asceticism of senescence and thus be liberated from the bodily mortifications that might have characterised their younger years. Bernard of Clairvaux asserted that 'the body helps the soul which loves God', emphasising the inherency of the body–soul dynamic in the medieval imaginary and interpreting ageing decline in eschatologically optimistic terms.[49] Authorities such as Bonaventure and Aquinas had regarded the body and soul as one being; the believed that pain of the body ignites disturbance of the soul and vice versa.[50] Trisha Olson notes that 'Rather than a prison that trapped the soul, the body was both integral to human identity and a conduit of religious experience. Thus in this period, the body in pain spoke to, reflected back, and shaped, the experience of pain in the soul.'[51] Kempe's old-body-in-pain, therefore, offers an opportunity for asceticism beyond any that she has hitherto experienced and thus represents the culmination of the pain-events of her life. Though she takes a different path from the conventional trajectory of the holy woman, straddling the earthly and the religious worlds in her humanity, she is now, more than ever, en route to spiritual satisfaction.[52] The medico-cultural prejudices against old women must nevertheless be persistently traversed, partly because she insists on remaining in that very world, and partly because those psychosomatic persecutions will be used as anamnestic fruit in the production of her life-text.

The Journey to Senescence

I wish to suggest that the accounts of Margery Kempe's overseas pilgrimages to northern Europe, dictated in 1438 when she is about sixty-five years old, vividly demonstrate the 'wise old woman' that Kempe has become and the reflective manner of the process of composition. For not only is the painful experience of travel amplified by her more infirm body, but the articulation of that pain to her scribal 'pain interpreter' (an issue that I discussed in the Introduction) is also underscored by a heightened verisimilitude that renders Book II tonally distinct from Book I. When Kempe's daughter-in-law sets out on her homeward voyage to Germany, Kempe is willing enough to accompany her as far as Ipswich; it is with a heavy heart, though, that she

---

[49] From Shahar, *Growing Old*, p. 54.
[50] See Trisha Olson, 'The Medieval Blood Sanction and the Divine Beneficance of Pain: 1100–1450', *Journal of Law and Religion*, 22 (2006/7), 63–129 (p. 83).
[51] Ibid., p. 128.
[52] Kempe follows in the footsteps of other holy women who also began their religious journey from the point of marriage and / or children, like Bridget of Sweden (c. 1303–1373), Marie of Oignes (1177–1213) and Elizabeth of Hungary (1207–31). See *Sancity and Motherhood: Essays on Holy Mothers in the Middle Ages*, ed. Anneke B. Mulder-Bakker (New York and London: Routledge, 2013).

acquiesces to God's command that she too should cross the sea. It is 1433, and Margery Kempe is sixty years old, described in the *Book* as 'a woman in gret age' (228). She has no leave from her confessor for travel to Germany; he was unconvinced that she should even journey to Ipswich due to her elderliness and an ongoing foot injury. He had objected that 'ʒe hirtyd but late ʒowr foote, & ʒe ar not ʒet al hool, & also ʒe arn an elde woman. ʒe may not gon' (226), relenting only after Kempe assured him that a young hermit would accompany her back to Lynn. Physical constraints and a lack of permission combine, then, to form Kempe's mental resistance to the command to travel that she feels in her heart. Moreover, she is 'not purueyd of gold ne of syluer sufficiently for to gon wyth as [she] awt to be' (227). Her economic situation in her widowhood is not fully clear; she is able to pay for a friar's chaperone services, but at other times requires the charity of others for clothing, food, and drink. Certainly, it is likely that whatever wealth she may have possessed was not wholly accessible to her in the required time frame; it is also possible that she chose to donate much of her inheritance in acts of charity.[53]

Female peregrination, whilst technically as permissible as male pilgrimage, was not only subject to the consent of Church and spouse but was also in some ways a transgression against the domestic sessility to which medieval women were bound. It is something that Terence Bowers has described as 'an offence against basic cultural axioms', reducing Kempe, he argues, to the status of a 'deviant, a threat to Christendom'.[54] Such deviance exposed women to ridicule; a woman on pilgrimage was removed from the 'male figures to whose authority she would normally defer', according to Niebrzydowski, which made female pilgrims 'easy targets for misogynistic satire'.[55] Cultural anxieties about female travel do indeed underlie Kempe's previous experience of travel; for example, when she went to Hessle she was branded a 'heretyk' and advised to 'forsake þis lyfe þat þu hast, & go spynne & carde as oþer women don' (129). Nonetheless, many women did undertake pilgrimage in the Middle Ages, often with different agendas from their male counterparts, as Susan Morrison has shown. She notes how 'the proportion of male to female pilgrims varied from shrine to shrine, often due to the type of miracle

---

[53] In Calais, a good woman provides her with a new smock and food (241). On her arrival in London, she is scarcely clad, 'for defawte of mony' (243). Although it is likely that Kempe would have inherited John's wealth (and the fact that her daughter-in-law stays with her for eighteen months indicates a retained family home for this to happen [225]), a husband was free to bequeath his property to anyone he chose. See Janet S. Loengard, '"Which may be said to be her own": Widows and Goods in Late-Medieval England', in *Medieval Domesticity*, ed. Kowaleski and Goldberg, pp. 162–76. Some widows were expected to transfer wealth and property to their sons during their lifetime. See Shahar, *Growing Old*, p. 140. Joel T. Rosenthal notes how widows as heads of households were, however, a fairly common phenomenon, in *Wife and Widow in Medieval England*, p. 43.
[54] Terence Bowers, 'Margery Kempe as Traveller', *Studies in Philology*, 97 (2000), 1–28, p. 3.
[55] Sue Niebrzydowski, 'The Middle-Aged Meanderings of Margery Kempe: Medieval Women and Pilgrimage', in *Medieval Life Cycles: Continuity and Change*, ed. Isabelle Cochelin and Karen Smyth (Turnhout: Brepols, 2013), pp. 265–85 (p. 269).

promised by the mythology of the saint worshipped there'. Furthermore, health and wellbeing were inherent aspects of female travel: 'gender-specific illnesses, mainly having to do with fertility and childbirth, are fundamental to understanding women's relationship to pilgrimage'.[56] Such health-giving motivations for female pilgrimage double the teleological benefits, since the journey itself and its devotional purpose are equally edifying.

Travel in itself posed a risk to health.[57] Some conditions would be exacerbated by movement and travel, and high-risk situations and mobility could make travellers susceptible to new infections and afflictions, including plague, famine, malnutrition, tuberculosis, and the sweating sickness.[58] Scientific explanations, both medieval and modern, help to uncover the inevitability of Kempe's suffering in her old-age peregrinations. Recent archaeological findings reveal that a large percentage of medieval women of menopausal age or beyond suffered from osteoporosis, a condition that, in fact, began to corrode the skeleton between the ages of thirty and forty.[59] Skeletal evidence shows high rates of osteoarthritis, which suggests that Kempe was likely to have had an orthopaedic, degenerative condition that would explain her broken foot and her struggle with walking. Medieval scientific texts indicate further conditions to which old women were prone. Retained menses after menopause were culturally understood as reasons not only for the corruption and 'poison' of old women, but also for their concomitant physical pain. *The Sickness of Women* describes the symptoms of retention as 'ache and dolour [suffering] with greuaunces and hevynessis from the navil dounward to their prevy membre and ache of their raynes [kidneys] and of their rige-bone [backbone] and of their forhede and of their necke and of their eyen [eyes]'.[60] Old-age dyscrasies are thus multifarious, and the 'greuaunces' are conflated specifically with *hevynesses*, a term that Kempe employs frequently to describe the burden and discomfort – no doubt both corporeal and psychological – of her final pilgrimage.[61]

[56] Susan S. Morrison, *Women Pilgrims in Late Medieval England: Private Piety as Public Performance* (London and New York: Routledge, 2000), p. 3 and pp. 128–41. See also Diana Webb, *Pilgrimage in Medieval England* (London and New York: Hambledon and London, 2000). On Kempe's domestic travel, see Mary C. Erler, 'Home Visits: Mary, Elizabeth, Margery Kempe and the feast of the Visitation', in *Medieval Domesticity*, ed. Kowaleski and Goldberg, pp. 259–76.

[57] See Brian Gushulak, 'Globalization, Migration, and Health: The History of Disease and Disparity in the Global Village', and Michel J. Deprez, 'The Pilgrimages of Christianity', in *Travel Medicine: Tales behind the Science*, ed. Annelies Wilder-Smith, Eli Schwarz, and Marc Shaw (Amsterdam and London: Elsevier, 2007), pp. 209–20 and pp. 263–7 respectively.

[58] See Youngs, *The Life Cycle in Western Europe*, pp. 26–7.

[59] See Classen, 'Introduction', in *Old Age in the Middle Ages and the Renaissance*, pp. 41–2.

[60] *Sickness of Women*, p. 487.

[61] For instance, Kempe feels 'heuy' en route to Aachen, as she is alone (236). She is in great despair and 'heuynes' when she temporarily loses the company of the poor friar on the way to Calais, feeling 'heuynes' again when she has no lodgings available for that night (240). She is 'sory & heuy' when she has no fellowship on her traverse to Canterbury (242).

Kempe's widowhood may have been perceived as putting her at risk of 'syncope' (*syncopen* – the weakening of the heart), a condition that *De secretis mulierum* considers common in women who suffer from uterine suffocation, itself more common in the widowed and chaste. The text further suggests that another term for 'syncope' is 'ecstasy' (*ecstasis*).[62] The symptoms of women suffering from suffocation are also described in the 'Book on the Conditions of Women', which states: 'Sometimes they suffer syncope, and the pulse vanishes so that from the same cause it is barely perceptible' ('Quandoque paciuntur sincopin, et ita pulsus euanescit quod penitus non sentitur ex eadum causa').[63] This strikingly connects the widow's pain with what might be interpreted to be ecstatic religious experience, perhaps conflating the faintings and collapsings of somatic suffering with those of spiritual rapture. Such medical texts, then, underscore the ontological interrelation of female pain and mystical experience perhaps most acutely at the elderly stage of life, when the pains of agedness and the biological contraindication of the state of widowhood might alter conscious processes and thus increase mystical perception.

* * *

Though Margery Kempe feels persistently 'comawndyd in hir hert' to travel overseas with her daughter-in-law, her concurrent reluctance stems from fear, brought about by her earlier, traumatic experiences of pilgrimage when great storms and tempests endangered her life: 'sche had ben in gret perell on þe see a-for-tyme & was in purpose neuyr to comyn þeron mor be hir owyn wille' (226).[64] Her pleas are nevertheless overruled by God's decree – 'I bydde þe gon in my name' (227) – and, despite the 'gret drede & heuynes' with which the prospect fills her, she accepts the mission. Her injured, elderly body and damaged foot must now endure the final, divinely decreed journey of her lifetime, a journey that will prove penitential to the highest degree. As an initially undesirable task, therefore, this final pilgrimage is characterised from its genesis by an agonised reluctance; reason, perhaps, for Rosalyn Voaden's suggestion that this journey is an aimless one, 'without clear purpose or destination'.[65] As an ultimate opportunity for epic edification, the northern European pilgrimage is a twofold test of endurance since Kempe must survive the arduous challenges faced by any pilgrim while at an advanced age, with a body 'diseased-by-default' and a psyche wracked with anxiety.

That anxiety is validated when the voyage is beset with 'swech stormys & tempestys þat þei wendyn alle to a ben perischyd' (229). The perilous condi-

---

[62] *De secretis mulierum*, trans. Lemay, p. 132. Albertus Magnus, *De secretis mulierum*, pp. 111–13.

[63] 'The Book on the Conditions of Women', in *The Trotula*, pp. 82–5.

[64] The voyage home from Rome, for example, is beset by 'gret tempestys and & dyrke wedyr' (102). On the dangers of sea travel see Rosalyn Voaden, 'Travels with Margery: Pilgrimage in Context', in *Eastward Bound: Travel and Travellers, 1050–1550*, ed. Rosamund Allen (Manchester: Manchester University Press, 2004), pp. 177–95.

[65] Voaden, 'Travels with Margery', in *Eastwood Bound*, ed. Allen, p. 188.

tions are so extreme that captaincy over the ship is relinquished, its fate and trajectory transferred into God's hands. The violence of the ordeal triggers in Kempe a rare crisis of faith as her elderly vulnerability and desperation manifest in an oppositionally strong prayer of divine challenge:

> A, Lord, for þi lofe cam I hedyr, & þu hast oftyn-tyme behite me þat I schulde neuyr perischyn neiþyr on londe ne in watyr ne wyth no tempest. Þe pepil hath many tyme bannyd me, cursyd me, & warijd [cursed] me for þe grace þat þu hast wrowt in me, desiryng þat I schulde deyin in myschef & gret disese, & now, Lord, it is lyke þat her banning comyth to effect, & I, vnworthy wretche, am deceyuyd and defrawdyd of þe promys þat þu hast mad many tyme on-to me, whech haue euyr trostyd in þi mercy & þi goodnesse, lesse þan þu þe sonar wythdrawe þes tempestys & schewe us mercy. Now may myn enmyis enyoyin [rejoice], & I may sorwyn yf þei haue her intent & I be deceyuyd (229).

In mortal peril once again, Kempe reverts to her worldly fear of the exclusion, spite, and curses to which she has been frequently subjected, now afraid that her enemies' desire 'þat I schulde deyin in myschef & gret disese' will in fact come to pass. Fragile and aged, in her infantile panic she angrily accuses God of fraudulence and deceit, demonstrating what Diane Watt sees as the 'spiritual entropy' of her tested faith.[66] Though she receives Godly reassurance, it is the appearance of the Virgin Mary – bearing the authoritative wisdom of a mother – that rings 'trewe' to Kempe, and sees her safely delivered to the coast of Norway, vulnerable and shaken.

In a striking, temporal juxtaposition of danger and salvation, Kempe symbolically arrives in Norway on Good Friday. Just as her brush with death and mortal isolation on the ship, in *imitatio Christi*, concludes on the Christian feast day of the Crucifixion, so she is redeemed and reintegrated back into the body of the Church on Easter Day, when, on land, she witnesses the raising of the cross and experiences an intense meditation. Through the liturgical exultation of the Resurrection, Kempe is reminded of the analgesia of Christ's Passion, her faith renewed in the promise of eschatological safety. It is therefore fitting that the episode closes with the kindness of the master of the ship, 'as sche had ben hys modyr' (231). He provides her with clothes from his own possession, realising that she is at risk of hypothermia. This act of charity stands as an affirmation both of God's renewed promise and of Kempe's aged distinction, for in assuming the role of a surrogate son the master acknowledges her mature status and ascetic merit as an elderly pilgrim. Indeed, such marks of respect were established by her daughter-in-law prior to their departure from Ipswich, when she planned her trip 'thorw hir eldmodrys consentyng' (225). Now transformed into an authoritative

---

[66] Diane Watt, 'Faith in the Landscape: Overseas Pilgrimages in *The Book of Margery Kempe*', in *A Place to Believe in: Locating Medieval Landscapes*, ed. Clare A. Lees and Gillian R. Overing (University Park: Pennsylvania State University Press, 2006), pp. 170–87 (p. 186).

widow and resolute pilgrim, Kempe's role as sagacious matriarch validates her senescent journey.

The limitations of her aged body are again tested when, after she has secured a guide to accompany her from Stralsund to Wilsnack, his fears of war and robbery increase and they are exposed to 'many perellys' (233).[67] Though she receives divine acroamatic reassurance, her affective response and boisterous sobbing causes the 'yrk[ar]' of the man, and he increases his walking pace so as to avoid her company, going 'so fast þat sche myth not folwyn wyth-owtyn gret labowr & gret *disese*' (233–4).[68] His impatience causes her great corporeal strain, the pressure to keep up creating a twofold infirmity where agedness and injury collide:

> þei passyd forth to-Wilsnak-ward wyth gret labowr. Sche myth not enduryn so gret jurneys as þe man myth, & he had no compassion of hir ne not wolde a-bydyn for hir. And þerfor sche labowryd as long as sche myth tyl þat sche *fel in sekenes* and myth no ferþer. It was gret merueyl & *myracle* þat a woman dys-ewsyd of goyng & also a-bowtyn iij scor 3er of age xuld enduryn cotidianly to kepyn hir jurney & hir pase wyth a man fryke & lusty to gon (234).

The extent of her 'sekenes' is such that a wain is ordered for her subsequent travel to the shrine of the Blood of Wilsnack, a passage that causes her 'gret penawns & gret disese' (234). That Kempe conflates *disese* with penance is indicative of the ascetic task that this travail presents, amplifying both the pain of every attritional step and her stoic endurance.[69] Indeed, the feat is described as nothing short of miraculous, a narrative subtext which clearly seeks to position the northern European expedition as a penitential endeavour of saintly proportion.[70] The *labowr* of her progress from Aachen to Calais is similarly reiterated; as her somatic failure increases she determinedly attempts to keep up with the party, yet finds herself lagging behind, 'to agyd & to

[67] Kempe informs us that 'þer was opyn werr be-twix þe Englisch & þo cuntreys' (233). As Diane Watt has exemplified, these are references to the Polish invasion of the Duchy of Pomerania, and to conflicts between England and the Teutonic Order and Hanseatic cities. Kempe's journey dissected these countries. See Watt, 'Faith in the Landscape', in *A Place to Believe in*, ed. Lees and Overing, p. 184.

[68] Whilst Kempe continues to 'sobbyn' and 'wepyn' (233) in ardent response to mystical conversation, she is not described as emitting loud 'cries' in Book II, as these were noted to cease at around the age of menopause. See *BMK*, p. 345, n. 233/34.

[69] MED s.v. disease: 1(b) that which inflicts hardship, misery or misfortune; grievance, harm, injury, wrong. MED s.v. penaunce: 5(a) Pain, suffering; affliction, hardship.

[70] There are several mentions of Kempe's apparent miracles in the *Book*. When she is hit by a piece of wood in St Margaret's Church in Lynn, she recovers immediately, described by God as 'a gret myracle' (22). In Chapter 67, her prayers avert a fire in the same local church, described as a 'myrakyl & specyal grace' (163). That these 'miracles' occur in her own parish church indicates a desire on the part of her scribe to establish Kempe as a beatified, local figure. On saint making, see Katherine Lewis, 'Margery Kempe and Saint Making in Later Medieval England', in *A Companion to The Book of Margery Kempe*, ed. Arnold and Lewis; and Diane Watt, *Medieval Women's Writing: Works by and for Women, 1100–1500* (Cambridge: Polity, 2007), pp. 116–35.

weyke to holdyn foot wyth hem. Sche ran & lept as fast as sche myth tyl hir myghtys failyd' (239). Kempe and the poor friar whose companionship she had purchased to secure her safety are forced to procure another wain in order that her pained and fatigued body might rest. But the respite is short-lived. Her misplaced trust in a 'worschepful woman' from London who rejects her, stating that she 'wyl not medelyn wyth þe', results in the loss of their transport, so Kempe and the friar must proceed on foot once again (240). Dissolving into 'gret diswer & heuynes', Margery Kempe is reduced to her lowest condition since her departure from England, memorialised with honest reflection. The asceticism of the travail is made extreme by the rugged terrain: they went 'wery weys & greuows in dep sondys [sands], hillys, & valleys tweyn days er þei comyn þedyr, suffering gret thrist & gret penawns, for þer wer fewe townys be þe wey þat þei went & ful febyl herberwe [lodgings]' (241). At pains to recall and communicate the penitential aspect of the journey – the thirst, the laborious hills, and the two days of survival in the outdoor elements – Kempe inscribes her anamnestic pain in her elderly, exposed body.

Nowhere, however, is there a more evocative and tormenting episode than that in Chapter 6 of Book II, when Kempe is compelled to join a party of poor folk en route to Aachen whose infestation with lice necessitates a systematic stripping and picking that causes Kempe not only intense humiliation, but also a distressing scourge of her own:

> Whan þei wer wyth-owtyn þe townys, hir felaschep dedyn of her clothys, &, sittyng nakyd, pykyd hem [the lice]. Nede compellyd hir to abydyn hem & prolongyn hir jurne & ben at meche mor cost þan sche xulde ellys a ben. Thys creatur was a-bauyd [afraid] to putte of hir cloþis as hyr felawys dedyn, & þerfor sche thorw hir comownyng had part of her vermyn & was betyn & stongyn ful euyl boþe day & nyght tyl God sent hir oþer felaschep. Sche kept forth hir felaschep wyth gret angwisch & disese & meche lettyng vn-to þe tyme þat þei comyn to Akun (237).

Faced with a choice between naked humiliation or the painful bites and stings of multitudinous lice, Kempe opts for physical pain over fleshly exposure; a testament to her ascetic ability to sustain discomfort, this sits paradoxically with her *in*ability to manage terror, as on the voyage to Norway.[71] Diane Watt views this episode as Kempe 'on the verge of being reduced to little more than an animal', and certainly the image of this elderly pilgrim on

---

[71] Margery Kempe's fear of rape and defilement as a threat to her spiritual health is a common thread throughout the later travels, when she appears to feel more vulnerable to attack. On the way to Aachen she encounters priests who insult her and show 'vn-clenly' behaviour, making her have 'drede for hir chastite' (236). On the road to Calais she is 'euyr a-ferd to a be rauishcyd er defilyd' (241). Some thirteenth-century theorists debated whether it was more sinful to fornicate with a beautiful young woman or an ugly old hag, 'on the basis of the pleasure quota', thus Kempe's fears may be justified. See Dyan Eliott, *Spiritual Marriage*, p. 136. See also Lois W. Banner, *In Full Flower: Aging Women, Power and Sexuality: A History* (New York: Alfred A. Knopf, 1992), pp. 164–384.

the margins of a group of delousing *homo sapiens* emphasises the elemental nature of the ordeal.[72] But moreover, her elected endurance of this *angwisch* and *disese* also evidences an acceptance of the implicit sacrificial asceticism of the journey, a faith in the eventual cure of the pestilence, and an empowered self-exclusion from the group that sets her more fixedly on her beatified path. This path, however, becomes so intensely arduous that she feels she will die: 'Sche was so wery & so ouyrcomyn wyth labowr to-Caleysward þat hir thowt hir spiryt xulde a departyd fro hir body as sche went in þe wey' (241). On the brink of annihilation, Margery Kempe is overcome with physical exhaustion and pain, her spirit wavering liminally somewhere between life and death. In this expedition it is, in Niebrzydowski's view, 'the going and her *spiritual response* to being there rather than the *seeing* that matters'.[73] While Kempe is indeed less concerned with the meticulous notation of places and visits during this later pilgrimage, and more with the spiritual sanctification of experiencing the holy sites, the ascetic, painful physicality of that very 'going' also facilitates the salvific conquering of her fragile flesh. This overcoming, this triumph over her very humanity, marks potent growth in her 'knowing' and the flowering of her elderly authority.

A Knowing Elder

It is no surprise that Book II opens with the story of Margery Kempe's conversion of her son, as we have seen, given that this section of the text is undoubtedly underpinned by an insistence upon Kempe's holy authority, if it is not a deliberate autohagiography. Yet while some responses to the *Book* have regarded Kempe's increased authority, particularly from her middle age, as predicated on a certain disembodiment, facilitating the elevation of her incarnated female flesh, I do not think that spiritual authority and feminine embodiment need necessarily be separated. As I have suggested, the distinct tonal immediacy of Book II and its anamnestic verisimilitude provide a direct-ness, a kind of dialogic 'hotline' to Kempe: rather than giving a contrived and sanctifying account of her travels, Book II instead foregrounds a highly audible *voice* which seizes the opportunity, in old age, to 'speke' of what she has achieved. Wynkyn de Worde's 1501 redaction of the *Book* is regarded by Rosalyn Voaden as edited to eliminate the woman herself, who thus becomes simultaneously invisible yet unambiguously holy in status. The 'revilement discourse' of the *Book* is removed, Voaden suggests, leaving a 'sanitized' version – a useful devotional text harnessed again by Henry Pepwell in 1521.[74] Liz

---

[72] Watt, 'Faith in the Landscape', in *A Place to Believe in*, ed. Lees and Overing, p. 185.
[73] Niebrzydowski, 'The Middle-Aged Meanderings of Margery Kempe', in *Medieval Life Cycles*, ed. Cochelin and Smyth, p. 281.
[74] Rosalynn Voaden, *God's Words, Women's Voices: The Discernment of Spirits in the Writing of Late-Medieval Women Visionaries* (York: York Medieval Press, 1999), pp. 147–54.

Herbert McAvoy has argued for Kempe's 'ageing "bodylessness"', while Barry Windeatt sees the *Book* as a 'life', and a 'stream-of-consciousness narrative' of recollected prayers.[75] Alastair Minnis similarly argues that Kempe 'makes a considerable show of staying within [the limits]'.[76] But Kempe's actively embodied form of didacticism is apparent from the opening of Book II, which establishes the clear caveat that the priest-scribe has written the *Secundus liber* 'aftyr hyr owyn tunge' (221). The tongue, in medieval thought, is inherently connected to the voice by providing its shape: 'A voys is þynnest ayer [air] ismyte [to taste] and schape wiþ wreste of þe tonge'.[77] Indeed, Bartholomaeus Anglicus attaches moral qualities to the human voice which cohere with its tone: one which is 'To heuy or to scharpe is euel and iblamed', while a 'swete voys and ordynat gladeþ and stirieþ to loue, and schewiþ out þe passiouns of þe soule, and witness þe strengþe and vertue of spiritualle members, and schewiþ purenesse and goodnesse of good disposicioun þereof'.[78] The tongue and the voice, then, are themselves the physiological tools of spiritual exhortation, and this, I therefore suggest, is the reason for the persistent emphasis on Kempe's edifying *speaking* and *doing* in Book II.

The son's salvation is engendered by his mother's fecund words. She 'cownselyd hym to leeuyn þe worlde'; she then, 'meuyd wyth scharpnes of spiryt, seyde' that God would punish him; she 'spake to hym a-geyn'; she spoke 'wyth scharp wordys of correpcyon' after he asked for her forgiveness; and finally she 'askyd' God 'for ȝeuenes of hys synne' (221–3). The value placed on his mother's words is reiterated in the next chapter when the son seeks her advice, asking if she 'wolde cownselyn hym' about whether to travel to England by land or sea, for he now 'trustyd meche in hys moderys cownsel', and was 'certifijd of hys moderys cownsel' (224). However, the theological milieu of the Middle Ages promoted the Pauline tenet that forbade women from teaching or preaching: 'I suffer not a woman to teach'.[79] This restriction on female religious teaching reverberated throughout late medieval culture, through the theological writings of Thomas Aquinas (c. 1225–1274) and Henry of Ghent (1217–93), and in the *Ancrene Wisse*, which stipulates that 'Ne preachi ȝe to na mon' (You should not preach to anyone).[80] Aquinas ques-

[75] Liz Herbert McAvoy, "[A] péler of holy cherch", in *The Prime of Their Lives*, ed. Mulder-Bakker, p. 19. Barry Windeatt, '"I Use but Comownycacyon and Good Wordys": Teaching and *The Book of Margery Kempe*', in *Approaching Medieval English Anchoritic and Mystical Texts*, ed. Dee Dyas, Valerie Edden, and Roger Ellis (Cambridge: D.S. Brewer, 2005), pp. 115–28 (p. 125).

[76] Alastair Minnis, 'Religious Roles: Public and Private', in *Medieval Holy Women in the Christian Tradition c. 1100–c. 1500*, ed. Alastair Minnis and Rosalynn Voaden (Turnhout: Brepols, 2010), pp. 47–82 (p. 58).

[77] *On the Properties of Things*, p. 211.

[78] Ibid., p. 213. MED s.v. air: (form: aer(e)). MED s.v. ismecchen (form: ismeiht): 1. To taste.

[79] 1 Timothy 2:12.

[80] *Ancrene Wisse*, ed. Millett, part 2, section 18, p. 29. Translation from *Ancrene Wisse: A Translation*, ed. Millett, p. 29.

tioned explicitly whether the grace of speech, wisdom, and knowledge pertains to women.[81] Restrictions on female preaching increased during the thirteenth century, after the Second Lateran Council (1139), when ecclesiastical ordination was narrowed in concept and the privileges of women were reduced.[82] While Hildegard of Bingen (1098–1179) was able to conduct several public preaching tours, by the time of Kempe's life female didacticism in the public sphere was prohibited. The wide readership of such sources testifies to the broad dissemination of anti-feminist discourse on the illegitimacy of women's public oration.[83] Windeatt sees Kempe as being more concerned, in fact, with learning than teaching, dictating her 'inward contemplative communing' more truthfully in the *Book* than she could have done in real life, since voicing such mystical dialogue in public might open her to further accusations of heresy.[84] Voaden, however, regards Margery Kempe's English travels in particular as 'a preaching tour that she believed to be divinely commanded', her white clothes making a bold hermeneutic statement of divine injunction. This preaching tour is, nonetheless, an 'underground' one which sees Kempe mounting 'an unofficial and invisible pulpit', justifying her exhortations through the tradition of preaching *ex beneficio* as opposed to *ex ordinatio*.[85]

The *Book* takes pains to elucidate Kempe's spiritual sagacity and counsel whilst at the same time remaining within the rigid boundaries of religio-cultural ideology: she may assertively 'speke', and 'shew' her spiritual *knowing*, but to step outside the vocal limits would be a dangerous heterodoxical move, as she has experienced before. She is thus described as 'schewyng hym [her son] & enformyng how owr Lord had drawyn hir thorw hys mercy & by what menys' (224), a process of 'shewing' that not only resonates with the *Showings* of Kempe's own spiritual advisor, Julian of Norwich, but also has connotations both of manifesting or showing, and of envisioning through revelation.[86] Kempe's somatic decline in old age is thus resoundingly counteracted with the recording of her *speaking*, *showing*, and *doing* in Book II; this is an account of active, measured, and demonstrative humanity fuelled with kinetic force, as opposed to the passive travelogue or hagiographic narrative it is sometimes

---

[81] Thomas Aquinas, *Summa theologiae* 2a2ae.177.2.

[82] Alastair Minnis, 'Religious Roles: Public and Private', in *Medieval Holy Women in the Christian Tradition*, ed. Minnis and Voaden, pp. 51–2.

[83] See McAvoy, "[A] péler of holy church", in *The Prime of Their Lives*, ed. Mulder-Bakker. See also Voaden, *God's Words, Women's Voices*; Theresa Tinkle, 'Contested Authority: Jerome and the Wife of Bath on 1 Timothy: 2', *The Chaucer Review*, 44 (2010), 268–93; and Warren S. Smith, 'The Wife of Bath and Dorigen debate Jerome', in *Satiric Advice on Women and Marriage: From Plautus to Chaucer*, ed. Warren S. Smith (Ann Arbour: University of Michigan Press, 2005), pp. 243–69.

[84] Barry Windeatt, 'I Use but Comownycacyon and Good Wordys', in *Approaching Medieval English Anchoritic and Mystical Texts*, ed. Dyas et al., pp. 115–28 (p. 126).

[85] Rosalynn Voaden, 'Wolf in Sheep's Clothing: Margery Kempe as Underground Preacher', in *Romance and Rhetoric: Essays in Honour of Dhira B. Mahoney*, ed. Georgiana Donavin and Anita Obermeier (Turnhout: Brepols, 2010), pp. 109–21.

[86] MED s.v. sheuing(e: 1(a) A manifestation; showing something. 2(a) A revelation, vision.

proposed as. Kempe is not removed from the narrative in authorial invisibility, but is, I argue, made an *audible* and visible 'auctrice' by the aged body whose very corporeality lies at the heart of her final validation.[87]

Old age, in fact, provides a physiological advantage for both contemplation and exhortation. Though there are many afflictions that accompany older age, medical texts also understand the aged body as dry, cool, and thus less superfluous. This is encapsulated by *The Knowing of Woman's Kind in Childing*, which posits that older women do not menstruate 'be-cause they be so dryed þat þe hote of þe blode is distroyde þat no *superhabundant humvre* may ryse in hem ne passe'.[88] The benefit of reduced superfluity is multiplied in religious women whose devotional activity creates somatic equilibrium where bodily matter is digested and utilised without waste or excess; in discussing women who do not menstruate, the text draws particular attention to 'tho þat syngvn & wake mekyll, as do þes religios, for of her wakynge & travelynge in syngynge her blode wastyth [diminishes] & defyet [digests] well here repast'.[89] The term 'travelynge' denotes hard physical labour or toil, especially in relation to a burden assumed for spiritual purposes.[90] Religious exertion thus uses up superfluous waste in the body, rendering older devout women's corporeal systems doubly efficient. The adaptation of the female body to its drier, aged biology, its cooling, drying, and pious exertion, illustrates an advanced stage of somatic maturation; the absence of waste and excess in senescence in fact emulates the idealised construction of the 'sealed up' Virgin Mary, whose untainted female flesh and silent composure are themselves imitated by fasting holy women who seek to curtail their own digestive leakage and menstruation.[91] Margery Kempe's measured ministry – like that of those other holy women, Bridget of Sweden and Catherine of Siena, who travel and offer spiritual counsel in their senescence – is perhaps then received with more acceptance because of the cultural understanding of medical ideas.[92] The 'flux' of crying and wailing with which she has been hitherto associated is transformed into a gentler weeping in her older years, as she transitions to the role of holy old woman whose voice might be empowered. Indeed, the *Ancrene Wisse* even sets such women apart: 'Na wepmon ne chastie ȝe, ne edwiten him his unþeaw bute he beo þe ouer-cuðre. *Halie alde* ancres hit mahe don summes weis, ah hit nis nawt siker þing, ne ne limpeð nawt to ȝunge' ('You should not rebuke any

---

[87] Thomas Hoccleve viewed the Wife of Bath as *auctrice*. See Alastair Minnis, 'The Wisdom of Old Women', in *Writings on Love in the English Middle Ages*, ed. Cooney, p. 100.

[88] My emphasis. *The Knowing of Woman's Kind in Childing*, p. 48.

[89] Ibid.

[90] MED s.v: 'travel(e).

[91] On female fasting and the 'sealed' female body see Caroline Walker Bynum, *Holy Feast and Holy Fast*, pp. 189–208.

[92] See for example, Bridget Morris, *St Birgitta of Sweden*; Rosalyn Voaden, *God's Words, Women's Voices*, pp. 73–108; and Beverly Mayne Kienzle, 'Catherine of Siena, Preaching, and Hagiography in Renaissance Tuscany', in *A Companion to Catherine of Siena*, ed. Carolyn Muessig, George Ferzoco, and Beverly Kienzle (Leiden: Brill, 2011), pp. 127–54.

man, or reproach him for his sin, unless he is over-familiar. *Holy old* anchoresses may to some extent, but it not a safe thing to do, and is not appropriate for the young').[93]

Furthermore, the question of prophecy and visionary experience, or 'spiritual gifts', posed some difficulties for the medieval Church and its stance on female preaching. As Alcuin Blamires has shown, spiritual gifts or talents (*gratia*) *should*, according to Aquinas and Henry of Ghent, be disseminated to others as part of a wider responsibility and recognition of that special grace embedded in the doctrine of 1 Peter 4:10.[94] Those select few who were empowered as 'prophetesses' were considered privileged ('electae et privilegiatae'), evidencing a theological disconnect between the prohibition of female preaching and the doctrinal imperative to share, and show, one's spiritual gifts.[95] Julian of Norwich explicitly states her divine obligation to speak of God: 'Botte for I am a woman shulde I therefore leve that I shoulde nought telle yowe the goodenes of God, sine that I sawe in that same time that it is his wille that it be knawen?'[96] But Julian is clear that she does not teach, but rather transmits her spiritual gifts according to *divine* will. Such precise delineations of holy women's freedom explains many of the indignant oppositions to Kempe's post-conversion exhortations. But the frequent interrogations with which she is beset over the course of the *Book* nearly always result in a recognition of her spiritual giftedness. During her interrogation by the Archbishop of York, her edifying tale is cause for the clerk to ask for her forgiveness and for her 'specyaly to prey for hym'. The archbishop himself ends the exchange with a request for 'hir to preye for hym' (128). The priest-scribe who, for a time, denounces her, realises her gift and 'louyd hir mor & trustyd mor to hir wepyng & hir crying þan euyr he dede be-forn' (152). And when Kempe is arrested for heresy and locked in an upper room of a house in Beverly, she leans from the upstairs window 'tellyng many good talys to hem þat wolde heryn hir'. The women, listening, 'wept sor & seyde wyth gret heuynes of her hertys, "Alas, woman, why xalt þu be brent?"' (130–1). The women who had doubted her are now affectively stirred, weeping and sighing at the fruits of Kempe's soul-sharing.[97] As she ages, and traverses into the events of Book II, the reduced superfluity of her senescent body and its cooling

[93] My emphasis. *Ancrene Wisse*, ed. Millett, part 2, section 18, p. 29. Translation from *Ancrene Wisse: A Translation*, ed. Millett, p. 29.

[94] 'As every man hath received grace, ministering the same one to another: as good stewards of the manifold grace of God'. See Blamires, 'Women and Preaching in Medieval Orthodoxy, Heresy and Saints' Lives', *Viator*, 26 (1995), pp. 140–1.

[95] Ibid., p. 148. Blamires paraphrases the thirteenth-century Franciscan Eustace of Arras's *Utrum mulier praedicando et docendo mereatur aureolam*.

[96] *The Writings of Julian of Norwich*, ed. Watson and Jenkins, p. 75.

[97] McAvoy nevertheless sees the physical location of Kempe at the window as evoking a 'preacher in the pulpit', which 'firmly regenders both orthodox preaching practices and the location of those practices'. McAvoy, "[A] péler", in *The Prime of Their Lives*, ed. Mulder-Bakker, p. 32.

and drying enhance her existing melancholic receptivity, authorising her by physiological, and holy, advantage.

Margery Kempe's journey towards *knowing* God and *knowing* pain, as a quasi Elder in the Church of the world, is born from the *experientia* that is regarded by Anneke Mulder-Bakker as a central source of learning for the illiterate woman; this is the acquired wisdom of *sapientia* and not *scientia* (the scholarly knowledge of books).[98] Kempe's transition into old age thus utilises the wisdom that she has internalised over many years of listening and living, a semi-literacy learned from practical experience and from the reading-aloud of books by her priests or confessors, which also usefully educate her in the hegemonic structures of misogynist ideology.[99] En route to Aachen, aged sixty or sixty-one, she visits a church of friars, where she witnesses the Sacrament, exposed in its crystal for the Octave of Corpus Christi (crystals being themselves imbued with esoteric properties of vision and female fecundity).[100] Her affective response and weeping anger the monk and chapmen, who consider her a hypocrite. Her retort, however, takes an erudite tone that is more aligned with learned clerks than with the unruly old woman such clerks would have her be. She justifies her tears with Latin scripture – 'Qui seminant in lacrimis' (They that sow in tears) and 'euntes ibant & flebant' (Going, they went and wept) – and when the men attempt to eject her from their company, she continues her persuasions in a measured tone, 'mekely & benyngly' (235–6).[101] Though her words do not prevent her eventual elimination from the group, they are emblematic of her memorial understanding of scripture and the Psalter, the Latin quotation

[98] Anneke Mulder-Bakker argues that female knowledge in the Middle Ages was gained by imitation and listening and that this knowledge was practical wisdom, preserved in the heart. Women were not supposed to offer out their knowledge without prior invitation. See 'The Metamorphosis of Woman: Transmission of Knowledge and the Problems of Gender', *Gender and History*, 12 (2000), 642–64 (p. 644). See also Brad Herzog, 'Portrait of a Holy Life: Mnemonic Inventiveness in *The Book of Margery Kempe*', in *Reading Memory and Identity in the Texts of Medieval European Holy Women*, ed. Margaret Cotter-Lynch and Brad Herzog (New York: Palgrave Macmillan, 2012), pp. 211–33.

[99] On the interplay between orality and literacy, see Diana R. Uhlman, 'The Comfort of Voice, the Solace of Script: Orality and Literacy in *The Book of Margery Kempe*, *Studies in Philology*, 91 (1994), 50–69.

[100] Roger Bacon's treatise on optics states that 'the crystalline humour is called the 'pupil'; and the visual power is located in it as subject' [Et humor cristallinus vocatur pupilla. Et in ae est virtus visiva sicut in subiecto]. From *Roger Bacon and the Origins of Perspectiva in the Middle Ages: A Critical Edition and Translation of Bacon's 'Perspectiva', with Introduction and Notes*, ed. David C. Lindberg (Oxford: Clarendon Press, 1996), cap. 3, pp. 31–2. Bartholomaeus Anglicus describes the instrument of the eye as the 'humour cristallin', which is 'clere and round, þat by þe clernes þerof þe eyȝe may byschine þe spirit and aier withoute'. He also describes the stone of 'cristalle' as a useful remedy for failed breastmilk: 'if it is ybete to poudre and dronke wiþ hony, it filleþ brestes and pappes fulle of melk if þe mylk faileþ byforehand bycause of colde'. *On the Properties of Things*, p. 108 and pp. 841–2.

[101] Psalms 125:5–6.

symbolic of her embarkation into the world of patriarchal scholasticism and her concomitant disruption of its guarded ownership.

Her spiritual maturity is further illustrated by her response to John, the guide who forsook her:

> Iohn, ȝe forsakyn me for non oþer cawse but for I wepe whan I se þe Sacrament & whan I thynke on owr Lordys Passyon. And, sithyn, I am forsakyn for Goddys cawse, I be-leue þat God xal ordeyn for me & bryngyn me forth as he wole hym-selfe, for he deceyuyd me neuyr, blissyd mote he be' (236).

The simple and understated explanation for her rejection by John – that he in fact forsook her for God – renders him illogical and over-reactive. In insisting on the presence of tears as signifiers of divine grace, and on their being a spiritual gift reflecting a privileged discernment of Christ's Passion, Kempe overturns the confrontational dynamic with her own elderly domination, replacing her earthly guide with God himself, who will instead 'bryngyn [her] forth'. The mystery of her compact with God thus forges a cognitive gulf between herself and her male onlookers, as she approaches a zenith in her assurance of divine providence. Her clerical companions might have the power to literally remove her from their retinue, but they are powerless to prevent this aged holy woman from stepping tenaciously into the realm of learned hegemony, or from directing their own sanctified discourse back at them in defiant acuity.[102]

Returning to London in 1434 Kempe is criticised once again in an episode that I have termed *Pike Gate*, gesturing towards the black humour of this poignant juxtaposition of pettiness and revilement. At a 'gret fest' her dinner companions, unaware of her identity, mockingly tell of an infamous woman from Lynn who hypocritically refuses to eat 'reed herring' and will instead eat only 'good pike'; Kempe recognises herself as the misrepresented subject (244).[103] By this time the tale has become proverbial, evidencing a regional mythology determined to construct her as a figure of unstable reliability, of 'womanish' indecision, through people's 'fals tunges': the very antithesis of her own speech as a tool for 'good wordys' (126). Responding now as an old woman, home from the travails of pilgrimage and secure in her faith in God's protection, she speaks with a spirit of measured authority, addressing her indicters with a tone of didactic chiding in which her matriarchal voice sounds clearly: 'ȝe awt to seyn no wers þan ȝe knowyn & ȝet not so euyl as ȝe knowyn' (244). Her instruction is heeded as the feasters are rebuked, 'desiryng thorw þe spirit of charite *her correccyon*' (245). Such a willing acceptance of

---

[102] Anne Clark Bartlett sees Kempe's 'incomplete literacy' as disrupting the antifeminist textual tradition as it 'garbles the message, and robs it of its authoritative status', terming such activity as 'strategic ignorance'. See Bartlett, *Male Authors, Female Readers: Representation and Subjectivity in Middle English Devotional Literature* (New York: Cornell University Press, 1995), pp. 19–23 (p. 23).

[103] See David Wallace's discussion of the London residency in *Strong Women*, pp. 122–8.

Kempe's didacticism by the guests underlines what they must perceive, now that they meet her in person, to be her aged wisdom; they recognise a deep faith born through the diachronic journey of suffering and spiritual education. No doubt encouraged by her exhortational efficacy, Kempe then goes about London speaking out boldly against sinners, her 'tunge' a vehicle for the spiritual profit of her quasi-parishioners:

> Sche spak boldly & mytily wher-so sche cam in London a-geyn swerars, bannars, lyars & swech oþer viciows pepil, a-geyn þe pompows aray boþin of men & of women. Sche sparyd hem not, sche flateryd hem not, neiþyr for her ʒiftys, ne for her mete, n[e] for her drynke. Hir spekyng profityd rith mech in many personys (245).

In kinaesthetic animation, she continues to *speak, do,* and *show* what she knows. Rather than being the passive narrative of a hagiographic travelogue, then, as Book II draws to its end Margery Kempe's emotive voice rings out louder, truer, and more certain. As an Elder of the universal Church she disseminates her chastisements throughout London as part of the Seven Spiritual Works of Mercy, focusing particularly on the sins occasioned by people's abuse of language: their swearing, cursing, and lying.[104] Refusing to moderate her words, she speaks plainly ('sche flateryd hem not'), an outspokenness won from her hard-earned experience and which dismantles the powerful words of slander that have frequently and painfully blighted her social interactions. No longer interested in the worldly frippery of 'ʒiftys, ne for her mete, n[e] for her drynke', she is unrelenting, the narrative listing of actions intoned with a speed indicative of her rapid dictation, her animated recall. Now she subverts the destructive language of slander with words of fruitful instruction – 'Hir speking profityd rith mech in many personys' – as she is herself metamorphosed from old ascetic pilgrim to Margery Kempe, the knowing Elder.

Yet Kempe's characteristic emotions continue to burst out humanely and inconveniently, further demonstrating that Book II is not the sanitised hagiography that is often suggested. Her efficacious ministry increases God's pleasure in her works and she is mystically told that she will enjoy 'hauyng joy & blysse wyth-owtyn ende', a blessing that revives her sobbing and weeping (for which she suffers further reproof), much to the irritation of the 'curatys & preistys of þe chirchis in London' (245). As a result 'Þei wold not suffyr hir to abydyn in her chirchys' (245), a denial of access that demonstrates continued ecclesiastical wariness of her womanly excess. But while her battle with the churchmen perpetuates, the common folk relate to her affective humanity, instinctively

---

[104] These are: teaching, counselling, chastising, comforting, suffering patiently, forgiving, and praying for enemies. Mary Beth L. Davis notes how Kempe suffers considerably for her chastisements. See '"Spekyn for Goddys Cawse": Margery Kempe and the Seven Spiritual Works of Mercy', in *The Man of Many Devices who Wandered Full Many Ways ... Festschrift in Honor of János M. Bak*, ed. Balázs Nagy and Marcell Sebök (Budapest: CEU Press, 1999), pp. 250–65.

trusting what is to be a devotional apotheosis: 'Mech of þe comown pepil magnifijd God in hir, hauyng good trost þat it was þe goodnes of God whech wrowt þat hy grace in hir sowle' (245). Their reception of her edifying words is testament to what Mary Erler sees as Kempe's 'apostolic vocation', as she draws on discourses of the holy mother to call disciples into her community ministry. Medieval female saints like Catherine of Siena, Margaret of Cortona, and Sibillina of Pavia attracted bands of followers as a type of spiritual family, referring to their followers as their 'children'.[105] In imitating the social role of the holy matriarch, then, Kempe bypasses anxieties over public teaching and once again fulfils the edict 'Crescite & multiplicamini' (increase and multiply), this time in elderly surrogacy and through the faithful followers who trust in the truth of her affective devotion.[106]

When she arrives at Syon in 1434 or 1435 for the Lammastide pardon ceremonies, the final destination of Kempe's arduous travel is coupled with a timely affirmation of her didacticism as a holy woman. As a metonym of the heavenly Jerusalem, Syon functions as an authorising site, since Kempe models her life on St Bridget's.[107] When a young man, moved by her affective response in the church there, asks the cause of her weeping, he addresses her as 'Modir', and confesses his desire to follow the path of God: '*Schewith modirly & goodly зowr conceit vn-to me as I trust vn-to зow*' (246). This man, in witnessing the spiritual suffering and fervour of an old woman at the close of the most epic journey of her life, recognises in her a matriarch and a teacher. As a surrogate mother, Kempe commends the man, revealing that her tears are the product of dismay at her sins, and of meditation on the Passion of Christ, by whose 'precyows blod schedyng sche was redemyd fro euyr-lestyng peyne' (246); we assume, moreover, that she here reproduces the spiritual conversion of her own worldly son. With the memories of the ascetic task of her journey inscribed in her mind and also in her frail and weary body, Kempe retains her faith in the promised healing of her pain in heavenly bliss. In a parallel to her own lifelong acts of surrogacy, she is now satisfied with the substitution of her pain in this life in return for its absence in the next. In communicating this lesson to the young man who trusts in her words, and thence to the amanuensis who records the events of Book II, her status as teacher is validated at the pivotal juncture of one journey's close and the start of another. This final, homiletic episode is situated near the end of Book II as an emblematic

---

[105] Mary Erler, 'Home Visits', in *Medieval Domesticity*, ed. Kowaleski and Goldberg, p. 275. St Anne was traditionally regarded as a maternal teacher. See Minnis, 'Religious Roles', in *Medieval Holy Women in the Christian Tradition*, ed. Minnis and Voaden, p. 48. On holy mother saints' teaching, see Herlihy, *Medieval Households*, pp. 122–4.

[106] Genesis 1:22.

[107] The Syon monastery, part of an overarching plan to found three monasteries around Richmond, was known as 'The King's Great Work at Sheen'. Syon Abbey was an important centre of contemplative piety in the fifteenth century. My thanks to Vincent Gillespie for his comments on this subject. See also Barry Windeatt, *The Book of Margery Kempe*, p. 418, n. 8269.

lesson in Kempe's journey towards, and final arrival at, her position as God's authorised representative on earth: an Elder in the Church of the world. On her return to Lynn to begin the inscription of her life at the end of Book II she is reconciled, with the 'Lord['s] halpe', with her confessor and friends (247). She is, then, authorised once again, beyond the leaves of her manuscript, to reproduce her life in the *Book* as a remembrance of disease and of deliverance: to go out and speak those 'good wordys' that 'spekyn of God' (126).

Afterword / Afterlife

Somewhere in the space beyond Margery Kempe's final prayer to her adopted children of the world is her physical death: silent, invisible, and beyond the margins of the *Book*. The absence of a real-death narrative enables a paradoxical permanence, a strategic drifting into the spiritual ether. The final prayer that calls for the salvation of the souls of all mankind is the last time that we hear Kempe's voice and an ultimate act of surrogacy: a call, in her extreme old age, for the spiritual work of her lifetime to be utilised and for her fruitfulness to be efficacious even beyond the grave. How fitting, then, that Kempe's final utterance is a prayer for the world: unconcerned with her own bodily decrepitude her disembodied voice becomes a universal wisdom removed from the confines of her pain-filled body and left to resonate in the realm beyond the leaves of her manuscript.[1] As her corporeality finally fails her utterly and she transitions to the next stage – beyond the bounds of the human life cycle – the spiritual perception and understanding that she has gained on her journey will enter a new phase of knowing, the heavenly perspicacity from which she has hitherto been separated.

The connections among vision, medicine, mysticism, life cycle, and reproduction are central to the final assimilation of what this book has attempted to unravel. Margery Kempe's particular form of spirituality makes no distinction between the corporeal and mystical, either in her reception of divine communication (seeing as 'verily' with her 'gostly eye' as with her 'bodily eye'), or in her visceral response *to* those visions or voices, as her devotion is articulated in a vociferously embodied way. What she *sees*, and how she *feels*, are the means through which she reaches at least a form of truth. As Jeffrey Hamburger has argued, 'Mysticism, at least mysticism understood as the experiential cognition of God ("cognitio Dei experimentalis"), cannot, it turns out, be imagined without recourse to the visible, however it is defined.'[2] In all its fleshly, fallible, tainted inadequacy, the body is the necessary vehicle of communion between humanity and God, the means through which we

---

[1] Windeatt has noted that *The Fifteen Oes* may have offered Kempe an example to emulate for her final prayers. See Windeatt, *BMK*, p. 421. See also Chapter 5, pp. 177–8 of this study. See also Josephine Koster, 'The Prayers of Margery Kempe and Subversive Self-Fashioning', in *Encountering The Book of Margery Kempe*, ed. Kalas and Varnam.

[2] Jeffrey F. Hamburger, 'Mysticism and Visuality', in *The Cambridge Companion to Christian Mysticism*, ed. Hollywood and Beckman, pp. 277–93 (p. 284).

perceive the world – the universe, even – and through which we *know*. And to know in the Middle Ages *is* to see, as Dallas Denery notes: 'Knowing something is somehow analogous to seeing something.'[3] To see, and indeed to suffer, are elemental and often painful human conditions, but they are ones that Margery Kempe clings to, bringing her closer, step by step, to a nexus with God as she strives to understand what they mean. This book has been largely about those transitions: from youth through to old age, from childbearing to surrogate reproductivity, from sickness to health – from life to death. But the final transition is yet to come, when Kempe's sickly flesh will become re-embodied, and 'hool a-ȝen' (66).

The Fourth Lateran Council, in 1215, clearly stated that all humankind is to be bodily resurrected:

> He will come at the end of time to judge the living and the dead, to render to every person according to his works, both to the reprobate and to the elect. *All of them will rise with their own bodies, which they now wear,* so as to receive according to their deserts, whether these be good or bad; for the latter perpetual punishment with the devil, for the former eternal glory with Christ.[4]

The *Ancrene Wisse* reiterates the same doctrine to its female audience:

> Vre alde curtel is þe flesch, þet we of Adam, ure alde feader, habbeð; þe neowe we schulen underuon of Godd, ure riche feader, I þe ariste of Domesdei, hwen ure flesch schal blikien schenre þen þe sunne, ȝef hit is totoren her wið wontreaðe ant wið weane.

> [Our old garment is the flesh, which we have from Adam, our ancestor; we shall receive the new one from God, our rich father, at the resurrection on the Day of Judgement, when our flesh will shine brighter than the sun, if it is torn here with suffering and with pain.][5]

While medieval scholastics debated the theory of Platonic dualism (that the person is the soul, to which the body is attached), the Aristotelian definition of the soul as a *form* of the body, that the person is human, not spiritual, helped to reconcile this contention, although the problematics of how the fragmented body would be reassembled on entering heaven remained.[6] John of Damascus (c. 675–749), who was widely quoted by medieval authors, stated that 'it is not a *re-surrectio* unless the same human being rises again' – a sentiment that echoes the assertion in the gospel of Luke that 'a hair of your head shall not

[3] Dallas G. Denery, *Seeing and Being Seen in the Later Medieval World: Optics, Theology and Religious Life* (Cambridge: Cambridge University Press, 2005), pp. 4–5.
[4] My emphasis. From The Fourth General Council of the Lateran, 1215 AD. 21: '1. Confession of Faith', in *Papal Encyclicals Online* <http://www.papalencyclicals.net> [accessed 8 May 2016]
[5] *Ancrene Wisse*, ed. Millett, part 6, section 7, p. 137. Translation from *Ancrene Wisse: A Translation*, ed. Millett, p. 137.
[6] Bynum, *Fragmentation and Redemption*, pp. 254–5.

perish'.[7] St Paul had taught that all bodies will be transfigured: 'We shall all indeed rise again: but we shall not all be changed … the dead shall rise again incorruptible: and we shall be changed'.[8] And some theologians, like Peter of Capua (d. 1214), suggested that it was a consequence not of divine grace but of the structure of human *nature* that body returned to soul after the Last Judgement.[9] Sanctified holy women in the Middle Ages were often subject to unusual deaths, their bodies embalmed and seen to be incorruptible, like that of Margaret of Cortona (c. 1247–1297), or their dissected bodies revealing relics embedded in their organs, like Clare of Montefalco's heart, mentioned in Chapter 2.[10] Another holy ecstatic, Margherita of Città di Castello (1287–1320), was opened up immediately after her death and several stones were discovered, impressed with images of Mary and the Christ Child. After her death, Marie of Oignies is recorded as clenching her teeth when the Prior of Oignies attempted to extract them as relics. When he asked for her pardon, she shook out a few teeth from her jaw for his use.[11] Hagiographies tell that the relic of Marie's finger healed others after her death, just as her physical presence had healed people during her lifetime.[12] Though medieval theology regarded saints' relics as problematic because of the dilemma of corporeal fragmentation and resurrection, stories, folktales, and some 'science' held that the body was in a sense alive after death; hagiographers describe dead saints sitting up to revere the crucifix, or exuding oil or milk to cure the sick.[13] But despite the powerful cultural value placed upon the dead bodies of medieval holy women, we do not have such material relics, or even legends, of Margery Kempe's afterlife. The lack of any posthumous narrative or beatific fragments is surprising, given how piously effusive and well known she was during her lifetime.[14]

Kempe has previously been understood to be have been admitted to the Guild of the Holy Trinity of Lynn in 1438, since that is the first record of her entry in the account rolls (the second entry is for the year 1438–9). The entry in the 1437–8 roll (Figures 5 and 6) states:[15]

[7] Bynum, *Fragmentation and Redemption*, p. 258. Luke 21:18.

[8] I Corinthians 15:51–3.

[9] Bynum, *Fragmentation and Redemption*, p. 254.

[10] See Katherine Park, *Secrets of Women*, pp. 39–76.

[11] Pope Boniface VIII's bull, *Detestande feritatis* of 1299, stipulated that no separation of bodily parts or evisceration after death was tolerable, although by the fifteenth century its provisions had been 'virtually forgotten'. See Elizabeth A.R. Brown, 'Death and the Human Body in the Later Middle Ages: The Legislation of Boniface VIII on the Division of the Corpse', *Viator*, 12 (1981), pp. 221–69 (p. 247 and p. 269).

[12] Bynum, *Fragmentation*, p. 285.

[13] Ibid., p. 266.

[14] Julian of Norwich, for example, would have been buried in an unmarked grave, as was customary for anchorites and anchoresses. However, Julian is honoured by a shrine in St Julian's Church, Norwich, and by a statue at the front of Norwich Cathedral.

[15] King's Lynn Borough Archives, KL/C38/16. I am indebted to Susan Maddock for her help in the locating and interpreting of the Holy Trinity Guild account rolls, and to Luke Shackell and the King's Lynn Borough Archives for allowing me access.

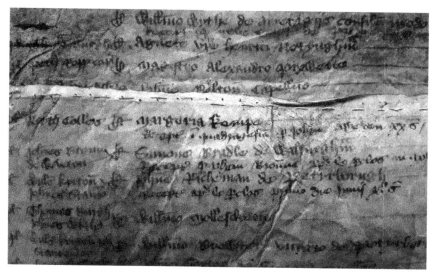

Figure 5. 1437–8 Trinity Guild account roll (KLBA, KL/C 38/16).

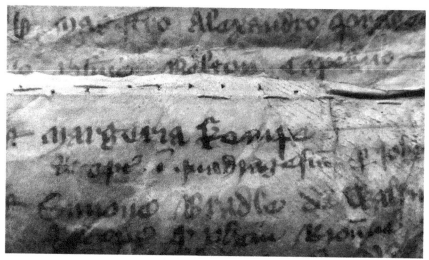

Figure 6. Detail of Margery Kempe's entry in the 1437–8
Trinity Guild account roll (KLBA, KL/C 38/16).

Pl[egius] B*ertholomeus Colles D[e] Margeria Kempe   xx s.
       Recept' in quadragesima per Iohannem Asheden xx s.

[Pledge Bartholomew Colles From Margery Kempe 20s.
         Received in Lent via John Asheden 20s.]

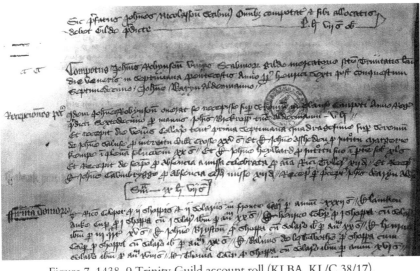

Figure 7. 1438–9 Trinity Guild account roll (KLBA, KL/C 38/17).

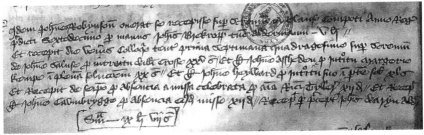

Figure 8. Detail of Margery Kempe's entry in the 1438–9
Trinity Guild account roll (KLBA, KL/C 38/17).

The entry in the 1438–9 roll (Figures 7 and 8) states it to be Kempe's full ('plenam'), or final, payment:[16]

        Et D[e] Iohanne Assheden pro Int[ro]itu Margerie
Kempe i[n] plena[m] soluc[i]o[n]em   xx s.

[And from John Assheden for the entry of Margery Kempe in full payment 20s.]

16 King's Lynn Borough Archives, KL/C 38/17. Credit as above.

Since the 'normal' admission fee for the Guild was 100 shillings, and if Margery Kempe made five equal payments of 20 shillings, she may well have made her first payment, and joined the Guild, in 1435 and not 1438 – so considerably earlier than was previously thought.[17] As the account roll shows, Kempe's final two payments were made via John Ashenden, an artificer-burgess, who was elected to the town's inner council in 1435 and elected Mayor of Lynn in 1440. It was not unusual for monies to be paid by an intermediary at this time.[18] What is unusual, however, is the late stage at which the Holy Trinity Guild of Lynn – said to be 'as masterful and wealthy as any in England' – began to accept women into its membership, which was not until the 1390s.[19] Most other guilds appear to have accepted women members (for 'spiritual benefits only') from much earlier in the fourteenth century.[20] Strikingly, it is Margery Kempe's own father, John de Brunham, who was the alderman of the Holy Trinity Guild at the time of the first recorded entry of women into the guild in the 1396–7 accounts.[21] Could a young, outspoken Margery Kempe, who had recently envisioned Christ visiting her in childbed, have influenced the decision of the Guild, via her father, to admit women to its membership? If she did, it was an early intervention into women's spiritual profit from which she would benefit in her afterlife.

Margery Kempe's entry to the Holy Trinity Guild thus occurs at about the same time as the revision of Book I and the dictation of Book II (in 1436 and 1438, respectively), and the synchronicity of these significant end-of-life activities should not be overlooked. In joining the Guild, Kempe would have benefited from increased funeral provision and the guarantee that prayers would be said for her soul; she may also have had her name entered onto a Bede Roll to be read out at Requiem masses and obits, thus ensuring her continuous presence in the memory of the community.[22] It is likely that

---

[17] The Holy Trinity Guild ordinances mention 100 shillings as the standard total admission fee. My thanks to Susan Maddock for this point.

[18] John Ashenden was married to Isabel Ashenden, who Susan Maddock speculates may have been related to Margery Kempe. See Susan Maddock, 'Society, status and the leet court in Margery Kempe's Lynn', in *Town Courts and Urban Society in Late Medieval England, 1250–1550*, ed. Richard Goddard and Teresa Phipps (Cambridge: D.S. Brewer, 2019), pp. 200–19.

[19] Alice Stopford Green, *Town Life in the Fifteenth Century* (London, 1894), vol. 1, p. 286. From Susan Maddock, 'Society, status and the leet court in Margery Kempe's Lynn', in *Town Courts and Urban Society*, p. 209.

[20] With thanks to Susan Maddock for this detail.

[21] The account roll for 1396–7 (KL/C 38/6) includes the first recorded entry of a female guild member. A detailed account of the evidence relating to the Brunhams' and neighbouring tenements in Briggate is in Susan Maddock, 'Mapping Margery Kempe's Lynn', *The Annual: The Bulletin of the Norfolk Archaeological and Historical Research Group*, 26 (2017), 3–14.

[22] Individuals could also ensure their posthumous remembrance by purchasing a specified number of masses. Donors could have their names engraved on plates, chalices, vestments, windows, church roofs and floor tiles. The wealthy elite could commission tomb effigies; 'transi tombs', which rather gruesomely depicted the cadaver in a state of decaying decomposition; or the 'double-decker' tombs which depicted the decaying body beneath a sculpture of the living body. See Youngs, *The Life Cycle in Western Europe, c. 1300–1500*, pp. 206–8.

these readings would have occurred in the chapel of the Holy Trinity Guild attached to St Margaret's Church in Lynn.[23] Her membership, then, symbolises her own preparation for dying according to the *Ars moriendi* tradition, at the same time as she prepares her *Book* as both a memorial of her spiritual life and a generative legacy for the future.

There is no record of Kempe's burial. She may have been buried in a tomb within St Margaret's Church, but much of the interior of St Margaret's was destroyed and rebuilt in the eighteenth and nineteenth centuries, after a storm in 1741 caused the south-western tower and spire to collapse onto the nave and aisles.[24] However, in 2014 workmen discovered the bones of a child in the Saturday market place in King's Lynn which dated from the twelfth or thirteenth century, when St Margaret's Church was being built. Later, close to the north-west tower of St Margaret's Church, a chapel named St John's and its charnel house were excavated, which had occupied the site from 1364 to 1779 (Figure 9).[25] Since the nineteenth century, historians had identified only two other chapels in Lynn – St James and St Nicholas – which lie some streets away from St Margaret's Church, and to which Kempe refers in the *Book* (58–9).[26] The chapel and charnel house of St John, by contrast, are adjacent to St Margaret's. In 1844, W. Taylor noted that 'The super-structure was a chapel dedicated to St John, and the basement story was the charnel, a consecrated vault, in which were carefully and decently deposited, the bones of the dead, disturbed in forming new graves, in the then extensive cemeteries of St Margaret's Church.'[27] The 2014 archaeological report records the existence of a possible box tomb in the charnel: 'It is thought that L1030 may have represented the surviving section of an inhumation burial within a brick and limestone 'box' tomb … This interpretation remains tentative, however.'[28] It is a risky temptation to speculate that such a 'box tomb' contains Margery Kempe's remains, but

[23] Goodman, *Margery Kempe and Her World*, p. 80 and p. 89.

[24] Ibid., p. 80.

[25] W. Taylor, *The Antiquities of King's Lynn, Norfolk* (London: Simpkin and Marshall, 1844), p. 62, in Antony R.R. Mustchin (report author), Kathren Henry and Gareth Barlow (fieldwork archaeologists), *Saturday Market Place, King's Lynn, Norfolk: Monitoring of Works under Archaeological Supervision and Control and Recording of Exposed Remains. Research Archive Report* (Archaeological Solutions, Ltd. Report no. 4718, November 2014), p. 3 and p. 6.

[26] See Goodman, *Margery Kempe and Her World*, p. xv and pp. 82–3. See also Katherine L. French, 'Margery Kempe and the Parish', in *The Ties that Bind: Essays in Medieval British History in Honor of Barbara Hanawalt*, ed. Linda E. Mitchell and Katherine L. French (Farnham: Ashgate, 2011), pp. 159–74.

[27] W. Taylor, *The Antiquities of King's Lynn, Norfolk* (London: Simpkin and Marshall, 1844), p. 59, from Clive J. Bond, *Interpretation of the Chapel of St John and Charnel House Excavated at the Saturday Market Place, King's Lynn*, p. 4. Unpublished Client Report: Borough Council of King's Lynn and West Norfolk, Apr 1, 2015, at: <https://www.academia.edu/18772746/Interpretation_of_the_Charnel_House_Saturday_market_Place_King_s_Lynn>. My grateful thanks to Clive Bond for supplying his report. The charnel house was apparently full of bones which were not excavated.

[28] Mustchin et al., *Saturday Market Place: Research Archive Report*, p. 14.

given her dedicated involvement in the parish of St Margaret's, it is probable that she is buried somewhere within the church, grounds, or charnel house.[29] If she did withdraw to an anchorhold, as Henry Pepwell's 1521 redaction of the *Book* would have us suppose in referring to her as a 'deuoute ancres', then she would, like her holy advisor Julian of Norwich, have been buried in an unmarked grave.[30] The location of Margery Kempe's bones, then, remains as elusive as do the many other aspects of her life that she omitted from the *Book* by selection or amnesia; it is a somehow fitting and ethereal dissolving of the very physical, rambunctious visibility of her earthly presence.

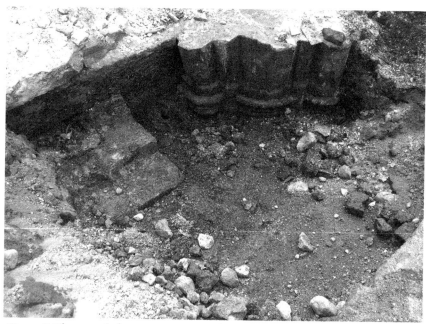

Figure 9. Photograph from excavations in the Saturday market place at King's Lynn in 2014, showing part of the charnel house beneath the chapel of St John, where human burials were discovered.

---

[29] On Kempe's close ties with the parish of St Margaret's Church, see Katherine L. French, 'Margery Kempe and the Parish', in *The Ties that Bind*, ed. Mitchell and French; and Laura Varnam, 'The Importance of St Margaret's Church in *The Book of Margery Kempe*: A Sacred Place and an Exemplary Parishioner', *Nottingham Medieval Studies*, 61 (2017), 197–243.

[30] See Santha Bhattacharji, *God is an Earthquake*, p. 23; and Liz Herbert McAvoy, '"Closyd in an hows of ston": Discourses of Anchoritism and *The Book of Margery Kempe*', in *Anchorites, Wombs and Tombs: Intersections of Gender and Enclosure in the Middle Ages*, ed. Liz Herbert McAvoy and Mari Hughes-Edwards (Cardiff: University of Wales Press, 2005), pp. 182–94. For the 1521 Pepwell redaction printed by Wynkyn de Word see Meech and Allen, *BMK*, pp. 353–7. All Saint's Church in south Lynn (within easy walking distance of St Margaret's Church) had a long-established anchorhold attached. See Goodman, *Margery Kempe and Her World*, pp. 81–2.

What does remain is *The Book of Margery Kempe*; the inscription of her life as a surrogate and healer, the 'very trewth schewyd in experiens' (220), and a sanctified undertaking for which she is thanked by Jesus, the Virgin, and many saints (219). But perhaps most crucially, Kempe is written into another book – the sacred 'Book of Life'. This, I argue, might in fact be regarded as Book III of the *Book* itself as her final rebirth in body, soul, and heavenly text:

> anon aperyd verily to hir sight an awngel al clothyd in white as mech as it had ben a lityl childe beryng an howge boke be-forn hym. Þan seyd þe creatur to þe childe, or ellys to þe awngel, 'A', sche seyd, 'þis is þe Boke of Lyfe'. And sche saw in þe boke þe Trinite & al in gold. Þan seyd sche to þe childe, 'Wher is my name?' Þe childe answeryd & seyd, 'Her is þi name at þe Trinyte foot wretyn', & þerwyth he was a-go, sche wist not how (206–7).

As Christ discloses in this magisterial vision, 'þi name is wretyn in Heuyn in þe Boke of Lyfe' (207).[31] Margery Kempe has therefore *already* entered heaven; resurrected through the gilded illumination of the 'Boke of Lyfe' she resides in hypostatic privilege at the foot of the Trinity. While we know of two, if not three, scribes of the *Book* (her adult son, the priest who was probably Robert Spryngolde, and the copier, 'Salthows'), there also, I suggest, exists a fourth scribe: God, the author of the 'Boke of Lyfe' that consolidates her painful knowledge in *imitatio Christi* to fulfil the teleology of her life as an 'unworthy' yet 'knowing' *creatur*. Margery Kempe is also now entered into the *Calendar of the Church of England* as 'Margery Kempe, Mystic, c. 1440 (E)', her life officially commemorated on 9 November each year, observed usually by 'a mention in prayers of intercession and thanksgiving'.[32] Though not sainted, and therefore not commemorated in the General Roman Calendar, this ecclesiastical recognition of Kempe's religious merit and authority provides a further, posthumous permanence. It is also an inscription into a fourth book – Book IV of *The Book of Margery Kempe*, even – as her life and spiritual perspicacity are authenticated and immortalised in fitting equivalence to those of her enduring life model, Bridget of Sweden, who is also 'commemorated' in the *Calendar*.[33] In April 2018 Kempe's memorialisation moved into the twenty-first century through a specially commissioned commemorative

---

[31] On this, see Liz Herbert McAvoy, '"[An] awngel al clothyd in white": Rereading the Book of Life as *The Book of Margery Kempe*', in *Women and Experience in Later Medieval Writing: Reading the Book of Life*, ed. Anneke B. Mulder-Bakker and Liz Herbert McAvoy (New York: Palgrave Macmillan, 2009), pp. 103–22 (pp. 117–18).

[32] Kempe was added to the Calendar in 1997. 'Commemoration' is the 'lowest' of the four observances, which are Principle Feasts, Festivals, Lesser Festivals, and Commemorations. For 'The Calendar', see *Exciting Holiness: Collects and Readings for the Festivals of the Calendars of The Church of England, The Church of Ireland, The Scottish Episcopal Church and The Church in Wales*, ed. Brother Tristam and Simon Kershaw, 3rd edn (Norwich: Canterbury Press, 2007), pp. 15–26.

[33] Bridget of Sweden is commemorated in England on 23 July each year. Other commemorated visionaries include Walter Hilton (24 March) and Mechtild of Madeburg (19 November). Julian of Norwich, Catherine of Siena, Hildegard of Bingen, and Elizabeth

bench in the Saturday market place near King's Lynn Minster (St Margaret's Church). As *The Manere of Good Lyvyng* attests, 'In dyeng in the paynes of this lyfe, all paynes be gon.'[34] Kempe has achieved, we hope, the 'good' death that underpinned the activities of most medieval people; a death which God declared would be free of pain: 'it xal be cawse þu xalt no peyn felyn whan þu art comyn owt of þis worlde & also þat þu xalt haue þe lesse peyn in thy deying, for þu hast so gret compassyon of my flesche I must need haue compassyon of þi flesch' (183).[35] In the Introduction I considered whether we can ever *know* pain. Like Kempe's esoteric mystical knowledge, her suffering is hers alone. Having given birth fourteen times in an age before anaesthesia, struggled with the pains of chronic illness, spiritual agony, and emptiness, suffered the tribulations of old age, and experienced infinite mourning for the Christ whose body bleeds freshly before her eyes, it seems safe to conclude that Margery Kempe does *know* pain.

As well as the painful inheritance of female flesh, this book has been concerned with the medical, mystical, mourning, and surrogacy phenomena that underlie the operations in Kempe's text. It is the story of a holy woman's marvellous experience, which resists 'diagnosis' just as much as she resists any other type of categorisation, as she seeks an eschatological truth, perceived 'verily'. In reaching back and pausing to observe some phases of her life – her melancholia, trauma, chaste marriage, transformed and gendered blood, surrogate reproductivity, pain surrogacy, aged asceticism, and matriarchal authority – we bear witness to the painful epistemology that provides Kempe's route towards God. The recipe for medicinal sweets at the end of the manuscript is thus the teleology of her spiritual healing, since she has journeyed from sickness to health and been 'restoryd her a-geyn', as it has 'openly be shewed aftyrward' (1–2). Without recourse to the medico–religious culture in which the *Book* was produced and understood, we disembody Kempe in the same, reductive manner as did Pepwell in 1521, since the voice that resounds fervently within and beyond the pages of her *Book* is one which emanates from a body through which experience begins. From her ears, eyes, heart, and mind, she perceives, feels, and knows God, translating his spiritual healing to the world.

In her final prayer, she continues in her quest to heal the pain of 'alle þat arn seke specialy, for alle laȝerys, alle bedred men and women', and for those 'þat arn in peynys of Purgatory'. For her own pains, she is grateful: 'I thank þe þat þu woldist letyn me suffryn any pane in þis world' (251). The memorial that is *The Book of Margery Kempe* is thus Kempe's apostolic gift to the world

---

of Hungary achieve the higher remembrance of 'Lesser Festival'. See 'Calendar', in *Exciting Holiness*, pp. 15–26.

[34] *The Manere of Good Lyvyng*, XLIII exhortation, p. 127.

[35] On good and bad deaths see Stephen Gordon, 'Disease, Sin, and the Walking Dead in Medieval England c. 1100–1350: A Note on the Documentary and Archaeological Evidence', in *Medicine, Healing and Performance*, ed. Gemi-Iordanou et al., pp. 124–58.

and her own embodied relic. Whilst her voice fades out after this final orison of hope, it remains an everlasting echo in the legacy of her rediscovered *Book*: her second resurrection. In the *shewing* of her healed body and soul, she has transformed pain into production, now able to *see* and to know, and to complete the flourishing in which much of her adult life was spent as she sought the gifts of vision, healing, and medicine.

Glossary of Medical Terms

aetiology: the branch of medicine related to the cause of disease.

analgesic: a treatment or remedy that relieves pain.

anamnestic: recalling to mind; aiding the memory or recollection.

apoplexy: a haemorrhage of the cerebrum or a stroke.

aposteme: a localized swelling such as a boil or tumour.

bile, black: also known as melancholy. One of the four bodily humours, having cold and dry qualities.

bile, yellow: also known as choler. One of the four bodily humours, having hot and dry qualities.

Christus medicus: Christ the Physician. The biblical understanding of Christ as a healer of bodies and souls, which was a ubiquitous notion in the Middle Ages.

complex: a whole made up of a number of often-interconnected parts; a complex or complicated whole.

complexion: the combined qualities or humours inherent in an individual person; a humoral type; a temperament.

diathesis: a condition of the body that renders it liable to certain special diseases or affections; a constitutional predisposition or tendency.

dyscrasia: the disruption of an individual's complexion or humoral balance.

dysmenorrhoea: painful menstruation.

fecundity: the faculty of reproduction; productiveness more widely.

flux: a 'flow'; normally with reference to diarrhoea. 'Bloody flux' is normally where blood is present in the excrement.

humour: one of four bodily fluids understood in ancient and medieval medicine to make up the physiology of human life. The humours are blood, phlegm, yellow bile, and black bile.

mania: mental illness marked by periods of great excitement or euphoria, delusions, and overactivity.

melancholic: designating or relating to the containment of black bile (melancholy).

melancholy: black bile. Also a state of disease caused by an excess of the humour black bile.

metapsychology: the study of mental processes and the mind–body relationship, beyond what can be studied experimentally.

naturals: in Galenic and medieval physiology, the unalterable 'givens' of the physical world and the human body: the elements, complexions, humours, organs, etc.

neural: relating to a nerve or the nervous system.

non-naturals: in Galenic and medieval medicine, the variable environmental and behavioural factors that influence the 'naturals': air, food and drink, sleep, rest, work, retention and elimination, emotional states.

phlebotomy: bloodletting.

phlegm: one of the four bodily humours, having cold and wet qualities.

psyche: the human mind, soul or spirit.

psychomotor: relating to the origination of movement in conscious mental activity.

psychophysical: the relationship between one's internal (psychic) and external (physical) worlds.

psychosis: a psychiatric disorder that causes individuals to perceive things differently from others and which may involve hallucinations or delusions.

psychosomatic: relating to the interaction of mind and body. Or, of a condition caused or aggravated by a mental factor such as internal conflict or stress.

puerperium: the period of approximately six weeks after childbirth, during which the mother's reproductive organs return to their original non-pregnant condition.

sanguine: the humour of blood; or a complexion dominated by blood.

somatic: of or relating to the body, bodily, corporeal, physical.

syncope: fainting.

temperament: the proper or balanced mixture of the four elements, qualities (hot, cold, wet, dry), or humours. Also one's generic 'type' or 'complexion'.

vapours: internal fumes produced by digestion.

Select Bibliography

Manuscripts

London, British Library, Additional MS 61823, *The Book of Margery Kempe*

Primary Texts

Aelred of Rievaulx, *De institutione inclusarum: Two Middle English Translations*, ed. John Ayto and Alexandra Barratt, EETS o.s. 287 (London, New York, and Toronto: Oxford University Press, 1984)

Albertus Magnus, *De secretis mulierum: Item de virtutibus herbarum lapidum et animalium* (Amsterdam: J. Janssonius, 1662)

Amis and Amiloun, ed. M. Leach, EETS o.s. 203, reprint edn (London: Oxford University Press, 2001); first edition published 1937

Ancrene Wisse: A Corrected Edition of the Text in Cambridge, Corpus Christi College, MS 402, with Variants from other Manuscripts, ed. Bella Millett with glossary and notes by Richard Dance, 2 vols, EETS o.s. 325 and 326 (Oxford: Oxford University Press, 2005–6)

Ancrene Wisse: Guide for Anchoresses, a Translation based on Cambridge, Corpus Christi College, MS 402, ed. Bella Millett (Exeter: University of Exeter Press, 2009)

Aquinas, Thomas, *Summa theologiae* <http://www.ccel.org/ccel/aquinas/summa>

———, *Summa theologiae: A Concise Translation*, ed. Timothy McDermott (Allen, Tex.: Christian Classics, 1989)

Aristotle, *Problems: Books 20–38, Rhetoric to Alexander*, vol. 2, ed. and trans. Robert Mayhew and David C. Mirhady (Cambridge, Mass., and London: Harvard University Press, 2011)

Augustine, 'On the words of the Gospel, Matt. xx. 30, about the two blind men sitting by the way side, and crying out, "Lord, have mercy on us, Thou Son of David"', *A Select Library of the Nicene and Post-Nicene Fathers of the Christian Church*, ed. Philip Schaff, vol. 6, Sermon 39 <http://www.ccel.org/ccel/schaff/npnf106.i.html>

———, 'Studium de mundando cordis oculo', *Opera Omnia*, vol. 6, Sermon 88 <http://www.augustinus.it/latino/discorsi/index2.htm>

Averroës, *Epitome of Parva Naturalia*, trans. Harry Blumberg (Cambridge, Mass.: Medieval Academy of America, 1961)

Avicenna, *The Canon of Medicine (al-Qānūn fī'l-tibb)*, vol. 1., trans. O. Cameron Gruner and Mazar H. Shah, adapted by Laleh Bakhtiar (Chicago: Kazi Publications, 1999)

——, *The Canon of Medicine (al-Qānūn fī'l-tibb)*, vol. 3, trans. Peyman Adeli Sardo, ed. Laleh Bakhtiar (Chicago: Kazi Publications, 2014)

The Book of the Craft of Dying, and other Early English Tracts Concerning Death, ed. Frances M.M. Comper (New York: Arno Press, 1977)

Bridget of Sweden, *The Liber celestis of St Bridget of Sweden: The Middle English Version in British Library MS Claudius B i, Together with a Life of the Saint from the Same Manuscript*, ed. Roger Ellis, vol. 1, EETS o.s. 291 (Oxford: Oxford University Press, 1987)

Burton, Robert, *The Anatomy of Melancholy* [1621], ed. Holbrook Jackson (New York: New York Review of Books, 2001)

Chaucer, Geoffrey, *The Canterbury Tales*, in *The Riverside Chaucer*, ed. Larry D. Benson (Oxford: Oxford University Press, 1987)

Constantine the African, *Viaticum*, in *Lovesickness in the Middle Ages: The Viaticum and its Commentaries*, ed. and trans. Mary Frances Wack (Philadelphia: University of Pennsylvania Press, 1990)

Cultures of Piety: Medieval English Devotional Literature in Translation, ed. Anne Clark Bartlett and Thomas H. Bestul (Ithaca, N.Y., and London: Cornell University Press, 1999)

Curye on Inglysch: English Culinary Manuscripts of the Fourteenth Century (Including the Forme of Cury), ed. Constance B. Hieatt and Sharon Butler, EETS s.s. 8 (London and New York: Oxford University Press, 1985)

The Cyrurgie of Guy de Chauliac, ed. Margaret S. Ogden, EETS o.s. 265 (London: Oxford University Press, 1971)

De secretis mulierum, Women's Secrets: A Translation of Pseudo-Albertus Magnus' 'De secretis mulierum' with Commentaries, ed. Helen Rodnite Lemay (Albany: State University of New York Press, 1992)

The Fifteen Oes, 'O Jhesu endless swetnes of louying soules …' (Westminster: William Caxton, 1491), STC 20195; available online through EEBO (login required)

The Fourth General Council of the Lateran, 1215 AD. 21, Papal Encyclicals Online <http://www.papalencyclicals.net>

Galen On the Usefulness of the Parts of the Body, ed. M.T. May, 2 vols (Ithaca, N.Y.: Cornell University Press, 1968)

Gerard of Berry, *Glosule super viaticum*, in *Lovesickness in the Middle Ages: The Viaticum and its Commentaries*, ed. and trans. Mary Frances Wack (Philadelphia: University of Pennsylvania Press, 1990)

Gilbertus Anglicus, *Compendium of Mediaeval Medicine*, in *System of Physic (GUL MS Hunter 509, ff. 1r–167v): A Compendium of Mediaeval Medicine Including the Middle English Gilbertus Anglicus*, ed. Laura Esteban-Segura (Bern: Peter Lang, 2012)

Guillaume de Lorris and Jean de Meun, *The Romance of the Rose*, trans. Charles Dahlberg, 3rd edn (Princeton: Princeton University Press, 1995)

Henry of Lancaster, *Le livre de seyntz medicines: The Book of Holy Medicines*, trans. Catherine Batt (Tempe: Arizona Center for Medieval and Renaissance Studies, 2014)

Hildegard of Bingen, *Causes and Cures: The Complete English Translation of Hildegardis Causae et curae Libri VI*, trans. Priscilla Throop (Charlotte: Medieval IMS, 2008)

——, *Epistolarivm: Pars Tertia CCLI–CCCX*, ed. L. Van Acker and M. Klaes-Hachmöller (Turnhout: Brepols, 2001)

——, *Hildegard von Bingen's Physica: The Complete English Translation of Her Classic Work on Health and Healing*, trans. Priscilla Throop (Rochester: Healing Arts Press, 1998)

——, *Hildegardis: Causae et curae*, ed. Paul Kaiser (Liepzig: In aedibus B.G. Teubneri, 1903)

——, *The Letters of Hildegard of Bingen*, vol. 3, trans. Joseph L. Baird and Radd K. Ehrman (New York and Oxford: Oxford University Press, 2004)

——, *On Natural Philosophy and Medicine: Selections from Cause et Cure*, trans. Margret Berger (Cambridge: D.S. Brewer, 1999)

——, 'Physica: cujus titulus ex cod. ms.: Subtilitatem Diversarum Naturarum Creaturam', *Opera Omnia*, ed. Jacques-Paul Migne, PL 197

The Infancy Gospels of James and Thomas, ed. Ronald F. Hock (Santa Ross, Calif.: Polebridge Press, 1995)

Jacobus de Voragine, *The Golden Legend: Readings on the Saints*, ed. William Granger Ryan and Eamon Duffy (Princeton: Princeton University Press, 2012)

Julian of Norwich, *The Writings of Julian of Norwich: A Vision Showed to a Devout Woman and A Revelation of Love*, ed. Nicholas Watson and Jacqueline Jenkins (Philadelphia: Pennsylvania State University Press, 2005)

Kempe, Margery, *The Book of Margery Kempe*, ed. Barry Windeatt (Cambridge: D.S. Brewer, 2004)

——, *The Book of Margery Kempe*, ed. Sandford Brown Meech and Hope Emily Allen, EETS o.s. 212, reprint edn (London: Oxford University Press, 1997); first edition published 1940

——, *The Book of Margery Kempe*, trans. Anthony Bale (Oxford: Oxford University Press, 2015)

The Knowing of Woman's Kind in Childing: A Middle English Version of Material Derived from the Trotula and other Sources, ed. Alexandra Barratt (Turnhout: Brepols, 2001)

The 'Liber de diversis medicinis' in the Thornton Manuscript (MS. Lincoln Cathedral A.5.2), ed. Margaret Sinclair Ogden, EETS o.s. 207 (London: Oxford University Press, 1938)

Love, Nicholas, *The Mirror of the Blessed Life of Jesus Christ: A Reading Text*, ed. Michael G. Sargent (Exeter: University of Exeter Press, 2004)

The Manere of Good Lyvyng: A Middle English Translation of Pseudo-Bernard's Liber de modo bene vivendi ad sororem, ed. Anne E. Mouron (Turnhout: Brepols, 2014)

Medieval Women's Guide to Health: The First English Gynecological Handbook, ed. Beryl Rowland (Kent, Ohio: The Kent State University Press, 1981)

Middle English Lyrics: Authoritative Texts, Critical and Historical Backgrounds, Perspectives on Six Poems, ed. Maxwell S. Luria and Richard L. Hoffman (New York and London: W.W. Norton, 1974)

Middle English Marian Lyrics, ed. Karen Saupe, TEAMS (Kalamazoo, Mich.: Medieval Institute Publications, 1997) <http://d.lib.rochester.edu/teams/publication/saupe-middle-english-marian-lyrics>

A Middle English Medical Remedy Book, Edited from Glasgow University Library, MS Hunter 185, ed. Francisco Alonso Almeida (Heidelberg: Universitätsverlag, 2014)

Morris, Richard, *Richard Morris's Prick of Conscience: A Corrected and Amplified Reading Text*, ed. Ralph Hannah and Sarah Wood, EETS o.s. 342 (Oxford: Oxford University Press, 2013)

Myrc, John, *Instructions for Parish Priests, Edited from Cotton MS. Claudius A II*, ed. Edward Peacock, EETS o.s. 31 (London: Trübner, 1868)

The Myroure of Our Ladye, ed. John H. Blunt, EETS e.s. 19 (London: Trüber, 1873)

'*The Nature of Women*, in London, British Library, MS Egerton 827, s. 14, ff. 28v–30v', ed. Monica Green, in *Women's Healthcare in the Medieval West* (New York and London: Routledge, 2000), pp. 83–8

The Pore Caitif, Edited from MS Harley 2336 with Introduction and Notes, ed. M.T. Brady (unpublished PhD thesis, Fordham University, 1954)

Rolle, Richard, *The English Writings*, trans. and ed. Rosamund S. Allen (New York: Paulist Press, 1988)

Secretum Secretorum: Nine English Versions, ed. M.A. Manzaloui, EETS o.s. 276 (Oxford: Oxford University Press, 1977)

The 'Sekenesse of Wymmen': A Middle English Treatise on Diseases in Women, Yale Medical Library, Ms. 47 fols. 60r–71v, ed. M.R. Hallaert, Scripta: Mediaeval and Renaissance Texts and Studies 8 (Brussels: Omirel, 1982)

Sex, Aging, and Death in a Medieval Medical Compendium: Trinity College Cambridge MS R.14.52; Its Texts, Language, and Scribe, ed. M. Teresa Tavormina, 2 vols (Tempe: Arizona Center for Medieval and Renaissance Studies, 2006)

Sickness of Women, ed. Monica H. Green and Linne R. Mooney, in *Sex, Aging, and Death in a Medieval Medical Compendium: Trinity College Cambridge MS R.14.52; Its Texts, Language, and Scribe*, ed. M. Teresa Tavormina (Tempe: Arizona Centre for Medieval and Renaissance Studies, 2006), II, 455–568

Shakespeare, William, *King Henry V*, ed. T.W. Craik, The Arden Shakespeare, 3rd ser., reprint edn (London: Thompson Learning, 2005)

Thomas of Cantimpré, *Liber de natura rerum* (Berlin: Walter De Gruyter, 1973)

Three Women of Liège: A Critical Edition of and Commentary on the Middle English Lives of Elizabeth of Spalbeek, Christina Mirabilis, and Marie D'Oignies, ed. Jennifer N. Brown (Turnhout: Brepols, 2008)

The 'Treatise on the Signs of Death' in Glasgow University Library, MS Hunter 513, ff. 105r–107v, transcribed and described by Teresa Marqués Aguado, The Málaga Corpus of Late Middle English Scientific Prose <http://hunter.uma.es/>

Trevisa, John, *On the Properties of Things: John Trevisa's Translation of Bartholomaeus Anglicus' De proprietatibus rerum*, ed. M.C. Seymour, 2 vols (Oxford: Oxford University Press, 1975)

The Trotula: A Medieval Compendium of Women's Medicine, ed. and trans. Monica H. Green (Philadelphia: University of Pennsylvania Press, 2001)

Two Fifteenth-Century Cookery-Books: Harleian MS 279 (ab. 1430) and Harl. MS 4016 (ab. 1450), with Extracts from Ashmole MS 1439, Laud MS 553 and Douce MS 55, ed. Thomas Austin, EETS o.s. 91, reprint edn (London: Oxford University Press, 2000); first edition published 1888

Secondary Texts

Amundsen, Darrel W., and Carol Jean Diers, 'The Age of Menopause in Medieval Europe', *Human Biology*, 45 (1973), 605–12

Alexandre-Bidon, Danièle, and Didier Lett, *Children in the Middle Ages: Fifth to Fifteenth Centuries*, trans. Jody Gladding (Notre Dame, Ind.: University of Notre Dame Press, 1999)

Allen, Rosamund, ed., *Eastward Bound: Travel and Travellers, 1050–1550* (Manchester: Manchester University Press, 2004)

Anadjar, Gil, *Blood: A Critique of Christianity* (New York: Columbia University Press, 2014)

Appleford, Amy, '"The comene course of prayer": Julian of Norwich and Late Medieval Death Culture', *Journal of English and Germanic Philology*, 107:2 (2008), 190–214

——, *Learning to Die in London, 1380–1540* (Philadelphia: University of Pennsylvania Press, 2015)

Arbesmann, R., 'The Concept of *Christus medicus* in St Augustine', *Traditio*, 10 (1954), 1–28

Arnold, John H., and Katherine J. Lewis, eds, *A Companion to 'The Book of Margery Kempe'* (Cambridge: D.S. Brewer, 2004)

Atkinson, Clarissa W., *Mystic and Pilgrim: The Book and the World of Margery Kempe* (Ithaca, N.Y.: Cornell University Press, 1983)

——, *The Oldest Vocation* (Ithaca, N.Y.: Cornell University Press, 1991)

Bale, Anthony, *The Book of Margery Kempe* (Oxford: Oxford University Press, 2015)

——, 'Richard Salthouse of Norwich and the Scribe of *The Book of Margery Kempe*', *Studies in the Age of Chaucer*, 52 (2017), 173–87

Banner, Lois W., *In Full Flower: Aging Women, Power and Sexuality: A History* (New York: Alfred A. Knopf, 1992)

Barratt, Alexandra, 'Spiritual Virgin to Virgin Mother: Confessions of Margery Kempe', *Paregon*, 17:1 (1999), 9–44

——, ed. *Women's Writing in Middle English*, 2nd edn (Harlow: Longman, 2010)

Bartlett, Anne Clark, *Male Authors, Female Readers: Representation and Subjectivity in Middle English Devotional Literature* (New York: Cornell University Press, 1995)

Bennett, Judith M., and Ruth Mazo Karras, eds, *The Oxford Handbook of Women and Gender in Medieval Europe* (Oxford: Oxford University Press, 2013)

Bestul, Thomas H., *Texts of the Passion: Latin Devotional Literature and Medieval Society* (Philadelphia: University of Pennsylvania Press, 1996)

Bhattacharji, Santha, *God is an Earthquake: The Spirituality of Margery Kempe* (London: Darton, Longman, and Todd, 1997)

Biddick, Kathleen, 'Genders, Bodies, Borders: Technologies of the Visible', *Speculum*, 68 (1993), 389–418

Bildhauer, Bettina, *Medieval Blood* (Cardiff: University of Wales Press, 2006)

Biller, Peter, and Alastair J. Minnis, eds, *Medieval Theology and the Natural Body* (York: York Medieval Press, 1997)

Biller, Peter, and Joseph Ziegler, eds, *Religion and Medicine in the Middle Ages* (York: York Medieval Press, 2001)

Biro, David, 'Is there Such a Thing as Psychological Pain? And Why It Matters', *Culture, Medicine and Society*, 34 (2010), 658–67

Bishop, Louise, *Words, Stones, Herbs: The Healing Word in Medieval and Early Modern England* (New York: Syracuse University Press, 2007)

Blaffer-Hrdy, Sarah, 'Fitness Tradeoffs in the History and Evolution of Delegated Mothering with Special Reference to Wet-Nursing', *Ethology and Sociobiology*, 13 (1992), 409–42

——, *Mother Nature: Maternal Instincts and the Shaping of the Species* (London: Vintage, 2000)

Blamires, Alcuin, 'Women and Preaching in Medieval Orthodoxy, Heresy, and Saints' Lives', *Viator*, 26 (1995), 135–52

Blumenfeld-Kosinski, R., and T. Snell, eds, *Images of Sainthood in Medieval Europe* (Ithaca, N.Y.: Cornell University Press, 1991)

Boffey, Julia, and Virginia Davis, eds, *Recording Medieval Lives: Proceedings of the 2005 Harlaxton Symposium* (Donington: Shaun Tyas, 2005)

Bourke, Joanna, *The Story of Pain: From Prayer to Painkillers* (Oxford: Oxford University Press, 2014)

Bowers, Barbara S., ed., *The Medieval Hospital and Medical Practice* (Aldershot: Ashgate, 2007)

Bowers, Terence, 'Margery Kempe as Traveller', *Studies in Philology*, 97:1 (2000), 1–28

Brenner, Elma, 'Recent Perspectives on Leprosy in Medieval Western Europe', *History Compass*, 8:5 (2010), 388–406

Brody, Howard, *Stories of Sickness*, 2nd rev. edn (New York: Oxford University Press, 2003)

Brooke, Christopher, *The Medieval Idea of Marriage* (Oxford: Oxford University Press, 2002)

Brother Tristam and Simon Kershaw, eds, *Exciting Holiness: Collects and Readings for the Festivals of the Calendars of the Church of England, the Church of Ireland, the Scottish Episcopal Church and the Church in Wales*, 3rd edn (Norwich: Canterbury Press, 2007)

Brown, Elizabeth A.R., 'Death and the Human Body in the Later Middle Ages: The Legislation of Boniface VIII on the Division of the Corpse', *Viator*, 12 (1981), 221–69

Brown, Peter, ed., *A Companion to Medieval English Literature and Culture, c. 1350–c. 1500* (Oxford: Blackwell, 2007)

Brundage, James A., '"Allas! That evere love was synne": Sex and Medieval Canon Law', *The Catholic Historical Review*, 72 (1986), 1–13

Bullough, Vern L., 'Marriage in the Middle Ages: Medieval Medical and Scientific Views of Women', *Viator*, 4 (1973), 485–501

——, and Cameron Campbell, 'Female Longevity and Diet in the Middle Ages', *Speculum*, 55:2 (1980), 317–25

——, and James A. Brundage, eds, *Sexual Practices in the Medieval Church* (New York: Prometheus, 1982)

Burgess, Clive, and Caroline M. Barron, eds, *Memory and Commemoration in Medieval England* (Donington: Tyas, 2010)

Burrow, J.A., *The Ages of Man: A Study in Medieval Writing and Thought* (Oxford: Clarendon Press, 1988)

Butler, Sara M., *Forensic Medicine and Death Investigation in Medieval England* (New York and London: Routledge, 2015)

Bynum, Caroline Walker, 'Death and Resurrection in the Middle Ages: Some Modern Implications', *Proceedings of the American Philosophical Society*, 142:4 (1998), 589–96

——, *Fragmentation and Redemption: Essays on Gender and the Human Body in Medieval Religion* (New York: Zone Books, 1989)

——, *Holy Feast and Holy Fast: The Religious Significance of Food to Medieval Women* (Berkeley: University of California Press, 1987)

——, *Jesus as Mother: Studies in the Spirituality of the High Middle Ages* (Berkley: University of California Press, 1982)

——, 'Why all the Fuss about the Body? A Medievalist's Perspective', *Critical Enquiry*, 22 (1995), 1–33

——, *Wonderful Blood: Theology and Practice in Late Medieval Northern Germany and Beyond* (Philadelphia: University of Pennsylvania Press, 2007)

Caciola, Nancy, *Discerning Spirits: Divine and Demonic Possession in the Middle Ages* (Ithaca, N.Y.: Cornell University Press, 2003)

Cadden, Joan, *Meanings of Sex Difference in the Middle Ages: Medicine, Science and Culture* (Cambridge: Cambridge University Press, 1993)

Carlson, Marla, *Performing Bodies in Pain: Medieval and Post-Modern Martyrs, Mystics, and Artists* (New York: Palgrave Macmillan, 2010)

Carruthers, Mary, *The Book of Memory: A Study of Memory in Medieval Culture* (Cambridge and New York: Cambridge University Press, 2008)

——, 'On Affliction and Reading, Weeping and Argument: Chaucer's Lachrymose Troilus in Context', *Representations*, 93:1 (2006), 1–21

——, and Elizabeth D. Kirk, eds, *Acts of Interpretation: The Text in Its Contexts 700–1600; Essays on Medieval and Renaissance Literature* (Norman, Okla.: Pilgrim Books, 1982)

Castelli, Elizabeth, 'Virginity and Its Meaning for Women's Sexuality in Early Christianity', *Journal of Feminist Studies in Religion*, 2 (1986), 61–88

Chappell, Julie, *Perilous Passages: The Book of Margery Kempe, 1534–1934* (New York: Palgrave Macmillan, 2013)

Christopher Catling, 'The Archaeology of Leprosy and the Black Death', *Current Archaeology*, 236 (2009), 22–9

Classen, Albrecht, ed., *Childhood in the Middle Ages: The Results of a Paradigm Shift in the History of Mentality* (Berlin and New York: De Gruyter, 2005)

——, ed., *Death in the Middle Ages and Early Modern Times: The Material and Spiritual Conditions of the Culture of Death* (Berlin: De Gruyter, 2016)

——, ed., *Old Age in the Middle Ages and the Renaissance: Interdisciplinary Approaches to a Neglected Topic* (Berlin and New York: De Gruyter, 2007)

Cleve, Gunnel, 'Semantic Dimensions in Margery Kempe's "whyght clothys"', *Mystics Quarterly*, 12 (1986), 162–70

Cochelin, Isabelle, and Karen Smyth, eds, *Medieval Life Cycles: Continuity and Change* (Turnhout: Brepols, 2013)

Cohen, Esther, *The Modulated Scream: Pain in Late Medieval Culture* (Chicago and London: University of Chicago Press, 2010)

——, and Leona Toker, Manuela Consonni, and Otniel E. Dror, eds, *Knowledge and Pain* (Amsterdam and New York: Rodopi, 2012)

Cohen, Jeffrey J., *Medieval Identity Machines* (Minneapolis: University of Minnesota Press, 2003)

——, and Bonnie Wheeler, eds, *Becoming Male in the Middle Ages* (New York and London: Garland Publishing, 2000)

Conboy, Katie, Nadia Medina, and Sarah Stanbury, eds, *Writing on the Body: Female Embodiment and Feminist Theory* (New York: Columbia University Press, 1997)

Conrad, L.I., and D. Wujastyk, eds, *Contagion: Perspectives from Premodern Societies* (Aldershot: Ashgate, 2000)

Cooney, Helen, ed., *Writings on Love in the English Middle Ages* (New York: Palgrave Macmillan, 2006)

Cotter-Lynch, Margaret, and Brad Herzog, eds, *Reading Memory and Identity in the Texts of Medieval European Holy Women* (New York: Palgrave Macmillan, 2012)

Covey, Herbert C., 'Perceptions and Attitudes towards Sexuality of the Elderly during the Middle Ages', *The Gerontologist*, 29 (1989), 93–100

Cox, Elizabeth, Liz Herbert McAvoy, and Roberta Magnani, eds, *Reconsidering Gender, Time and Memory in Medieval Culture* (Cambridge: D.S. Brewer, 2015)

Cressy, David, 'Purification, Thanksgiving and the Churching of Women in Post-Reformation England', *Past & Present*, 141 (1993), 106–46 d'Avray, David, *Medieval Marriage: Symbolism and Society* (Oxford: Oxford University Press, 2005)

Davis, Isabel, Miriam Müller, and Sarah Rees Jones, eds, *Love, Marriage, and Family Ties in the Later Middle Ages* (Turnhout: Brepols, 2003)

Demaitre, Luke, 'The Art and Science of Prognostication in Early University Medicine', *Bulletin of the History of Medicine*, 77 (2003), 765–88

——, 'The Idea of Childhood and Child Care in Medical Writings of the Middle Ages', *Journal of Psychohistory*, 4 (1977), 461–90

——, *Leprosy in Premodern Medicine: A Malady of the Whole Body* (Baltimore: John Hopkins University Press, 2007)

Dinshaw, Carolyn, *Getting Medieval: Sexualities and Communities, Pre- and Postmodern* (Durham, N.C.: Duke University Press, 1999)

——, *How Soon Is Now? Medieval Texts, Amateur Readers, and the Queerness of Time* (Durham, N.C., and London: Duke University Press, 2012)

——, and David Wallace, eds, *The Cambridge Companion to Medieval Women's Writing* (Cambridge: Cambridge University Press, 2003)

Donnelly, Colleen, 'Menopausal Life as Imitation of Art: Margery Kempe and the Lack of Sorority', *Women's Writing*, 12 (2005), 419–32

Douglas, Mary, *Collected Works*, vol. 2: *Purity and Danger: An Analysis of Concepts of Purity and Danger*, reprint edn (London and New York: Routledge, 2003); first edition published 1966

Dyas, Dee, Valerie Edden, and Roger Ellis, eds, *Approaching Medieval English Anchoritic and Mystical Texts* (Cambridge: D.S. Brewer, 2005)

Edwards, Anthony S.G., ed., *Middle English Prose: A Critical Guide to Major Authors and Genres* (New Brunswick, N.J.: Rutgers University Press, 1984)

Elliott, Dyan, *Fallen Bodies: Pollution, Sexuality, and Demonology in the Middle Ages* (Philadelphia: University of Pennsylvania Press, 1999)

——, *Proving Woman: Female Spirituality and Inquisitional Culture in the Later Middle Ages* (Princeton and Oxford: Princeton University Press, 2004)

——, *Spiritual Marriage: Sexual Abstinence in Medieval Wedlock* (Princeton: Princeton University Press, 1993)

Erler, Mary, 'Margery Kempe's White Clothes', *Medium Aevum*, 62 (1993), 78–83

Evans, Ruth, and Lesley Johnson, eds, *Feminist Readings in Middle English Literature: The Wife of Bath and all Her Sect* (Abingdon: Routledge, 1994)

Falconer, Rachel, and Denis Renevey, eds, *Medieval and Early Modern Literature, Science and Medicine*, Swiss Papers in English Language and Literature 28 (Tübingen: Gunter Narr, 2013)

Fanous, Samuel, and Vincent Gillespie, eds, *The Cambridge Companion to Medieval English Mysticism* (Cambridge: Cambridge University Press, 2011)

Farley, Mary Hardman, 'Her own creatur: Religion, Feminist Criticism, and the Functional Eccentricity of Margery Kempe', *Exemplaria*, 11 (1999), 1–21

Farmer, S., and B.H. Rosenwein, eds, *Monks and Nuns, Saints and Outcasts: Religion in Medieval Society; Essays in Honor of Lester K. Little* (Ithaca, N.Y.: Cornell University Press, 2000)

Fildes, Valerie, *Breasts, Bottles and Babies: A History of Infant Feeding* (Edinburgh: Edinburgh University Press, 1986)

Finucci, Valeria, and Kevin Brownlee, eds, *Generation and Degeneration: Tropes of Reproduction in Literature and History from Antiquity to Early Modern Europe* (Durham, N.C., and London: Duke University Press, 2001)

Fletcher, Alan J., 'Death Lyrics from Two Fifteenth-Century Sermon Manuscripts', *Notes and Queries* n.s. 23, 221 (1976), 341–2

——, *Late Medieval Popular Preaching in Britain and Ireland: Texts, Studies, and Interpretations* (Turnhout: Brepols, 2009)

Florschuetz, Angela, 'Women's Secrets: Childbirth, Pollution, and Purification in Northern *Octavian*', *Studies in the Age of Chaucer*, 30 (2008), 235–68

Foucault, Michel, *Madness and Civilisation* (London and New York: Routledge, 1961)

Fradenburg, Louise, and Carla Freccero, eds, *Premodern Sexualities* (New York and London: Routledge, 1996)

Freeman, Phyllis R., Carley Rees Bogarad, and Diane E. Sholomskas, 'Margery Kempe, a New Theory: The Inadequacy of Hysteria and Postpartum Psychosis as Diagnostic Categories', *History of Psychiatry*, 1 (1990), 169–90

French, Roger, Jon Arrizabalaga, Andrew Cunningham, and Luis Garcia, eds, *Medicine from the Black Death to the French Disease* (Aldershot: Ashgate, 1998)

Freud, Sigmund, *On Murder, Mourning and Melancholia*, trans. Shaun Whiteside (London: Penguin Classics, 2005)

Fuller, Robert C., *Spirituality in the Flesh: Bodily Sources of Religious Experience* (Oxford: Oxford University Press, 2008)

Fuss, Diana, *Essentially Speaking: Feminism, Nature and Difference* (New York: Routledge, 1989)

Galloway, Andrew, ed., *The Cambridge Companion to Medieval English Culture* (Cambridge: Cambridge University Press, 2011)

Garcia-Ballester, Luis, Roger French, Jon Arrizabalaga, and Andrew Cunningham, eds, *Practical Medicine from Salerno to the Black Death* (Cambridge: Cambridge University Press, 1994)

Gemi-Iordanou, Effie, et al., eds, *Medicine, Healing and Performance* (Oxford: Oxbow Books, 2014)

Gertsman, Elina, ed., *Crying in the Middle Ages: Tears of History* (London: Routledge, 2012)

——, ed., *Visualising Medieval Performance: Perspectives, Histories, Contexts* (Abingdon and New York: Routledge, 2016)

Gibson, Gail McMurray, 'Scene and Obscene: Seeing and Performing Late Medieval Childbirth', *The Journal of Medieval and Early Modern Studies*, 29 (1999), 7–24

——, *Theatre of Devotion: East Anglian Drama and Society in the Late Middle Ages* (Chicago and London: University of Chicago Press, 1989)

Gillespie, Vincent, 'Dead Still / Still Dead', *The Mediaeval Journal*, 1 (2011), 53–78

——, 'Strange Images of Death: The Passion in Later Medieval English Devotional and Mystical Writing', *Analecta Cartusiana*, 117 (1987), 110–59

Glasscoe, Marion, ed., *The Medieval Mystical Tradition in England: Papers Read at Dartington Hall, July 1984* (Cambridge: D.S. Brewer, 1984)

——, ed., *The Medieval Mystical Tradition in England: Papers Read at Dartington Hall, July 1992* (Cambridge: D.S. Brewer, 1992)

——, ed., *The Medieval Mystical Tradition in England: Papers Read at the Exeter Symposium, July 1980* (Exeter: Exeter University Press, 1980)

——, ed., *The Medieval Mystical Tradition in England, Ireland and Wales: Exeter Symposium VI; Papers Read at Charney Manor, July 1991* (Cambridge: D.S. Brewer, 1999)

Glaze, Florence Eliza, and Brian K. Nance, eds, *Between Text and Patient: The Medical Enterprise in Medieval and Early Modern Europe* (Florence: Sismel, 2011)

Glucklich, Ariel, *Sacred Pain: Hurting the Body for the Sake of the Soul* (Oxford: Oxford University Press, 2001)

Goddard, Richard, and Teresa Phipps, eds, *Town Courts and Urban Society in Late Medieval England, 1250–1550* (Cambridge: D.S. Brewer, 2019)

Goldberg, P.J.P., ed., *Woman is a Worthy Wight: Women in Medieval English Society, 1200–1500* (Stroud: Sutton, 1992)

Goodman, Anthony, *Margery Kempe and Her World* (London and New York: Longman, 2002)

Green, Monica, 'Bibliography on Medieval Women, Gender, and Medicine (1985–2009)', Digital Library of Sciència.cat (2010), Universitat de Barcelona: <http://www.sciencia.cat/biblioteca/documents/GreenCumulativeBibFeb2010.pdf>

——, 'From "Diseases of Women" to "Secrets of Women": The Transformation of Gynaecological Literature in the Later Middle Ages', *Journal of Medieval and Early Modern Studies*, 30 (2000), 5–39

——, *Making Women's Medicine Masculine: The Rise of Male Authority in Pre-Modern Gynaecology* (Oxford: Oxford University Press, 2008)

——, 'Obstetrical and Gynaecological Texts in Middle English', *Studies in the Age of Chaucer*, 14 (1992), 53–88

Grosz, Elizabeth, *Volatile Bodies: Toward a Corporeal Feminism* (Bloomington and Indianapolis: Indiana University Press, 1994)

Hanawalt, Barbara, and David Wallace, eds, *Bodies and Disciplines: Intersections of Literature and History in Fifteenth-Century England* (Minneapolis and London: University of Minnesota Press, 1996)

Harding, Wendy, 'Medieval Women's Unwritten Discourse on Motherhood: A Reading of Two Fifteenth-Century Texts', *Women's Studies*, 21 (1992), 197–209

Heffernan, Thomas J., ed., *The Popular Literature of Medieval England* (Knoxville: University of Tennessee Press, 1985)

Hellwarth, Jennifer Wynne, *The Reproductive Unconscious in Medieval and Early Modern England* (New York and London: Routledge, 2002)

Henderson, John, *The Renaissance Hospital: Healing the Body and Healing the Soul* (New Haven and London: Yale University Press, 2006)

Herlihy, David, *Medieval Households* (Cambridge, Mass.: Harvard University Press, 1985)

Hirsch, John C., 'Author and Scribe in *The Book of Margery Kempe*', *Medium Aevum*, 44 (1975), 145–50

Hogg, James, 'Mount Grace Charterhouse and Late Medieval Spirituality', *Analecta Cartusiana*, 82 (1980), 1–43

Holloway, Julia Bolton, Joan Bechtold, and Constance S. Wright, eds, *Equally in God's Image: Women in the Middle Ages* (New York: Peter Lang, 1990)

Hollywood, Amy, 'Acute Melancholia', *Harvard Theological Review*, 99 (2006), 381–406

——, and Patricia Z. Beckman, eds, *The Cambridge Companion to Christian Mysticism* (Cambridge: Cambridge University Press, 2012)

Holmes, Martha Stoddard, 'Thinking through Pain', *Literature and Medicine*, 24 (2005), 127–41

Howes, Laura L., 'On the Birth of Margery Kempe's Last Child', *Modern Philology*, 90 (1992), 220–5

Jacquart, Danielle, and Claude Thomasset, *Sexuality and Medicine in the Middle Ages*, trans. Matthew Adamson (Cambridge: Polity Press, 1988)

Jantzen, Grace, *Becoming Divine: Towards a Feminist Philosophy of Religion* (Manchester: Manchester University Press, 1998)

Jones, E.A., ed., *The Medieval Mystical Tradition in England: Exeter Symposium VIII; Papers Read at Charney Manor, July 2011* (Cambridge: D.S. Brewer, 2013)

Jones, Peter Murray, and Lea T. Olsan, 'Performative Rituals for Conception and Childbirth in England, 900–1500', *Bulletin of the History of Medicine*, 89 (2015), 406–33

Kachel, A. Friederike, L.S. Premo, and Jean-Jacques Hublin, 'Grandmothering and Natural Selection Revisited', *Proceedings: Biological Sciences*, 278 (2011), 1939–41

Kalas Williams, Laura, '"Slayn for Goddys lofe": Margery Kempe's Melancholia and the Bleeding of Tears', *Medieval Feminist Forum: A Journal of Gender and Sexuality*, 52 (2016), 84–100

——, 'The *Swetenesse* of Confection: A Recipe for Spiritual Health in London, British Library, Additional MS 61823, *The Book of Margery Kempe*', *Studies in the Age of Chaucer*, 40 (2018), 155–90

Kalof, Linda, ed., *A Cultural History of the Human Body in the Medieval Age* (London and New York: Bloomsbury, 2010)

Katajala-Peltomaa, Sari, and Susanna Niiranen, eds, *Mental (Dis)Order in Later Medieval Europe* (Leiden and Boston: Brill, 2014)

Kemp, Simon, *Medieval Psychology* (New York: Greenwood Press, 1990)

Ker, Neil, ed., *Medieval Libraries of Great Britain: A List of Surviving Books*, 2nd edn (London: Butler and Tanner, 1964)

Kerby-Fulton, Kathryn, ed., *Women and the Divine in Literature before 1700: Essays in Memory of Margot Louis* (Victoria: ELS Editions, 2009)

——, and Maidie Hilmo, and Linda Olson, eds, *Opening up Middle English Manuscripts: Literary and Visual Approaches* (Ithaca, N.Y.: Cornell University Press, 2012)

——, John J. Thompson, and Sarah Baechle, eds, *New Directions in Medieval Manuscript Studies and Reading Practices: Essays in Honor of Derek Pearsall* (Notre Dame, Ill.: University of Notre Dame Press, 2014)

Kern-Stähler, Annette, Beatrix Busse, and Wietse de Boer, eds, *The Five Senses in Medieval and Early Modern England* (Leiden: Brill, 2016)

Kieckhefer, Richard, *Unquiet Souls: Fourteenth-Century Saints and Their Religious Milieu* (Chicago: University of Chicago Press, 1984)

Kirkwood, Thomas B.L., and Daryl P. Shanley, 'The Connections between General and Reproductive Senescence and the Evolutionary Basis of Menopause', *Annals of the New York Academy of Sciences*, 1204 (2010), 21–9

Klapisch-Zuber, Christiane, *Women, Family and Ritual in Renaissance Italy*, trans. Lydia Cochrane (Chicago and London: University of Chicago Press, 1985)

Kleinman, Arthur, *The Illness Narratives: Suffering, Healing and the Human Condition* (New York: Basic Books, 1988)

Klibansky, Raymond, Erwin Panofsky, and Fritz Saxl, *Saturn and Melancholy: Studies in the History of Natural Philosophy, Religion and Art* (London: Nelson, 1964)

Knowles, David, *The English Mystical Tradition* (London: Burns and Oates, 1961)

Kowaleski, Maryanne, and P.J.P. Goldberg, eds, *Medieval Domesticity: Home, Housing and Household in Medieval England* (Cambridge: Cambridge University Press, 2008)

Kroll, Jerome, and Bernard Bachrach, 'Visions and Psychopathology in the Middle Ages', *The Journal of Nervous and Mental Disease*, 170 (1982), 41–9

Krötzl, Christian, Katariina Mustakallio, and Jenni Kuuliala, eds, *Infirmity in Antiquity and the Middle Ages: Social and Cultural Approaches to Health, Weakness and Care* (Farnham and Burlington, Vt.: Ashgate, 2015)

Krug, Rebecca, *Margery Kempe and the Lonely Reader* (Ithaca, N.Y., and London: Cornell University Press (2017)

Lakoff, George, and Mark Johnson, *Philosophy in the Flesh: The Embodied Mind and Its Challenge to Western Thought* (New York: Basic Books, 1999)

Lees, Clare A., and Gillian R. Overing, *A Place to Believe in: Locating Medieval Landscapes* (Philadelphia: Pennsylvania State University Press, 2006)

Lewis, Mary E., and Rebecca Gowland, 'Brief and Precarious Lives: Infant Mortality in Contrasting Sites from Medieval and Post-Medieval England (AD 850–1859)', *American Journal of Physical Anthropology*, 134 (2007), 117–29

Leyser, Conrad, and Lesley Smith, eds, *Motherhood, Religion, and Society in Medieval Europe, 400–1400* (Farnham: Ashgate, 2011)

Lindblom, U., et al., 'Pain Terms: A Current List with Definitions and Notes on Usage', *Pain*, 24 (1986), Supplement 1, S1–S226

Lochrie, Karma, *Margery Kempe and Translations of the Flesh* (Philadelphia: University of Pennsylvania Press, 1991)

Lomperis, Linda, and Sarah Stanbury, eds, *Feminist Approaches to the Body in Medieval Literature* (Philadelphia: University of Pennsylvania Press, 1997)

Lynch, Joseph H., *Godparents and Kinship in Early Medieval Europe* (Princeton: Princeton University Press, 1986)

MacDonald, A.A., H.N.B. Ridderbos, and R.M. Schulusemann, eds, *The Broken Body: Passion Devotion in Late-Medieval Culture* (Groningen: Egbert Forsten, 1998)

MacKendrick, Karmen, 'The Multipliable Body', *Postmedieval: A Journal of Medieval Cultural Studies*, 1 (2010), 108–14

MacLehose, William F., *A Tender Age: Cultural Anxieties over the Child in the Twelfth and Thirteenth Centuries* (New York: Columbia University Press, 2008)

Makowski, Elizabeth M., 'The Conjugal Debt and Medieval Canon Law', *Journal of Medieval History*, 3:2 (1977), 99–114

McAvoy, Liz Herbert, *Authority and the Female Body in the Writings of Julian of Norwich and Margery Kempe* (Cambridge: D.S. Brewer, 2004)

——, '"Flourish like a garden": Pain, Purgatory and Salvation in the Writing of Medieval Religious Women', *Medieval Feminist Forum: A Journal of Gender and Sexuality*, 50 (2014), 33–60

——, 'Margery's Last Child', *Notes and Queries*, 46:2 (1999), 181–3

——, *Medieval Anchoritisms: Gender, Space and the Solitary Life* (Cambridge: D.S. Brewer, 2011)

——, and Mari Hughes-Edwards, eds, *Anchorites, Wombs and Tombs: Intersections of Gender and Enclosure in the Middle Ages* (Cardiff: University of Wales Press, 2005)

——, and Diane Watt, eds, *The History of British Writing, 700–1500* (Basingstoke and New York: Palgrave Macmillan, 2011)

McCaffery, Margo, *Nursing Practice: Theories Related to Cognition, Bodily Pain, and Man–Environment Interactions* (Los Angeles: UCLA Student Store, 1968)

McCann, Daniel, *Soul-Health: Therapeutic Reading in Later Medieval England* (Cardiff: University of Wales Press, 2018)

McClanan, Anne L., and Karen Rosoff Encarnación, *The Material Culture of Sex, Procreation, and Marriage in Premodern Europe* (New York: Palgrave, 2002)

McCracken, Peggy, *The Curse of Eve, the Wound of the Hero: Blood, Gender, and Medieval Literature* (Philadelphia: University of Pennsylvania Press, 2003)

McEntire, Sandra, ed., *Margery Kempe: A Book of Essays* (New York and London: Garland, 1992)

McNamara, Jo Ann, 'Sexual Equality and the Cult of Virginity in Early Christian Thought', *Feminist Studies*, 3 (1976), 152–4

McNamer, Sarah, *Affective Meditation and the Invention of Medieval Compassion* (Philadelphia: University of Pennsylvania Press, 2010)

Medcalf, Stephen, ed., *The Later Middle Ages* (London: Methuen, 1981)

Melzack, Ronald, and Patrick Wall, *The Challenge of Pain*, 2nd edn (London: Penguin, 1996)

Merback, Mitchell B., *The Thief, the Cross and the Wheel: Pain and the Spectacle of Punishment in Medieval and Renaissance Europe* (London: Reaktion Books, 1999)

Miller, Sarah Alison, *Medieval Monstrosity and the Female Body* (New York and Oxon: Routledge, 2010)

Mills, Robert, *Suspended Animation: Pain, Pleasure and Punishment in Medieval Culture* (London: Reaktion Books, 2005)

Minnis, Alastair, *Translations of Authority in Medieval English Literature: Valuing the Vernacular* (Cambridge: Cambridge University Press, 2009)

———, and Rosalynn Voaden, eds, *Medieval Holy Women in the Christian Tradition, c. 1100–c. 1500* (Turnhout: Brepols, 2010)

Mitchell, Linda E., and Katherine L. French, eds, *The Ties that Bind: Essays in Medieval British History in Honor of Barbara Hanawalt* (Farnham: Ashgate, 2011)

Mitchell, Maria, *The Book of Margery Kempe: Scholarship, Community, and Criticism* (New York: Peter Lang, 2005)

Mitchell, Piers D., 'Retrospective Diagnosis and the Use of Historical Texts for Investigating Disease in the Past', *International Journal of Paleopathology*, 1 (2011), 81–8

Mongan, Olga Burakov, 'Slanderers and Saints: The Function of Slander in *The Book of Margery Kempe*', *Philological Quarterly*, 84 (2005), 27–47

Montford, Angela, *Health, Sickness, Medicine and the Friars in the Thirteenth and Fourteenth Centuries* (Aldershot and Burlington, Vt.: Ashgate, 2004)

Mooney, Catherine, ed., *Gendered Voices: Medieval Saints and Their Interpreters* (Philadelphia: University of Pennsylvania Press, 1995)

Morris, Bridget, *St Birgitta of Sweden* (Woodbridge: Boydell Press, 1999)

———, and Veronica O'Mara, eds, *The Translation of the Works of St Birgitta of Sweden into the Medieval European Vernaculars* (Turnhout: Brepols, 2000)

Morris, David, *The Culture of Pain* (Berkley and Los Angeles: University of California Press, 1991)

Moscoso, Javier, *Pain: A Cultural History*, trans. Sarah Thomas and Paul House (Basingstoke: Palgrave Macmillan, 2012)

Mowbray, Donald, *Pain and Suffering in Medieval Theology: Academic Debates at the University of Paris in the Thirteenth Century* (Woodbridge: Boydell Press, 2009)

Muessig, Carolyn, 'Signs of Salvation: The Evolution of Stigmatic Spirituality before Francis of Assisi', *Church History*, 82:1 (2013), 40–68

Mulder-Bakker, Anneke B., 'The Metamorphosis of Woman: Transmission of Knowledge and the Problems of Gender', *Gender and History*, 12 (2000), 642–64

———, ed., *The Prime of Their Lives: Wise Old Women in Pre-Industrial Europe* (Leuven, Paris, and Dudley: Peeters, 2004)

——, ed., *Sancity and Motherhood: Essays on Holy Mothers in the Middle Ages* (New York and London: Routledge, 2013)

——, and Liz Herbert McAvoy, eds, *Women and Experience in Later Medieval Writing: Reading the Book of Life* (New York: Palgrave Macmillan, 2009)

Neel, Carol, ed., *Medieval Families: Perspectives on Marriage, Household, and Children* (Toronto and London: University of Toronto Press, 2004)

Neugebauer, Richard, 'Medieval and Early Modern Theories of Mental Illness', *Archives of General Psychiatry*, 36 (1979), 477–83

Newman, Barbara, *From Virile Woman to Woman Christ: Studies in Medieval Religion and Literature* (Philadelphia: University of Pennsylvania Press, 1995)

——, 'Intimate Pieties: Holy Trinity and Holy Family in the late Middle Ages', *Religion and Literature*, 31 (1999), 77–101

Niebrzydowski, Sue, '*Asperges me, Domine, hyssopo*: Male Voices, Female Interpretation and the Medieval English Purification of Women after Childbirth Ceremony', *Early Music*, 39 (2011), 327–34

——, *Bonoure and Buxom: A Study of Wives in Late Medieval English Literature* (Bern: Peter Lang, 2006)

——, ed. *Middle Aged Women in the Middle Ages* (Cambridge: D.S. Brewer, 2011)

Nightingale, Pamela, 'Some New Evidence of Crises and Trends of Mortality in Late Medieval England', *Past & Present*, 187 (2005), 33–68

Ober, William B., 'Margery Kempe: Hysteria and Mysticism Reconciled', *Literature and Medicine*, 4 (1985), 24–40

Olsan, Lea T., 'Charms and Prayer in Medieval Medical Theory and Practice', *Social History of Medicine*, 16 (2003), 343–66

——, 'The Language of Charms in a Middle English Recipe Collection', *ANQ: A Quarterly Journal of Short Articles, Notes and Reviews*, 18 (2005), 29–35

Olson, Linda, and Kathryn Kerby-Fulton, eds, *Voices in Dialogue: Reading Women in the Middle Ages* (Notre Dame, Ill.: University of Notre Dame Press, 2005)

Olson, Trisha, 'The Medieval Blood Sanction and the Divine Beneficence of Pain: 1100–1450', *Journal of Law and Religion*, 22 (2006/7), 63–129

Orlemanski, Julie, 'How to Kiss a Leper', *Postmedieval: A Journal of Medieval Cultural Studies*, 3 (2012), 142–57

——, 'Jargon and the Matter of Medicine in Middle English', *Journal of Medieval and Early Modern Studies*, 42 (2012), 395–420

Pablo de, Angel González, 'The Medicine of the Soul: The Origin and Development of Thought on the Soul, Diseases of the Soul and Their Treatment, in Medieval and Renaissance Medicine', *History of Psychiatry*, 5 (1994), 483–516

Park, Hwanhee, 'Domestic Ideals and Devotional Authority in *The Book of Margery Kempe*', *The Journal of Medieval Religious Cultures*, 40 (2014), 1–19

Park, Kathryn, *Secrets of Women: Gender, Generation, and the Origins of Human Dissection* (Brooklyn, N.Y.: Zone Books, 2006)

Parsons, John Carmie, and Bonnie Wheeler, eds, *Medieval Mothering* (New York and London: Garland, 1996)

Paxton, Frederick S., 'Signa Mortifera: Death and Prognostication in Early Medieval Monastic Medicine', *Bulletin of the History of Medicine*, 67 (1993), 631–50

Petroff, Elizabeth, *Medieval Women's Visionary Literature* (Oxford: Oxford University Press, 1986)

Phillips, Kim, ed., *A Cultural History of Women in the Middle Ages* (London and New York: Bloomsbury, 2013)

Pierce, Joanne M., '"Green Women" and Blood Pollution: Some Medieval Rituals for the Churching of Women after Childbirth', *Studia Liturgica*, 29:2 (1999), 191–215

Porter, Laurel, and Laurence M. Porter, eds, *Aging in Literature* (Troy, Mich.: International Book Publishers, 1984)

Powell, Hilary, 'The "Miracle of Childbirth": The Portrayal of Parturient Women in Medieval Miracle Narratives', *Social History of Medicine*, 25 (2012), 795–811

Radden, Jennifer, *The Nature of Melancholy: From Aristotle to Kristeva* (Oxford: Oxford University Press, 2000)

Rawcliffe, Carole, *Leprosy in Medieval England* (Woodbridge: Boydell Press, 2006)

——, *Medicine for the Soul: The Life, Death and Resurrection of an English Medieval Hospital, St Giles's, Norwich, c. 1249–1550* (Stroud: Sutton, 1999)

Renevey, Denis, and Christiania Whitehead, eds, *Writing Religious Women: Female Spiritual and Textual Practices in Late Medieval England* (Cardiff: University of Wales Press, 2000)

Resnick, Irven M., 'Medieval Roots of the Myth of Jewish Males Menses', *The Harvard Theological Review*, 93 (July 2000), 241–63

Rey, Roselyn, *The History of Pain*, trans. Louise Elliott Wallace, J.A. Cadden, and S.W. Cadden (Cambridge, Mass., and London: Harvard University Press, 1993)

Riddle, John M., *Contraception and Abortion from the Ancient World to the Renaissance* (Cambridge, Mass.: Harvard University Press, 1992)

Riehle, Wolfgang, *The Middle English Mystics* (London, Boston, and Henley: Routledge and Kegan Paul, 1981)

——, *The Secret Within: Hermits, Recluses, and Spiritual Outsiders in Medieval England* (Icatha, N.Y., and London: Cornell University Press, 2014)

Robertson, Elizabeth, and Christine M. Rose, eds, *Representing Rape in Medieval and Early Modern Literature* (New York: Palgrave, 2001)

Roffey, Simon, and Phil Marter, 'Treating Leprosy: Inside the Medieval Hospital of St Mary Magdalen, Winchester', *Current Archaeology*, 267 (2012), 12–18

Rose, Mary Beth, ed., *Women in the Middle Ages and Renaissance* (Syracuse, N.Y.: Syracuse University Press, 1986)

Rosenthal, Joel T., ed., *Medieval Women and the Sources of Medieval History* (Athens: University of Georgia Press, 1990)

Rubin, Miri, *Corpus Christi: The Eucharist in Late Medieval Culture* (Cambridge: Cambridge University Press, 1991)

——, *Mother of God: A History of the Virgin Mary* (London: Penguin Books, 2010)

Ruether, Rosemary Radford, ed., *Religion and Sexism: Images of Women in the Jewish and Christian Traditions* (New York: Wipf and Stock, 1974)

Salih, Sarah, *Versions of Virginity in Late Medieval Europe* (Cambridge: D.S. Brewer, 2001)

Saunders, Corrine, and Jamie Kinstry, eds, 'Medievalism and the Medical Humanities', special issue, *Postmedieval: A Journal of Medieval Cultural Studies*, 8 (2017)

Scanlon, Larry, ed., *The Cambridge Companion to Medieval English Literature, 1100–1500* (Cambridge: Cambridge University Press, 2009)

Scarry, Elaine, *The Body in Pain* (New York and Oxford: Oxford University Press, 1985)

Sears, Elizabeth, *The Ages of Man: Medieval Interpretations of the Life Cycle* (Princeton: Princeton University Press, 1986)

Shahar, Shulamith, *Childhood in the Middle Ages* (London and New York: Routledge, 1990)

——, *Growing Old in the Middle Ages: 'Winter clothes us in shadow and pain'* (London and New York: Routledge, 1997)

——, 'Who Were Old in the Middle Ages?', *Social History of Medicine*, 6 (1993), 313–34

Siggins, Lorraine D., 'Mourning: A Critical Survey of the Literature', *International Journal of Psycho-Analysis*, 47 (1966), 14–25

Skemer, Don, *Binding Words: Textual Amulets in the Middle Ages* (Philadelphia: Pennsylvania State University Press, 2006)

Sobecki, Sebastian, '"The writyng of this tretys": Margery Kempe's Son and the Authorship of Her Book', *Studies in the Age of Chaucer*, 37 (2015), 257–83

Soergel, Philip M., and Andrew Barnes, eds, *Sexuality and Culture in Medieval and Renaissance Europe* (New York: AMS Press, 2005)

Sperling, Jutta Gisela, ed., *Medieval and Renaissance Lactations: Images, Rhetorics, Practices* (London and New York: Routledge, 2013)

Staley, Lynn Johnson, *Margery Kempe's Dissenting Fictions* (Philadelphia: Pennsylvania State University Press, 1994)

——, 'The Trope of the Scribe and the Question of Literary Authority in the Works of Julian of Norwich and Margery Kempe', *Speculum*, 66 (1991), 820–38

Stiller, Nikki, *Eve's Orphans: Mothers and Daughters in Medieval English Literature* (Westport, Conn., and London: Greenwood Press, 1980)

Stolberg, Michael, 'A Woman's Hell? Medical Perceptions of Menopause in Preindustrial Europe', *Bulletin of the History of Medicine*, 73 (1999), 404–28

Stork, Nancy P., 'Did Margery Kempe Suffer from Tourette's Syndrome?', *Mediaeval Studies*, 59 (1997), 261–300

Swanson, R.N., *Religion and Devotion in Europe, c. 1215–1515* (Cambridge: Cambridge University Press, 1995)

Szarmach, Paul E., ed., *An Introduction to the Medieval Mystics of Europe* (Albany: State University of New York Press, 1984)

Tarvers, Josephine, 'The Alleged Illiteracy of Margery Kempe: A Reconsideration of the Evidence', *Medieval Perspectives*, 11 (1996), 113–24

Thurston, Herbert, 'Margery the Astonishing', *The Month*, 168 (1936), 446–56

Toussaint-Samat, Maguelonne, *A History of Food*, trans. Anthea Bell (Chichester: Wiley Blackwell, 2009)

Towler, Jean, *Midwives in History and Society* (London: Croom Helm, 1986)

Turner, Marion, ed., *A Handbook of Middle English Studies* (Oxford: Wiley-Blackwell, 2013)

——, ed., 'Medical Discourse in Premodern Europe', special issue, *Journal of Medieval and Early Modern Studies*, 46 (2016)

Uhlman, Diana R., 'The Comfort of Voice, the Solace of Script: Orality and Literacy in *The Book of Margery Kempe*', *Studies in Philology*, 91 (1994), 50–69

Van Ginhoven, Brian, 'Margery Kempe and the Legal Status of Defamation', *The Journal of Medieval Religious Cultures*, 40:1 (2014), 20–43

Varnam, Laura, 'The Crucifix, the Pietà, and the Female Mystic: Devotional Objects and Performative Identity in *The Book of Margery Kempe*', *Journal of Medieval Religious Cultures*, 41 (2015), 208–37

——, 'The Importance of St Margaret's Church in *The Book of Margery Kempe*: A Sacred Place and an Exemplary Parishioner', *Nottingham Medieval Studies* 61 (2017), 197–243

Voaden, Rosalynn, *God's Words, Women's Voices: The Discernment of Spirits in the Writing of Late-Medieval Women Visionaries* (York: York Medieval Press, 1999)

——, ed., *Prophets Abroad: The Reception of Continental Holy Women in Late-Medieval England* (Cambridge: D.S. Brewer, 1996)

——, and Diane Wolfthal, eds, *Framing the Family: Narrative and Representation in the Medieval and Early Modern Periods* (Tempe: Arizona Center for Medieval and Renaissance Studies, 2005)

Voigts, Linda E., and Michael R. McVaugh, 'A Latin Technical Phlebotomy and Its Middle English Translation', *Transactions of the American Philosophical Society*, 74:2 (1984), 1–69

Wack, Mary Frances, *Lovesickness in the Middle Ages: The 'Viaticum' and Its Commentaries* (Philadelphia: University of Pennsylvania Press, 1990)

Walker, Sue Sheridan, ed., *Wife and Widow in Medieval England* (Ann Arbor: University of Michigan Press, 1993)

Wall, Patrick, *The Science of Suffering* (London: Weidenfeld and Nicholson, 1999)

Wallace, David, *Strong Women: Life, Text, and Territory, 1347–1645* (Oxford: Oxford University Press, 2011)

Wallace, Edwin R., and John Gach, eds, *History of Psychiatry and Medical Psychology: With an Epilogue on Psychiatry and the Mind–Body Relation* (New York: Springer, 2008)

Wallis, Faith, ed., *Medieval Medicine: A Reader* (Toronto: University of Toronto Press, 2010)

Warner, Marina, *Alone of All Her Sex: The Myth and the Cult of the Virgin Mary* (London: Weidenfeld, 1976)

Watson, Andrew G., *Medieval Libraries of Great Britain: A List of Surviving Books, Supplement to the Second Edition* (London: Royal Historical Society, 1987)

Watt, Diane, 'Margery Kempe', Oxford Bibliographies Online <DOI: 10.1093/obo/9780199846719-0034>

———, *Medieval Women's Writing: Works by and for Women, 1100–1500* (Cambridge: Polity, 2007)

Webb, Diana, *Pilgrimage in Medieval England* (London and New York: Hambledon and London, 2000)

Williams, Norman Powell, *The Ideas of the Fall and of Original Sin: A Historical and Critical Study* (London: Longmans, 1927)

Williams, Tara, '"As thu wer a wedow": Margery Kempe's Wifehood and Widowhood', *Exemplaria*, 21:4 (2009), 345–62

———, 'Manipulating Mary: Maternal, Sexual, and Textual Authority in *The Book of Margery Kempe*', *Modern Philology*, 107 (2010), 528–55

Winstead, Karen A., 'The Conversion of Margery Kempe's Son', *English Language Notes*, 32 (1994), 9–13

Wood, Charles T., 'The Doctor's Dilemma: Sin, Salvation, and the Menstrual Cycle in Medieval Thought', *Speculum*, 56 (1981), 710–27

Wood, Diana, ed., *Women and Religion in Medieval England* (Oxford: Oxbow Books, 2003)

Yoshikawa, Naoë Kukita, 'Holy Medicine and Diseases of the Soul: Henry of Lancaster and *Le livre de seyntz medicines*', *Medical History*, 53 (2009), 397–414

———, *Margery Kempe's Meditations: The Context of Medieval Devotional Literature, Liturgy, and Iconography* (Cardiff: University of Wales Press, 2007)

———, ed., *Medicine, Religion and Gender in Medieval Culture* (Cambridge: D.S. Brewer, 2015)

Youngs, Deborah, *The Life Cycle in Western Europe, c. 1300–1500* (Manchester: Manchester University Press, 2006)

Zimmerman, Susan, 'Leprosy in the Medieval Imaginary', *Journal of Medieval and Early Modern Studies*, 38:3 (2008), 559–87

Ziolkowski, Jan, ed., *Obscenity: Social Control and Artistic Creation in the European Middle Ages* (Leiden and Boston: Brill, 1998)

———, 'Old Wives' Tales: Classicism and Anti-Classicism from Apuleius to Chaucer', *The Journal of Medieval Latin*, 12 (2002), 90–113

Index

Aachen 137 n.46, 165, 196 n.61, 199, 200, 206
Adam 34–6, 75 n.61, 212
affective piety 11–12, 16, 18, 41, 45–47, 51, 119–20, 140, 150, 162, 176, 180–2, 190, 199, 205–6, 208–9
affective receptivity 24, 31, 33, 45–7, 58
age *see also* life-course
aged asceticism 26, 183, 190, 194, 220
ageing, process of 33, 101, 103, 193
Ages of Man 15, 33, 164
    middle age 25, 97–126, 149, 201
    old age (senescence) 26, 33, 98 n.7, 99, 101–4, 156, 183–209, 211–12, 220
Aldobrandino of Siena 103, 117 n.89, 185
Aleyn of Lynn, Master 7
Allen, Hope Emily 5, 59 n.1, 89 n.114, 90 n.119–20, 114 n.78, 118 n.92, 135 n.42, 168 n.31
al-Qānūn fī'l-tibb 19, 34 n.25
Amis and Amiloun 151
analgesia 25, 63, 90–4, 171, 198
Anatomy of Melancholy, The 38
anchoritism 50 n.83, 63 n.40, 80–1, 109, 120, 124, 143, 150, 160, 181 n.76, 187, 205, 213 n.14, 218, 218 n.30
Ancrene Wisse 108, 109 n.55, 143, 187, 202, 204–5, 212
Angela of Foligno 49 n.80, 60–1, 100 n.13, 145
Anselm of Canterbury 85, 119
Aquinas, Thomas 24, 31, 37, 62 n.13, 75, 108, 186, 194, 202–5
Aristotle 24, 47, 101
ars moriendi 167, 217
asceticism 18, 25, 26, 31, 54, 57, 61, 62, 79–83, 88, 161, 185, 194, 200, 220
    aged asceticism see under age
    fasting 61, 66, 79–80, 85–6, 88, 188, 204

hair-shirt 72, 80, 96
    on pilgrimage *see* pilgrimage
    self-abasement 62, 142, 144–7, 200
    suffering slander 94–6, 150, 154, 208
Augustine 36–7, 128, 155 n.121, 163–4, 185, 188
authority, of Margery Kempe 11 n.23, 16, 23, 66, 82, 96, 97 n.3, 99, 101, 134, 146, 148, 183, 192, 195, 201, 207, 219–20
authorship 6, 9–16, 101, 159 n.127, 165, 178 n.69, 183–4, 204, 219
Autumn 15, 36
Averroës 47
Avicenna 19, 24, 34, 42, 45 n.62, 101, 115, 122, 130, 188

baptism 133 n.33, 135
barrenness 38, 53, 54 n.99, 98, 105 n.38
Bartholomaeus Anglicus 2, 24, 34, 70, 107, 122, 130, 147, 164, 185, 189, 202, 206 n.100
Beatrice of Nazareth 30, 48, 107
Bernard of Clairvaux 24, 69, 85, 94, 119 n.95, 142, 194
Bernard of Gordon 77, 103, 113
birth *see also* childbirth 34, 191
    of Jesus 12, 14, 111–16, 175
    spiritual birth 25, 55, 81, 93, 107, 137, 152, 219
Bishop's Lynn 7, 41, 45, 57, 59, 64, 71 n.47, 73, 81, 113 n.77, 114 n.78, 117, 121, 123, 134, 136 n.42, 144 n.76, 149, 153, 158 n.125, 167, 168, 174, 177 n.65, 195, 199 n.70, 207, 210, 213, 216–18, 220
black bile 15, 26, 32–6, 42, 44–5, 47–9, 143, 161, 172
blindness 36 n.33, 37, 68, 107, 147
blood 25, 32–5, 39 n.43, 49, 50–1, 55, 63, 71 n.45, 97, 100, 105–10, 120, 153, 172, 175, 186, 188, 220
    blood piety 50, 106

245

blood relics 107, 199
Christ's blood 55, 63, 72, 85, 93
   n.129, 106, 108, 120, 179–82
menstrual blood 35, 38, 83, 98, 100,
   104, 105, 108–10, 131–2, 136
   n.45, 150–1, 188
Bonaventura 85 n.101, 190
Book of Margery Kempe, The
   Book II as distinct feature 16, 26,
     148, 183–4, 190, 191, 194, 201–3,
     205, 208–10, 216
   British Library, Additional MS 61823
     17, 18 n.2, 46, 137, 169, 220
   chronology of 15, 92 n.125, 117
     n.91, 119, 124 n.119, 165 n.20
Book of the Craft of Dying, The 167
brain 17, 20, 34, 35, 37, 42
Brakleye, Thomas 124
breasts *see also under* milk 42, 111, 116,
   119, 121, 132–3
Breviarium Bartholomei 139
Bridget of Sweden 14, 39 n.42, 61,
   80, 83 n.89, 99 n.8, 100 n.13, 112
   n.69, 116 n.86, 121, 129, 142, 145,
   148, 177, 184, 190, 194 n.52, 204,
   219
Brunham, John 64, 113 n.77, 216
Burton, Robert 38, 48, 58

Calais 195 n.53, 196 n.61, 199, 200
Calvary, Mount 51, 52, 56, 105
Canon of Medicine, The 19, 34 n.25
Catherine of Siena 26, 81, 119 n.95,
   162–5, 175, 179, 204, 209, 219 n.33
Causea et Curae 34
Celibacy *see* chastity
chastity 25, 62, 73, 74 n.57, 61–2,
   75–8, 84, 90, 92, 95–6, 98, 105, 114,
   123, 150, 170
   vow of 14, 25, 59 n.1, 62, 79, 84,
     87–9, 92, 94, 105, 117 n.91, 127,
     154, 155 n.121, 156
   white clothes as symbolic of 90
     n.120, 94–6, 203
childbearing 12, 61, 72, 73, 75, 78
   n.77, 80, 84, 93, 96, 100–1, 106, 120
   n.103, 129, 137, 140, 191, 212
childbirth *see also* birth 9, 23, 25, 55,
   56 n.106, 61–73, 77–8, 81, 84, 89,
   92, 103, 111–16, 125 n.20, 127, 135
   n.39 & n.41, 136–40, 146, 148, 182,
   188 n.27, 196, 220
   postpartum, state of being 9, 63–4,
     69–73, 89, 116, 127, 134–7, 140,

     141, 146, 148, 150, 160 n.132,
     169, 178
children
   of Margery Kempe 10, 25, 80, 89,
     113 n.77, 114–16, 124, 125, 148,
     189, 211, 219
   orphans 118, 120, 123
Christ
   body of 14, 16, 57, 60, 91, 93, 106,
     108, 127, 142, 144, 157, 161, 174,
     177, 179–82
   -child 25, 108, 112, 117, 119–21,
     123, 137, 174, 213
   crucifixion of 24, 52, 54, 107, 124,
     141, 161, 174–7, 181, 198
   as mother 91, 119, 120
   scourging of 177, 140
   wounds of 17, 47, 49–63, 69, 70,
     107, 144, 146–7, 163, 177–9
Christina Mirabilis 132
Christine de Pizan 100, 183, 193
Christus Medicus 6, 25, 54, 63, 88,
   127–9, 133
Church
   body of 160
   Elder 26, 206, 208, 210
   Fathers 24, 74, 79, 188
   liturgy 14, 71, 127
Churching *see also* purification 71, 127,
   136
Cistercians 69
Clare of Montefalco 69–70, 83 n.89,
   213
coldness, of body 2, 33, 37, 44, 47–9,
   53, 65, 77, 94, 101, 102, 131, 170,
   172, 187–9
commemoration, of Margery Kempe
   164, 219
compassion 12, 40 n.45, 55, 90–1,
   111–12, 120–1, 135, 146, 152, 199
Compendium medicinae 21, 24, 33, 76
   n.65
confession 42, 49, 63, 64, 66, 68, 69, 93
   n.129, 128, 152, 167
Constantine the African 24, 35, 88
constitution (physiological) 15, 21, 24,
   31, 33, 34, 37, 45, 47, 49, 53, 67, 77,
   85, 94, 101, 122
contamination 60, 82, 83, 109, 136
   n.45, 142, 144, 146
Crucifixion *see under* Christ
Cyrurgie of Guy de Chauliac 34, 65,
   143, 172

Danzig   153, 184
darkness   20, 34, 36–7, 47, 68
De Institutione Inclusarum   119–20
De Interioribus   19
De Medicina Animae   36, 49
De Melancholia   24
De Mulierum Affectibus   43
De Proprietatibus Rerum   2, 24, 34
De retardation accidentum senectutis   103
De Secretis Mulierum   22, 23, 49 n.81, 65,
      67, 78, 83–4, 94, 143, 170, 186, 197
death
   burial   66, 164, 182, 217, 218
   deathbed   161, 164, 167, 173–4, 182
   death surrogacy see surrogacy
   living death   26, 55, 162, 166, 174,
      176, 180
   prophecy of   164–7
   rituals   66, 174
dealbation   108
desire   24, 29, 30, 35–8, 42, 48, 52, 54,
      57–8, 61–2, 69, 76, 110, 114, 116,
      121–2, 129, 137, 141, 144, 146, 150,
      161–2, 165, 174, 178, 198
diagnosis   6, 8, 9, 13, 16, 39, 42, 45, 58,
      71, 149, 150, 220
Discretio Spirituum   9, 162,
disease   25, 34–5, 42, 45 n.66, 49, 65
      n.18, 74, 78–9, 109, 128, 145–7,
      149–50, 169, 183, 188, 199 n.69, 210
Dominicans   7, 22, 24, 55, 61 n.7, 69
      n.37, 117
Dorothy of Montau   61
dragges   2, 4 n.8, 10
dryness (of body)   2, 26, 33, 37, 47–9,
      52, 53, 58, 85, 99, 101–4, 116, 132,
      179, 181, 187, 188, 204, 206

Easter   52, 124, 198
Ebner, Margaret   30, 48
ecstasy   46, 47, 60, 93, 106, 161, 176,
      197, 213
Eden, Garden of   12
elements   33, 200
Elizabeth of Hungary   43 n.55, 49 n.80,
      61, 145, 184, 190, 194 n.52
Elizabeth of Spalbeek   42, 50
England   7, 11, 21, 23–4, 39, 43 n.55,
      114, 124, 153 n.113, 200, 202, 216,
      219,
epilepsy   9, 32, 46, 83
falling evil, the   46, 109
Eucharist   2, 26, 72, 93, 106–7, 128,
      140, 145, 161, 167, 174

Eve   12, 82, 116 n.86
even christen   26, 58, 119, 160, 167, 173
exsanguination   180–1
eyes   1 n.3, 8, 20, 32, 35–6, 50–4, 83,
      111, 114, 135 n.41, 147, 149, 162,
      171–2, 179, 186–7, 190, 196, 206
      n.100, 211, 220,
evil eye, the   187, 190

Fall of Man   83
fasting *see under* asceticism
fear   34, 37, 39, 52, 57, 63, 65–6, 68,
      82, 84, 86, 94, 96, 144 n.77, 146,
      162, 169 n.33, 187, 188 n.25,
      197–200
fecundity *see also* fruitfulness; fertility
      19, 25, 53, 55, 78, 89, 97, 99–100,
      103–5, 107, 110–11, 125–6, 158,
      161, 191, 206, 223
fertility *see also* fecundity; fruitfulness
      61, 98, 104, 107, 109–10, 196
Fifteen Oes, The   177, 178 n.68 & n.69,
      211 n.1
fire   33, 42, 68, 143, 174, 199 n.70
flesh   74, 91, 107, 109, 133, 156, 172
      n.42, 211–12
   of Christ   72, 91, 93, 127, 140, 142,
      160, 168, 180–1
   female   6, 8, 12–13, 26, 46, 58, 60,
      67, 69–70, 84, 93, 161, 168, 175,
      189, 200–1, 204, 212, 220
   injury to   54, 55, 60, 69–70, 160,
      180–1, 200
   purification of   85
fostering   25, 100, 117, 120, 122–4, 130
Foucault, Michel   147
Freud, Sigmund   9, 29, 38, 58, 114
Fruitfulness *see also* fecundity; fertility
      34, 47, 53, 54 n.99, 62, 76, 81, 84,
      96, 100, 104–5, 125–6, 136 n.44,
      139, 158, 194, 205, 208, 211

Galen   19–20, 24, 33, 43, 45 n.66, 77,
      84, 101, 108, 153, 171, 223, 224
Gate Control Theory   17
Gerard of Berry   37
Germany   22, 158 n.125, 184 n.5, 191,
      194–5
Gertrude of Helfta   69
Gilbertus Anglicus   21, 24, 33, 76 n.65,
      149, 186
God
   Godhead, the   32, 62, 90–2, 94, 105
      n.39, 121, 134, 157, 157 n.123, 165

Manhood, the   90, 93, 105 n.39, 121, 157, 165, 182
the Physician *see Christus Medicus*
Godparent   25, 100, 118, 122–3, 135 n.88
Good Friday   52, 54, 198
grandchild   152, 191
Guy de Chauliac   34, 65, 143, 172

Hailes   207
handmaid   111, 118, 123, 137, 140–1
health   2, 6–7, 10, 13–14, 31, 34–5, 43 n.55, 54, 62, 76, 82, 84, 94, 99, 106, 108, 112 n.72, 116, 117 n.89, 122–3, 130, 137, 142, 144, 146, 152, 160, 169, 180, 196, 200 n.71, 212, 220
heart   12, 20, 34, 36, 42, 44, 50 n.88, 51–2, 69–70, 72–3, 78, 81, 88, 100, 109, 116, 163, 179, 194–5, 197, 204, 206 n.98, 213, 220
heat, of body   37, 44, 77–8, 82, 94, 101–3, 106, 130–1, 169, 186–7
heaven   32, 53, 59–60, 68 n.33, 81, 91 n.123, 92, 120, 133, 142, 146–7, 157, 209, 211–12, 219
Hedwig of Silesia   61
Henry of Lancaster   127 n.4, 128, 141
Hildegard of Bingen   24, 34–5, 45, 48, 98, 101, 103–4, 150–2, 203, 219 n.33
Hilton, Walter   43 n.55, 49 n.80, 190, 219 n.33
Hippocrates   24, 32, 43, 45, 92, 171–2
Holy Land   51, 94 n.135, 105, 107, 115–16
Holy Trinity Guild   123, 213 n.15, 216–17
hospital   7, 118 n.93, 129, 144–5, 147–8, 150
Hugh of Saint-Victor   36, 88
Hugo of Folieto   36, 49
humour   15, 24, 32–3, 35–38, 42, 44, 48, 54, 78, 83, 85, 102, 109, 144 n.77, 149 n.99, 172, 186, 190, 206 n.100, 207, 223, 224
husband   25, 35, 59–60, 73, 76, 78–80, 82, 85–9, 94, 113 n.77, 121, 134, 140, 145, 154–9, 166, 182 n.81, 185, 187, 191, 195
hysteria   9, 43, 56

Ibn al-Jazzar   35
Ibn Rushd *see* Averroës
Ibn Sīnā *see* Avicenna

iconography   16, 18, 40, 69 n.37, 106–7, 116, 119, 157, 174, 176 n.58, 191
Ida of Louvain   140
Il Dialogo della Divina Provvidenza   163
imitatio Christi   50, 60, 96, 110, 129, 150, 198, 219
imitatio Mariae   96, 117, 176
Ipswich   158 n.125, 194–5, 198
Isidore of Seville   84

Jacques de Vitry   43 n.54, 150, 162
Jerusalem   49, 52, 55, 70, 94 n.135, 105 n.39, 117 n.91, 209
John of Mirfield   139
Jordanus de Turre   149
Julian of Norwich   x, 20, 53, 56, 119, 160, 168, 171, 174, 181, 184, 190, 203, 205, 213 n.14, 218, 219 n.33

Kempe, John   59–60, 62, 64, 79–80, 84–8, 90, 96, 127, 153–9, 195 n.53
Knowing of Woman's Kind in Childing, The   22, 43–5, 65, 67, 70, 77–9, 82, 84, 102, 109, 110 n.62, 112, 116, 122–3, 130–1, 138–9, 169, 204

labour   16, 54–5, 56 n.106, 65–8, 70–2, 78, 111–12, 131, 135, 137 n.46, 148, 156, 159, 192, 199, 201, 204
lamentation   35, 42, 44, 46, 49, 52, 55, 58, 117, 121, 162, 175–6, 181–2
Lammastide   26, 90 n.119, 209
Le Livre de Seyntz Medicines   127 n.4, 128, 141
leprosy   25, 83, 134, 141–52, 156
Liber de Diversis Medicinis   132 n.30, 172–4
life-course *see also* age   13–5, 89, 98–102, 164–5, 174, 188, 211, 216
life cycle *see* life-course
light   20, 36, 42, 68, 92, 111, 172
London   123, 168, 195 n.53, 200, 207–8
Love, Nicholas   93, 111, 176
lovesickness   35, 37, 52–3
Lydwine of Schiedam   162

madness   34, 45, 147, 181
Magnus, Albertus   22
Manere of Good Lyvyng, The   142–3, 220
Man of Sorrows   106, 111
Margaret of Cortona   42, 209, 213
Marie of Oignies   18, 49 n.80, 61, 145, 184, 190, 194 n.52, 213
marriage   35, 59–96, 170, 185, 194 n.52

debt   25, 60, 62, 73, 77–80, 82, 84,
    86, 88, 156
doctrine of   61, 74–5, 84, 154–5
spiritual   25, 73–5, 83, 87–9, 93–4,
    96, 220
to Godhead *see also under* God   32,
    62, 90–2, 94, 121, 134, 157
to Manhood *see also under* God   90,
    93, 157–8, 160
martyrdom   19, 26, 45, 83, 86, 104,
    143, 161–2
Mary Magdalene   85, 182
Mater Dolorosa   50, 175
maternity   6, 8, 12–13, 25, 51, 63, 65,
    81, 89, 98–100, 104, 106–7, 112–14,
    117, 119, 121, 124–5, 129, 134, 138,
    140–1, 152, 174–5, 177, 181–2, 209
    n.105
medicine   6–8, 21–3, 25, 27, 32–3, 72,
    79, 84, 106, 108, 127–30, 135 n.41,
    139–41, 153, 159, 167–8, 211, 221,
    223, 224
Meditationes vitae Christi   111, 176, 179
melancholia   6, 14–5, 24, 26, 29–38,
    42–58, 63, 65, 68, 72, 73, 77–8, 92,
    103, 121, 161, 172, 186, 206, 220,
    223
melancholy *see* melancholia
memory   13, 15–16, 26, 30, 48, 52, 73,
    156, 163, 177, 183–4, 190, 200, 206,
    209, 216–7, 219, 220, 223
menopause   25, 62, 75, 98–107, 110,
    118 n.92, 121 n.104, 151, 158, 170,
    188, 192, 196, 199 n.68
menses *see* menstruation
menstruation   25, 35, 38, 61 n.6, 78,
    82–4, 99, 100–2, 105–6, 108–10,
    113, 120, 136 n.45, 143, 150–1, 170,
    186–8, 196, 204, 223
midwife   70, 111–12, 135–40
milk
    breastmilk   50 n.87, 108, 110, 113,
        116, 119, 120, 121, 130–3, 138,
        174, 191, 206 n.100
    of nursing   98, 111, 112 n.72, 113,
        116, 119–22, 129, 130–3, 138,
        141, 191
Mirabilis, Christina   132
miracles (of Margery Kempe)   135, 199
Mirror of the Blessed Life of Jesus Christ, The
    93, 111, 176
monstrosity   48, 67, 84
motherhood   14, 62–3, 65, 73–5, 81,
    84, 89, 91, 100, 105, 110, 112, 114,

117, 119, 120 n.101, 121, 123–4,
    130, 133, 134 n.35, 137, 139, 143,
    148–9, 151–3, 157, 175–7, 182, 185,
    187, 191, 192 n.39, 198, 209
of Christ *see* Christ as mother
Mount Calvary *see* Calvary, Mount
mourning   6, 26, 29–30, 40, 46, 48–9,
    52–3, 55–8, 65, 105, 142, 161, 220
multispectral imaging   ix, 1, 4
Musico   22, 110 n.62
Myroure of Oure Ladye, The   40, 80 n.81
mysticism   4, 6–8, 12, 14–18, 24–6,
    30–1, 34, 39, 42, 47–50, 53, 56–9,
    62–3, 65, 68, 73–4, 81, 85, 90–5,
    99–100, 106, 111–12, 117–18, 121,
    123, 129, 137, 141, 144, 147, 157,
    160–6, 171–5, 177 n.64 & n.67, 180,
    182, 184, 186, 190–1, 197, 199 n.68,
    203, 208, 211, 219–20

nativity   111
Non omnes quidem   22
Norway   198–200
Norwich   10, 53, 55, 89, 95, 124–5,
    168, 176, 190
nurse *see also* wet nurse   25, 112–13,
    115–24, 128–41, 145, 155

olfaction   92
Original Sin   12, 34, 67, 74, 79, 110,
    136 n.45

pain   6–20, 25–7, 29–32, 39, 43, 47–8,
    51–62, 65–73, 85–99, 106, 108–12,
    127–9, 131, 133, 140–52, 153–63,
    168–85, 189–90, 194, 196–201, 206,
    208–12, 219–21, 223
    paradox   25, 62–3, 73–9, 96
    removal   25, 88, 110, 133, 140, 144,
        147, 152
    surrogacy   25–6, 60, 79–82, 117, 126,
        127–60, 161, 177, 219–20
Palm Sunday   56
Passion, The   26, 30, 41–2, 47, 51–2,
    90–1, 108, 111, 117, 128, 140, 142,
    159–60, 161–81, 198, 207, 209
Passion visions   26, 51–2, 140, 161–81,
    198, 209
pathologisation   4, 6, 9, 12–13, 16,
    23–4, 29, 31, 36, 38–9, 41–2, 47, 58,
    106 n.41, 116, 135 n.41, 138, 185–6,
    188–90
penance   79–81, 85, 156, 184, 199
Pepwell, Henry   81, 201, 218, 220

pestilence   66, 118 n.92, 201
Philip of Clairvaux   50
Philip of Novara   103
phlebotomy   42, 108, 180, 181 n.76, 224
phlegm   1 n.1, 2, 32–4, 77, 103, 223, 224
Physica, The   24, 151 n.105, 152 n.108
physician   6–7, 19–21, 23, 34, 45, 54, 73, 88, 102, 127–30, 133–4, 135 n.41, 136 n.44, 137–9, 141, 145, 149, 152, 155, 158, 160, 174, 223
physiology   8, 15–16, 26, 31–3, 36–8, 39 n.43, 47, 50 n.88, 76, 79, 92–3, 98, 101–2, 105, 122, 129, 161, 169, 171, 173, 178, 181, 202, 204, 206, 223
pietà   55, 175–6
pilgrimage   39, 51, 57, 66 n.22, 71 n.47, 94, 105, 107, 113–15, 117 n.91, 121–5, 137 n.46, 146 n.87, 153, 185, 189–90, 194–201, 207–8
  methods of   194, 196–201
  asceticism of   185, 198–201, 208–9
Plato   43, 212
poison   60, 78, 83, 110, 186, 196
pollution   60, 61 n.6, 76, 82–3, 109–10, 144, 151
Pore Caitif, The   40, 61, 68, 75–6, 83, 93, 104, 133, 161
preaching   126, 128, 173, 202–5
pregnancy   14, 61 n.6, 65, 67, 72–3, 77, 84, 89 n.116, 115, 125, 224
Prickyng of Love, The   50
purgation   20, 38, 82, 84, 109–12, 172, 180–1
purification *see also* Churching   49, 62, 70–2, 85, 108–10, 127, 136–7, 143, 182
Purification Day   136

Queste del saint graal   151

rapture   30–1, 47–9, 68, 92–3, 129, 161–2, 176, 180, 197
Raymond of Capua   163
recipe   ix, xii, 1–5, 10, 27, 53 n.98, 98, 130–2, 137, 139–40, 169, 220
Regimen sanitatis   108, 113, 130, 150
relics   16, 70, 107, 137 n.46, 164, 213, 221
reproduction   6, 12–13, 25–6, 35, 62, 65, 72, 74, 76–8, 80, 89, 92, 96–106, 110, 113–16, 121, 124–6, 133, 136–7, 146, 148, 152–3, 155, 159, 183–5, 188 n.25, 191–2, 211–12, 220, 223, 224
Repyngdon, Philip   88
resurrection   14, 159, 165, 198, 212–13, 219, 221
retrospection   8, 9 n.18, 16, 26, 64, 92, 183, 193
Richard Salthouse   10, 219
Rolle, Richard   42, 43 n.55, 85, 177 n.67, 190
Roman de la rose   187
Rome   25, 31 n.11, 39, 40 n.45, 53, 90, 94 n.135, 105 n.39, 113–14, 116, 117 n.91, 118, 120–4, 133, 141, 157, 190, 197 n.64

sacraments   60 n.6, 61, 88, 90, 93, 106–7, 119–20, 127, 132 n.33, 140, 145, 165, 167, 206–7
Sacred Disease, The   32, 45
Sacred Heart, The   69
salvation   2, 12, 16, 30, 40, 49, 60, 72, 75, 86, 96, 104, 108–9, 121, 123, 135, 137, 143, 147, 149–50, 153, 168, 176–7, 188, 190, 198, 201–2, 211
Santiago de Compostela   57, 94 n.135, 146 n.87
Scarry, Elaine   7, 16, 18, 69
scribe   2, 9–10, 15, 20, 43 n.54 & n.55, 92, 135, 152 n.111, 153, 171, 190, 194, 199 n.70, 202, 205, 219
seasons   15, 33, 108
Secretum Secretorum   187
Sekenesse of Wymmen, The see Sickness of Women, The
Senescence *see under* age
senses   36 n.30, 48, 82, 86, 92–3
sex
  sexuality   12, 78, 82, 84, 89, 92, 101 n.21, 114, 151, 156, 184, 186–7, 193
  sexual intercourse   35, 38, 60, 62, 65, 66 n.22, 67, 74, 75–80, 84–8, 91, 94, 113, 122, 125, 127 n.2, 144 n.76, 149, 151, 156, 170, 187
sickness   6–7, 13–14, 20, 26, 32, 35, 39, 45, 47, 51 n.89, 53, 55 n.102, 56 n.106, 57–8, 62–8, 70 n.41, 73, 76–8, 81, 92, 106–9, 117 n.89, 127–9, 130, 136, 142–5, 147, 150–3, 155, 160, 165, 167–72, 196, 212–13, 220
  as result of sin   6–7, 65–72, 128, 142–4, 148–51

Sickness of Women, The 22, 67, 102, 109, 130–1, 138, 189, 192, 196
sight *see* vision
Signa Mortifera 26, 171–3, 179, 181
Signs of Death *see Signa Mortifera*
speech 36, 90, 92, 122, 202–3, 205, 207–10
spices 2, 4, 53 n.98, 98, 137–8, 141
spiritual gifts 24, 39, 42, 46–7, 52–3, 81, 92, 105, 142, 168, 190, 205, 207, 220–1
Spryngolde, Robert 10, 184, 219
St Agatha 104, 133
St Agnes 83, 104
St Ambrose 83, 104
St Anne 136 n.45, 137, 209 n.105
St Elizabeth 137, 140 n.63, 141, 145 n.81
stigmata 31, 49–51, 69–70, 73
St John the Baptist 137
St Margaret 72, 137 n.46, 139
St Margaret's Church 114 n.78, 127, 134, 135 n.42, 166, 169 n.33, 199 n.70, 217–20
St Stephen's Church 55, 89, 115
suffocated womb *see under* uterus
suicide 69–70, 87
Summa Theologiae 24
surrogacy
 death 26, 154, 159, 161, 163–5, 174–82
 foster parent 100, 115, 120, 124–5
 image substitution 25, 69, 100, 114, 117, 121, 137
 maternal 12, 13, 25, 96, 97–100, 105, 110–11, 113–25, 129–33, 138–41, 152–3, 174–7, 181, 185, 191, 198, 209, 212, 219–20
 pain surrogacy see under pain
 surrogate substitution 6, 8, 19, 122, 141, 155, 158
 of *The Book of Margery Kempe* 211
Suso, Henry 18, 69 n.37
sweetness 2, 4–5, 49, 53 n.98, 60, 91 n.122, 119, 130, 137 n.47, 141, 157, 220
synaesthesia 92
Syon Abbey 26, 40, 142, 163 n.8, 178 n.69, 209
System of Physic 24

taste 60, 92, 140, 202
teaching *see also* preaching 26, 63, 84, 95, 97, 124–5, 128, 149–50, 171 n.41, 185, 190–3, 202–5, 208–9

tears 2 n.4, 9, 24, 29–58, 70, 85, 105, 112, 114, 121, 148, 154, 180, 182, 190, 206–7, 209
temperament 33, 38, 77, 122, 223–4
Thomas of Cantimpré 110, 132, 162, 164
touch 25, 35, 82–8, 95–6, 100, 117, 147
Trevisa, John 24
Trinity, Holy 92, 219
Trotula, The 21, 23, 43 n.55, 94
 'The Book on the Conditions of Women' 21, 44, 77–8, 87, 98, 102 n.26, 112–13, 115–16, 123 n.113, 130–2, 138, 169–70, 188–9, 197
 'On Treatments for Women' 21, 62, 72, 76, 113, 138, 189
 'On Women's Cosmetics' 21

union
 Christic 46, 58, 63, 74, 90–4, 129, 134, 145, 157, 160–1, 211
 marital 80, 94, 127 n.2
uterus 21, 35, 43–5, 69, 70, 72, 76–8, 81, 92, 104, 108, 111, 119, 125, 130–1, 136 n.45, 140, 152, 169, 170, 188–9, 192
 uterine prolapse 45, 169–70, 188–9
 uterine precipitation *see under* uterine prolapse
 uterine suffocation 43–6, 78, 88, 94, 169–70, 197

Vanna of Orvieto 162, 182
vapours 38, 47, 224
Viaticum, The 24, 35, 37
Vincent of Beauvais 103, 185
Virgin Mary 25, 40–1, 50–1, 53, 55, 61, 67, 70, 71 n.47, 75, 82, 108, 111–12, 114–17, 119, 121, 123, 128–9, 132–4, 136–7, 140–1, 151, 161, 174–7, 181–2, 191, 198, 204, 213, 219
 as physician 128–41
virginity *see* chastity
vision 2, 26, 31–2, 36, 41, 44–5, 49, 51, 52–5, 56, 59, 66 n.22, 68, 71–2, 80, 85, 89 n.116, 92–4, 92, 99 n.8, 106–7, 111–12, 114, 117–18, 120–1, 123, 128, 133, 136–7, 140–2, 146–7, 149, 151, 160–5, 170–1, 175–82, 190, 203, 205–6, 211, 216, 219, 221

weeping *see* tears
wet nurse *see also* nurse   25, 112–17,
    120 n.101, 122, 124 n.118, 130, 133,
    138, 141 n.66
widowhood   26, 38, 45, 61, 76, 78,
    80, 87, 90, 94, 100, 129, 136 n.44,
    153–4, 158–60, 170, 185, 193, 195,
    197, 199
wifehood   13, 59, 62–3, 70, 73–4, 80–2,
    85–8, 90, 95, 100, 105, 114, 117,
    122, 129, 134, 153–60
Wife of Bath   97–8, 103, 154–5, 187,
    204 n.87
Wilsnack   107, 199

wine   53 n.98, 67 n.25, 84, 120, 131,
    134, 137, 140, 141 n.64, 191
womb *see* uterus
wounds *see also* Christ   17, 24, 29–36,
    47–58, 63–5, 67 n.25, 68–73, 107,
    119, 128, 133, 141, 143–4, 146–7,
    163, 177–8, 189
Wynkyn de Worde   27, 163 n.8, 201,
    218 n.30

yellow bile   32–3, 223

Zād al-Musāfir   35

Printed and bound by CPI Group (UK) Ltd, Croydon, CR0 4YY

09/06/2025

14685710-0003

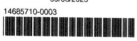